201 SECRETS to Healthy LIVING

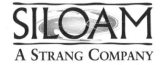

SILOAM
A STRANG COMPANY

Most Strang Communications Book Group products are available at special quantity discounts for bulk purchase for sales promotions, premiums, fund-raising, and educational needs. For details, write Strang Communications Book Group, 600 Rinehart Road, Lake Mary, Florida 32746, or telephone (407) 333-0600.

201 Secrets to Healthy Living
Published by Siloam
A Strang Company
600 Rinehart Road
Lake Mary, Florida 32746
www.strangbookgroup.com

Scripture quotations marked AMP are from the Amplified Bible. Old Testament copyright © 1965, 1987 by the Zondervan Corporation. The Amplified New Testament copyright © 1954, 1958, 1987 by the Lockman Foundation. Used by permission.

Scripture quotations marked KJV are from the King James Version of the Bible.

Scripture quotations marked NAS are from the New American Standard Bible. Copyright © 1960, 1962, 1963, 1968, 1971, 1972, 1973, 1975, 1977 by the Lockman Foundation. Used by permission. (www.Lockman.org)

Scripture quotations marked NIV are from the Holy Bible, New International Version. Copyright © 1973, 1978, 1984, International Bible Society. Used by permission.

Scripture quotations marked NKJV are from the New King James Version of the Bible. Copyright © 1979, 1980, 1982 by Thomas Nelson, Inc., publishers. Used by permission.

Scripture quotations marked NLT are from the Holy Bible, New Living Translation, copyright © 1996, 2004. Used by permission of Tyndale House Publishers, Inc., Wheaton, IL 60189. All rights reserved.

Scripture quotations marked TLB are from The Living Bible. Copyright © 1971. Used by permission of Tyndale House Publishers, Inc., Wheaton, IL 60189. All rights reserved.

Cover design by Amanda Potter
Design Director: Bill Johnson

Library of Congress Cataloging-in-Publication Data:

201 secrets to healthy living / compiled by Siloam editors ; [authors, Lisa Bevere ... et al.].
    p. cm.
 Includes bibliographical references.
 ISBN 978-1-59979-856-1
 1. Self-care, Health. 2. Medicine, Popular. 3. Health--Religious aspects--Christianity. I. Bevere, Lisa. II. Siloam (Publisher) III. Title: Two hundred and one secrets to healthy living. IV. Title: Two hundred one secrets to healthy living.
 RA776.95.A14 2010
 613--dc22

                    2009035979

This book contains the opinions and ideas of its authors. It is solely for informational and educational purposes and should not be regarded as a substitute for professional medical treatment. The nature of your body's health condition is complex and unique. Therefore, you should consult a health professional before you begin any new exercise, nutrition, or supplementation program or if you have questions about your health. Neither the authors nor the publisher shall be liable or responsible for any loss or damage allegedly arising from any information or suggestion in this book.

The statements in this book about consumable products or food have not been evaluated by the Food and Drug Administration. The recipes in this book are to be followed exactly as written. The publisher is not responsible for your specific health or allergy needs that may require medical supervision. The publisher is not responsible for any adverse reactions to the consumption of food or products that have been suggested in this book.

While the authors have made every effort to provide accurate telephone numbers and Internet addresses at the time of publication, neither the publisher nor the authors assume any responsibility for errors or for changes that occur after publication.

10 11 12 13 14 — 9 8 7 6 5 4 3 2 1
Printed in Canada

CONTENTS

SECTION 3: WEIGHT LOSS

Section 4: Detoxing

Section 5: Fitness

SECTION 6: DISEASES AND DISORDERS

SECTION 7: PAIN RELIEF

Section 8: Secrets to Longevity

Section 9: Women's Health

WHAT IS WELLNESS?

from the editors of Siloam

WE BELIEVE WELLNESS *is* attainable for you, which is why we want to present the material in this book in a way that is understandable, reachable, and even fun for you to pursue. Let's face it; very few of us will ever have the body of Brad Pitt or the beauty of Jennifer Aniston, but it is possible to reach a state of wellness that is just right for you.

Most people probably think of wellness in primarily physical terms—in which case good nutrition, hydration, clean air, exercise, and rest are the main issues. Some would add in a mental factor, as in the "mind-body connection," and emphasize that true wellness is only possible when a person is healthy in both body and mind. But we would add that spiritual health is also essential.

In fact, at Siloam, we think that true wellness involves *four* arenas of life: body, mind, spirit, and social relationships. This is because we are all persons with bodies, minds, and spirits who live in the context of relationships—whether we are speaking of one-on-one friendships or our relationship to the entire human race.

Our basis for making this statement is our Judeo-Christian perspective. You will find many of the health-producing practices promoted in our books in the teachings of Moses and the Old Testament prophets and in the teachings of Jesus and the writers of the New Testament. The Old Testament word for *wellness* is *shalom*, which is often translated "peace" even though its much broader meaning is "whole." The New Testament word is *soteria*, which is often translated "salvation." This word is best understood in the context of healing, health, and wellness.

Many Americans feel overwhelmed by the constant barrage of information regarding what to eat, what not to eat, how to exercise, and how to avoid contracting disease. That's why *201 Secrets to Healthy Living* is designed to cut through the onslaught of wellness approaches, diet plans, and workout programs to provide you with a treasure trove of the best advice from twenty-seven of our leading Siloam health authors. We want to motivate you to move from feeling overloaded by wellness ideas to the realization that you can live a whole, happy, and healthy life.

Our goal is to reinforce the health-enhancing habits you already practice and show you how to improve in areas that need it—some of which you might not have even considered to be related to wellness. To do this, we encourage you to read through the book at whatever pace works for you. Some of you will read it from beginning to end to add to your overall knowledge about healthy living; others will find it helpful to read specific secrets pertaining to the health situation you are dealing with. Whichever way you choose to read this information, we want you to experience an increased sense of wellness in your life.

You'll find that every secret in this book is supported by modern scientific evidence. Where appropriate, we've cited studies and other research so that you can look them up on your own. You can refer to the individual credentials of each contributing author on pages 246–249. The combined experience of the Siloam authors featured on these pages represents more than three hundred years of experience and almost two hundred published books, many of which were published by Siloam. Because of this, you know that you are about to read advice you can trust. And we hope that in the future, you will keep turning to Siloam for natural, Bible-based solutions for all of your health care needs.

Adapted from David B. Biebel and Harold G. Koenig, *Simple Health* (Lake Mary, FL: Siloam, 2005), 2–6.

HEALTH-CARE BASICS

BE PROACTIVE

by David B. Biebel, DMin, and Harold Koenig, MD

SOME PEOPLE BELIEVE providers of medical and dental care or various government agencies are responsible for their health care, but that is only part of the truth. The other side involves individuals taking a proactive stance in maintaining good health.

AN OUNCE OF PREVENTION

1. Make and keep regular medical and dental checkups. Use a date you'll remember as a reminder—for example, on New Year's Day, celebrate another year of good health by making a note to call your doctor's office tomorrow.
2. Stay informed and up-to-date regarding products and practices that enhance health.
3. Practice the healthful habits you are learning about in this book, and avoid anything that might threaten your health.
4. Monitor your own weight and blood pressure; perform self-examinations regularly.
5. Make your home safe from pollution, toxins, allergens, and infectious bacteria.
6. Take responsibility for your own health and the health of those you care about.

A POUND OF CURE

1. Take care of any developing dental issues as soon as possible.
2. Be aware of your insurance coverage—and its limits. For example, mercury-free fillings might not be covered, but paying extra for the less-toxic filling material will benefit your health in the long run.
3. Know your rights and responsibilities as a patient. You have the right to full information about the outcomes of the care, treatment, and services you receive. You have the right to refuse treatment and seek a second opinion.
4. Make yourself part of your own treatment team. Become a consumer of health-care information. Ask questions, read health-care journals and magazines, and search the Internet to find information on treatment options.
5. Know the medications you're taking and why; know their possible side effects and interactions with other prescription or over-the-counter medications or supplements you are using.

David B. Biebel and Harold G. Koenig, *Simple Health* (Lake Mary, FL: Siloam, 2005), 79–97.

WHEN IT'S TIME TO SEE A DOCTOR

by Reginald Cherry, MD

I HAVE BEEN ASKED, "When I'm sick, should I call my pastor or my doctor?" My answer to this is: Call both! There doesn't have to be a conflict of interest between the two. Consult a doctor to find out exactly what you're are dealing with, and then call your pastor with the specifics so that he will know exactly how to pray.

When you visit your doctor, don't be afraid to have tests done. This is not a lack of faith. Many tests that doctors perform can help in determining the cause and/or scope of a disease. The information that medical tests provide can empower your prayers against the illness because they provide specifics against which you can target your prayers. However, some tests can also be difficult or uncomfortable to undergo, so the first prayer you should pray is that you know which tests to undergo.

Ask God to give His peace (Col. 3:15) when you pray about certain tests that you are facing. If you feel a continual sense of anxiety or dread every time you think or pray about a certain procedure, it may not be the path God would have you take. But if His peace begins to flood your heart about a certain test or procedure, you can be assured that the divine "umpire" is ruling in your heart, indicating the right course of action for you to take.

"WHAT IF I'M HOSPITALIZED FOR AN ILLNESS?"

Being in the hospital can be a frightening and often confusing experience. First of all, it is important to resolve the misconception that being in the hospital is contradictory to walking in faith as a believer. Sometimes medical intervention is a necessary step in the healing process. God's presence goes with you into the hospital just as He goes with you everywhere else. You can exercise your faith in a hospital bed as effectively as you can at home.

What many patients fail to realize is that information is key to making right decisions for their health. Ask your doctor questions. Be sure you understand what courses of treatment are available to you and what the effects—both pro and con—are for each possible treatment. Becoming as informed as possible about your disease will help you feel more comfortable in making decisions, and you will know better how to pray.

Sometimes patients have trouble determining when their doctor will make his or her rounds in the hospital so that they can be prepared to ask the questions they need answered. One suggestion I have given is to call the doctor's office (perhaps early in the morning when the office begins to answer the phones) and ask what time he or she will be visiting your particular hospital on that day. Make a list of questions to ask him or her so that nothing important is forgotten.

Finally, remember that the doctor will always present you with the worst-case scenario. That's his or her job. Instead of thinking of him or her as the bearer of bad news, begin to view him as a messenger of God sent to tell you the truth, to show you how to pray, and to give you the options you need to understand in order to discover your pathway to healing. An original definition of a physician was a teacher. We need to think of our doctors in that way: They are teachers sent by God to show us the things that we can do in the natural to help prevent or treat a condition. And the knowledge they give us will help us to know more specifically how to pray.

Reginald Cherry, *Bible Health Secrets* (Lake Mary, FL: Siloam, 2003), 26–28.

FAITH AND DIVINE HEALING

by Scott Hannen, DC

FAITH IS A reality that reflects our core beliefs. Someone who is facing surgery places his or her faith in the surgeon. If the patient did not have faith in the surgeon, he would not submit to the procedure. What we do or don't do depends on where we place our faith.

Unless we understand what faith is, we may think we have faith without experiencing the reality of it. For example, here are four kinds of faith:

1. Religious faith says, "Lord, I know You can help me today." It rests in the knowledge of God's ability without believing His willingness to do it.

2. Weak faith says, "Lord, if it is Your will, please help me." It rests in faulty knowledge or lack of knowledge of the Word of God, hence not knowing the will of God—His desire—to help.

3. No faith says, "I cannot be helped." This attitude of unbelief needs to be repented of so that you can experience the "measure of faith" God gives to everyone (Rom. 12:3, KJV).

4. Strong faith says, "I can do all things through Christ which strengtheneth me" (Phil. 4:13, KJV).

Where do you see yourself in this list? I can honestly tell you that if you picked any one of those choices except number four, you need to make some honest changes in your approach to God. Strong faith only sees what God has spoken. It has no other option. F. F. Bosworth stated, "If your faith is saying anything other than what God's Word declares, you are only walking in mental reasoning, which is hostile to God (Rom. 8:7)."[1] Hebrews 11:6 says, "But without faith it is impossible to please him: for he that cometh to God must believe that he is, and that he is a rewarder of them that diligently seek him" (KJV).

In order to receive divine healing, you have to know who God is and diligently seek Him as the loving Father who promises healing and health.

Sometimes it takes years to see God's plan fully unfold in people's lives. Yet if they remain faithful and adhere to His Word, they will eventually prosper in every area. When it comes to healing, these same principles apply. The health condition may not turn around right away, but as you place your faith in God for healing, the Bible says He will be faithful to heal you. It may take some time before you experience complete healing. You may have to demonstrate your faith in the design of your Creator and in the inherent recuperative powers that He placed inside of every created being.

Scott Hannen, *Healing by Design* (Lake Mary, FL: Siloam, 2003, 2007), 153–155.

CHOOSING A PHYSICIAN: IS CHIROPRACTIC CARE RIGHT FOR YOU?

by Scott Hannen, DC

HERE ARE MY recommendations for choosing the right physician for the problem you are having. Of course, my first rule is to ask the doctor if he or she is a Christian. After you are satisfied with that answer, I recommend that you see a qualified doctor according to the following criteria:

CHOOSING A PHYSICIAN

TYPE OF PHYSICIAN	TREATMENT FOR
Medical doctor (MD) or osteopathic physician (DO)	Emergency medicine (acute care, stabilization care, surgery, physical therapy, rehabilitation)
Chiropractic doctor (DC)	Biomechanical and structural problems: spinal, joints, muscle spasm, nervous system imbalances, nutrition and diet; source of alternative medicines
Naturopathic doctor (ND): A licensed ND (not the ND mail order or Internet degree) from an accredited naturopathic school	Herbal and nutrient therapies: alternative treatments, colonic irrigations, herbal detox and internal cleansing
Homeopathic doctor (DHM): A certified practitioner	Chronic disorders, detoxification, supports all other therapies listed above, no known side effects

Note: Many physicians have taken postgraduate courses and are certified to practice treatments from several of the therapies listed above.

As a chiropractic physician, it is my greatest joy to remove pain and sickness permanently for my patients. May I suggest that the next time you find yourself dealing with pain, suffering, or an unsolved health problem, you consider a chiropractic physician? I am sure you will be pleasantly surprised with the results.

Regardless of which type of physician you visit, remember to seek the primary cause for the symptoms instead of just looking for relief by treating the symptoms. Although conventional medical science does address many of these factors, sadly, the end result of their proposed treatment often remains the same: drugs or surgery. There are many times when these interventions and procedures are necessary. But it is my conviction that we need to take a more whole-person approach based on the patient's individual needs. As physicians, we should do thorough examinations and make recommendations that address needs for the entire body, not just the obvious symptoms.

If your physician does not approach your situation from a whole-person perspective and help uncover the primary cause for your illness, try chiropractic. In my opinion, it is the best-kept secret in health care because it is based on finding the primary cause to bring about healing, which then brings long-term health benefits.

Scott Hannen, *Healing by Design* (Lake Mary, FL: Siloam, 2003, 2007), 29–32.

HEALTH-CARE SCREENINGS EVERYONE SHOULD HAVE
by Janet Maccaro, PhD, CNC

WHEN IT COMES to your health care, prevention and early detection of disease should be the cornerstone of your wellness plan.

Described here are general screening guidelines—some for everyone and some just for women. Of course, every person's needs are unique, so discuss your screening status with your doctor. He or she may suggest additional tests or a different schedule.

SCREENINGS EVERYONE NEEDS

- *Clinical skin exam:* Beginning at age forty, you should have a head-to-toe skin check for irregular moles and other signs of skin cancer once a year.
- *Colorectal cancer screenings:* Starting at age fifty, all adults should have a fecal occult blood test performed annually and a sigmoidoscopy every three to ten years to check for polyps or cancerous lesions. If you are at high risk for colorectal cancer, your physician may suggest a colonoscopy instead.
- *Glaucoma screening:* Get this eye test beginning at age forty. If you have normal vision, you should get an eye exam every three to five years.
- *Electrocardiogram (ECG):* You should get a baseline ECG by age forty. This painless test uses electrodes to record your heart's electrical impulses, and it evaluates heart function; it can identify injury or abnormality.
- *Blood pressure screening:* Your blood pressure should be checked at least once every two years. If your blood pressure is elevated, steps should be taken to control it; more frequent monitoring may be required.
- *Cholesterol test:* If your LDL, HDL, triglyceride, and total cholesterol levels fall within the desirable range, this simple blood test, which helps assess your risk of cardiovascular disease, should be performed every five years.

FOR WOMEN ONLY

- *Total thyroxin test (T4):* This blood test assesses thyroid function; women should talk to a physician about getting the test done around menopause.
- *Bone density test:* Every woman needs a baseline test at menopause to detect osteoporosis or assess your risk for the disease in the near future.
- *Clinical breast exam:* Your physician should examine your breasts each year to look for lumps, swollen lymph nodes, and other irregularities.
- *Mammogram:* A baseline mammogram is recommended by age forty, followed by mammograms every two years and annually after age fifty.
- *Pap smear:* You should have this test at least once every three years and annually after age fifty.

Janet Maccaro, *A Woman's Body Balanced by Nature* (Lake Mary, FL: Siloam, 2006), 172–174.

AN INTRODUCTION TO NATURAL HEALING PROTOCOLS
by Janet Maccaro, PhD, CNC

I T IS THE premise of natural medicine that the body has a God-given, built-in ability to heal itself and that the role of the physician is to aid or enhance this process with natural therapies such as dietary changes, herbs, vitamins, and minerals. Natural medicine is noninvasive. It supports the body by feeding, balancing, and cleansing.

Proponents of natural medicine view the person as a whole being—body, mind, and spirit—and seek to educate patients by involving them in their own health care. They become active participants in their personal well-being. Studies have shown that when people take an active part in their wellness protocol, healing is swifter, more successful, and complete.

The following widely used natural healing protocols will enable you to be proactive when it comes to your health.

- *Massage:* This systematic and scientific manipulation of the soft tissues of the body helps to relieve pain and muscle tension; prepare muscles for exercise or movement to their fullest capacity; and prevent, treat, and heal many conditions. However, massage is not recommended in cases of cancer, high fever, infection, high blood pressure, phlebitis, varicose veins, diabetes, broken bones, cysts, or bruises. In addition, use caution with swollen limbs, employing gentle massage only above the swelling.
- *Hydrotherapy:* This practice of using hot or cold water therapeutically helps to improve many conditions, including stress, arthritis, headaches, menstrual problems, muscle pain, asthma, and back pain.
- *Osteopathy:* This treatment of mechanical problems of the skeletal system is also an effective treatment for many other conditions, including osteoarthritis, back pain, breathing problems, digestive problems, strain from sports injuries, sciatica, and stress.
- *Reflexology:* This technique involves manipulating reflex points on the hands or feet that correspond to different organ systems of the body. It helps to control pain and promote well-being. Reflexology is useful especially in the following conditions: liver problems, kidney disorders, heart disease, digestive complaints, menstrual problems, sinusitis, and stress.
- *Myotherapy:* This muscle treatment uses manual or electrical stimulation of trigger points in order to relieve pain. It is very effective in treating chronic musculoskeletal pain, sports injuries, and TMJ.
- *Macrobiotic diet:* This therapeutic diet involves the use of brown rice and specific vegetables to rebalance the body, to help heal degenerative disease, and to promote health. Macrobiotic diet therapy has been used extensively for cancer, arthritis, stress, digestive disorders, and depression.
- *Orthomolecular therapy:* This therapy uses vitamins therapeutically. This means larger doses are used to treat specific diseases such as cancer, diabetes, aging, high blood pressure, colds, flu, PMS, menopause, and more.
- *Light therapy:* This therapy is used in the treatment of seasonal affective disorder (SAD), depression, and anxiety. It involves the use of sunlight or light boxes to lift mood.

- *Acupressure:* This treatment involves pressing certain points on the body in order to relieve pain and remove circulatory blockages. It is very effective for the relief of back pain, muscle pain, head and neck aches, and in respiratory problems like asthma. This technique is thousands of years old.
- *Acupuncture:* This technique is similar to acupressure but uses very fine needles placed strategically along meridians that correspond to different nerves, muscles, or organs. It is really quite painless and is remarkable in the fact that it can either stimulate or sedate any area of the body to reestablish balance. Much success has been shown over thousands of years in the treatment of headaches, back pain, liver and kidney problems, smoking, insomnia, allergies, anxiety, depression, and much more.
- *Colonic therapy:* Colonics involve the insertion of a small hose into the rectum, which then sends water throughout the entire length of the colon to gently clean out toxins. Usually done in a series of four to six sessions, colonic therapy has been very successful in the treatment or alleviation of constipation, diverticulitis, Candida overgrowth, and more.
- *Chiropractic:* Also known as joint manipulation therapy, chiropractic is very effective in treating stress-related pain, muscular pain, injury pain, sciatica, and more by adjusting subluxations that occur throughout the entire skeletal system.
- *Homeopathy:* This gentle two-hundred-year-old system of healing uses extremely diluted medicines or remedies that are designed to activate the body's own healing ability. The remedies are derived from minerals, plants, or animals and act as a catalyst for the immune system to eradicate the root cause of a particular illness.

Janet Maccaro, *Natural Health Remedies* (Lake Mary, FL: Siloam, 2003, 2006), 47–50.

TEN FOODS THAT STRENGTHEN YOUR IMMUNE SYSTEM

by Janet Maccaro, PhD, CNC

GOD HAS PROVIDED us with everything we need, not only in our physical bodies but also in nature. I want to share with you some of my favorite immune system fortifiers and boosters that my clients have come to love as well. They truly make a difference. Just try any one of the following gifts from God's garden, and experience a higher level of health.

TEN FUNCTIONAL FOODS THAT BUILD IMMUNITY

1. *Soy.* Twenty-five grams of soy protein a day may help lower cholesterol and reduce heart disease risk. Soy may also fight osteoporosis.
2. *Tomatoes.* Cooked, canned, or as ketchup, tomatoes are protective against prostate cancer when ten servings are consumed each week. Tomatoes contain lycopene, which neutralizes harmful free radicals that can damage cells and trigger cancer.
3. *Oats.* Oats have been shown to reduce the risk of heart disease.
4. *Grapes.* Polyphenols or flavonoids in red grapes may lower the risk of stroke and heart disease.
5. *Tea.* One cup of green or black tea per day could cut the risk of heart attack by 44 percent.
6. *Citrus.* Fruit and juices contain high levels of vitamin C, potassium, and folic acid.
7. *Fresh herbs.* Herbs are used to enhance the natural flavor of foods, thereby discouraging the overuse of butter and salt.
8. *Spinach.* One serving of spinach per week can protect against colon cancer, twice weekly to prevent cataracts. Its vitamin K content helps to build strong bones.
9. *Vegetables (cruciferous).* Eaten two to three times a week, these help prevent colon and lung cancer.
10. *Vegetables (beta-carotene).* These are protective against heart disease, stroke, and some cancers.

Turn to the next secret for some great-tasting recipes featuring the immune-boosting foods from this list.

Janet Maccaro, *90-Day Immune System Makeover* (Lake Mary, FL: Siloam, 2000, 2006), 174, 182.

IMMUNE-BOOSTING RECIPES

by Janet Maccaro, PhD, CNC

N OW THAT YOU have learned how to eat for maximum immunity, it is time to add these delicious recipes to your eating plan. Notice how each recipe incorporates ingredients that boost immune function. *Bon appétit!*

Green Tea Chicken Salad

3 Tbsp. sesame oil
4 boneless, skinless chicken breasts
3 Tbsp. green tea leaves
½ cup cold spring water, plus ⅛ cup rice vinegar
½ tsp. Bragg's Liquid Aminos

⅛ tsp. stevia powder extract (or to taste)
¾ cup olive oil
½ cup slivered almonds (toasted)
1 can sliced water chestnuts, drained
1 head of romaine lettuce, torn into pieces

In a large skillet over medium heat, heat 2 tablespoons of sesame oil. Sauté chicken breasts until cooked, about 5 to 7 minutes on each side. Set them aside to cool. To make the dressing, steep green tea leaves in water and vinegar for at least 30 minutes. Strain and discard the leaves. Add the remaining sesame oil, Bragg's Liquid Aminos, stevia, and olive oil; mix well. Tear the cooked chicken breasts into pieces. Combine with toasted slivered almonds, water chestnuts, and romaine lettuce. Add dressing and serve immediately. Serves 4.

Broiled Fish Steaks With Tomato–Bell Pepper Relish

4 medium plum tomatoes or 1 can (14 oz.) whole tomatoes, well drained, coarsely chopped
1 small red bell pepper
3 scallions
¼ cup fresh basil leaves
2 Tbsp. olive oil

2 Tbsp. apple cider vinegar
½ tsp. black pepper
¼ tsp. sea salt
4 tuna, cod, or halibut steaks, about ¾-in. thick

Preheat the broiler. Line broiler pan with foil and lightly grease the foil. In a food processor, coarsely chop the bell pepper, scallions, and basil. Transfer the vegetable mixture to a bowl. Stir in the chopped tomatoes, olive oil, vinegar, black pepper, and sea salt; stir well. Place the fish steaks on the prepared broiler pan. Strain the excess liquid from the tomato–bell pepper relish into a small bowl. Brush the fish with some of the liquid and broil 4 inches from the heat for 4 minutes. Turn the fish over and brush with more of the liquid; broil until the fish flakes when tested with a fork, about 4 minutes longer. Serve the steaks topped with the tomato–bell pepper relish. Serves 4.

Janet Maccaro, *90-Day Immune System Makeover* (Lake Mary, FL: Siloam, 2000, 2006), 162–169.

PROTECT YOURSELF FROM COLDS AND FLU
by Reginald Cherry, MD

For years, scientists have been working on the elusive "cure" for the common cold, which they have yet to discover. Fortunately, there are several natural ways to prevent it and to help protect yourself from ever catching a cold or coming down with the flu in the first place.

Echinacea

Echinacea is familiar to many people as a popular immune-boosting herb. It ranks near the top of the list when it comes to countering colds or the flu. This herb not only prevents viral infections, but it can also fight them if they try to attack the body. Studies have demonstrated that it can shorten the duration of the common cold and help prevent the flu from developing.

Echinacea should not be taken on a daily basis for an extended period of time because tolerance can develop and cause it not to work as effectively. Echinacea should be used for four to eight weeks and then discontinued for at least two weeks. The recommended dosage is 2 to 3 teaspoons of the tincture daily, or you can take the standard-dose capsules and follow the directions on the label.

Garlic

Another important herb to use during the cold and flu season is garlic, which can fight viruses as well as bacteria. It is also effective for reducing the duration of colds and the flu. Again, garlic works by stimulating the immune system function. I recommend taking the capsule form daily, checking the label to be certain a capsule is the equivalent of one clove of fresh garlic.

Lesser-known herbs

There are several lesser-known herbs that are helpful for colds and the flu. For example, *thyme* has antiviral as well as antibacterial properties and can be made into a tea or taken as syrup. Another herb available at health food stores, known as *elder*, is a decongestant and an anti-inflammatory that has traditionally been taken in the form of a hot tea. *Lemon balm* is a helpful herb for easing headaches and the aching associated with flu's symptoms.

Be certain also that you are on a good supplement program with a multivitamin and mineral supplement that includes B complex, zinc, and vitamin E, as well as chromium and selenium. All of these nutrients support immune system function. Remember the old chicken soup recipe? If you come down with symptoms, it can help to clear out mucus.

The body often develops a fever during a bout with the flu. Fevers stimulate the body's immune system and help it to overcome the virus and bacterial infection. Of course, a fever that is too high can be dangerous, as we know. Be sure to force fluids, particularly if you have developed a fever. It is very important to do all you can to strengthen your body's defenses against these viral infections.

Reginald Cherry, *Bible Health Secrets* (Lake Mary, FL: Siloam, 2003), 76–78.

MYTHS ABOUT COLDS AND FLU

by Leslie Ann Dauphin, PhD

CAN YOU COUNT the number of times you or someone in your family has been sick with a cold? Don't try. I know the answer to that question. Colds are probably the most common of all infectious diseases, hence the name common cold. What about the flu? It is equally common. Each year we [at the CDC] dread the countdown to the approaching flu season.

Why is it that people know the symptoms and the time of year they occur but very little else that is true about these two diseases? Since they are the most common infectious diseases, I would like to clarify some misconceptions about them.

COLDS

The myth

Many people have the misconception that colds are caused by cold weather and that not dressing properly for the weather conditions will lead to the illness.

The truth

First, colds are caused by viruses. In order to get sick from the viruses that cause colds, you must come into contact with them. They must attach to your cells and multiply within your cells to cause infection. Although not dressing properly for the weather conditions is probably not a good idea, there is no direct evidence that a person can contract a cold because of it.

FLU

The myths

Many people have the same misconceptions about the flu as they do for colds. One is the belief that the flu can be contracted from cold weather conditions. Another is that you must be sick to be susceptible to the flu. There is also the belief that the symptoms of a cold can become so severe that the cold can develop into or become the flu.

The truth

The flu is also a respiratory infection caused by viruses. Just as with cold viruses, you must be exposed to the flu virus to become infected. It is not transmitted via cold weather, nor is it necessary to be sick to become infected. Unless a person is infected with both cold and flu viruses, it is unlikely that a cold will develop into the flu. It is more likely that the symptoms of a severe cold and the flu are so similar that it is difficult for many people to distinguish between the two diseases.

Almost every winter, flu viruses cause epidemics leading to both the hospitalization and death of many people worldwide. The CDC estimates that 10–20 percent of Americans are infected with the flu virus each year. Of those, an average of 114,000 is hospitalized each year for complications associated with the infection. The most startling reports, however, are related to the number of deaths that occur each year: an estimated 36,000 Americans die each year from complications of the flu.

Leslie Ann Dauphin, *The Germ Handbook* (Lake Mary, FL: Siloam, 2005), 29–32.

AVOIDING GERMS

by Leslie Ann Dauphin, PhD

O NE OF THE best ways to prevent infectious diseases is so simple that many people don't consider the health benefits. It is hand washing. Hand washing is effective and takes very little time. Below is the CDC's recommendation for effective hand washing.[1]

- First, wet your hands and apply liquid or clean bar soap. Place the bar soap on a rack and allow it to drain.
- Next, rub your hands together vigorously and scrub all surfaces, including between your fingers and under your fingernails.
- Continue for twenty seconds or about the length of a short tune. The soap combined with the scrubbing action helps dislodge and remove germs. Rinse well, then dry your hands.

KEEPING YOUR ENVIRONMENT "GERM FREE"

Part of taking care of yourself is taking care of your environment. It is important to take care of areas where you spend your time—workplace, home, or automobile. I would like to offer some suggestions that may help. First, remember that there is a difference between cleaning and disinfecting. Cleaning is the removal of dirt, while disinfecting is killing germs. I am sure you would like to do both in your environment.

To clean your environment, use detergents (soap). These products are very effective at removing dirt and may also be effective at killing some, but not all, germs.

To disinfect your environment, use bleach-based products. An inexpensive and effective way to kill germs in your environment is to use 10 percent bleach as a disinfectant. Ten percent bleach is effective at killing almost all germs. You may purchase a squirt bottle and make a disinfectant using one part bleach to nine parts water. Note: The bleach solution will lose its effectiveness after a while, so make a fresh disinfectant batch routinely, at least once a week. Also, be careful around other household members and pets.

Sterilization is another method of killing germs. Dishwashers and clothes washers have heating coils, so the water in them gets much hotter than the water from your kitchen sink. Many germs don't like high temperatures. Your dishwasher and clothes washer are two of the best things you can use to sterilize dishes, utensils, bedding, towels, and clothing in your home. Most dishwashers and clothes washers have a cycle for sanitizing. Note: Please use water conservatively. It is wasteful to run a dishwasher or clothes washer that is less than half full.

Once a week:

- Use disinfectant wipes to clean frequently used items like refrigerator door handles, telephone receivers and buttons, remote controls, gaming controls, etc.
- Soak sponges in bleach water in the sink overnight to disinfect both the sponge and the sink.

Leslie Ann Dauphin, *The Germ Handbook* (Lake Mary, FL: Siloam, 2005), 13–15, 89–91.

MANAGE YOUR STRESS

by David B. Biebel, DMin, and Harold Koenig, MD

EVERYONE HAS STRESS. Some of us have a little. Some of us have a lot. Wouldn't you like to live a calmer, more stress-free life? Try following one or more of these simple solutions to stress management.

Develop a hobby.

Hobbies reduce stress because of the emotional and sociological benefits of connecting with people who have similar interests. The benefits of creative hobbies are found in the process, not what you do with the results.

Seek and enjoy solitude.

Whether you get outside or simply turn off the phone, find a quiet place, lie down, or listen to nature sounds or relaxing music, the important thing is that for at least thirty minutes, once or twice a day, you take a break and unwind.

Look for the humor in the situation.

Stress often comes from how we interpret and judge the world we live in. But humor can be used to think about a situation in a different way.

Pray and connect yourself to the Eternal.

Prayer can be an effective antidote for stress. Christian meditation begins when you quiet your soul before your Creator and think about Him. When you invite God's company on your day's journey, you can have ceaseless communion and perpetual dialogue with your Creator.

Exercise.

Take a walk or exercise every day. Exercise has an extremely calming effect.

Ditch the perfectionism.

Get the perfectionism monkey off your back—you don't have to please your parents anymore or even meet the unrealistic expectations of yourself or others.

Catch some Zs.

Be sure you get enough sleep—seven to eight hours per night is recommended.

Get by with a little help from your friends.

Enlist the help of friends who understand and love you, and stay close to them.

You are what you eat.

Good nutrition, including a diet rich in whole foods—fruits, vegetables, grains, dairy, and protein—will help you establish and maintain optimum physical health.

Pet the dog.

Pet your pet—but if your only pet is a goldfish and it purrs, perhaps you're more stressed than you thought. (That's a joke.)

David B. Biebel and Harold G. Koenig, *Simple Health* (Lake Mary, FL: Siloam, 2005), 31, 39–45.

MANAGING A GOOD NIGHT'S SLEEP

by David B. Biebel, DMin, and Harold Koenig, MD

A GOOD NIGHT'S SLEEP cannot be overrated when it comes to living a happy, healthy life. If you are not getting enough sleep, then you have a lot in common with about seventy million Americans. Each year more than fifteen hundred Americans die in an estimated one hundred thousand automobile accidents that are attributed to drowsy driving. Thousands of industrial and other work-related accidents result from drowsiness. Even when no accidents occur, workers who are always tired have trouble concentrating, are not as good at problem solving, make more mistakes, and forget more important matters than their peers.

Many serious medical conditions seem related to lack of sleep, though it is not clear whether lack of sleep is the cause or effect in some of these:

- High blood pressure
- Heart failure, heart attacks, and strokes
- Obesity
- Depression, mood disorders, and other types of mental impairment[1]

Not only does lack of sleep affect you physically, but it also makes it difficult to manage stress, relate well to other people, and maintain a positive outlook on life.

A ZZZZZ's QuiZZZZZZ

Check any of the following that are true of you:

- ❑ Most nights, I do not get more than five or six hours of sleep.
- ❑ Quite often when I'm driving, I have to fight to stay awake.
- ❑ I often wake up during the night, and when I do, it's hard to fall asleep again.
- ❑ I sometimes have a hard time staying awake and alert at work.
- ❑ It is hard for me to concentrate for very long.
- ❑ I seldom feel refreshed in the morning.
- ❑ Even if I'm tired, I sometimes have a hard time falling asleep.
- ❑ I'm not as good at solving problems as I used to be.
- ❑ I often need a stiff drink, a sleeping pill, or some other substance in order to fall asleep.
- ❑ I need caffeine to get myself going in the morning and keep myself going during the day.
- ❑ Sometimes when I wake up at night, I feel as if I'm gasping for air.

This ZZZZZZ's quiz is not a scientific tool by any means, but if you checked three or more of these, you should probably consult your physician.

David B. Biebel and Harold G. Koenig, *Simple Health* (Lake Mary, FL: Siloam, 2005), 53–54.

HEALTHY EATING and DRINKING

FROM KERNEL TO COLONEL—THE WESTERN DIET

by Hans Diehl, DrHSc, and Aileen Ludington, MD

THE STATISTICS ARE pretty convincing. We weren't meant to die in such numbers from heart attacks, strokes, diabetes, and colon and breast cancer. Significant cardiovascular disease began to emerge in America after World War I. It became really rampant after World War II when people could afford diets rich in animal products and when the food industry began producing highly processed foods crammed with calories and emptied of nutrition.

Could this be coincidental?

Hardly. This problem is unique to westernized peoples. Rural populations in China, Japan, and Southeast Asia who had little access to rich and processed foods experienced few heart attacks. Similarly, most people in rural Africa and South and Central America had little fear of diabetes and cardiovascular disease. Yet in North America, Australia, New Zealand, and the increasingly affluent countries in Europe and Asia, where diets are rich in fat, heart disease, cancer, diabetes, obesity, and hypertension are epidemic.

The villains, low fiber and high fat, take their toll by damaging the body's vital oxygen-carrying arteries and by upsetting important metabolic functions. Because of thickened, narrowed arteries, thousands of Americans have heart attacks every day, a large portion of the population has high blood pressure, and so many more are crippled from strokes. Because of disordered metabolisms from unbalanced lifestyles, obesity is epidemic and diabetes is running rampant.

How did these dietary changes come about?

Before the twentieth century, the American diet consisted mostly of foods grown in local gardens and nearby farms, supplemented with a few staples from the general store and meat from barnyard animals and range-fed cattle. Our grandparents didn't have thousands of beautifully packaged and highly promoted food products waiting at the supermarket. Fast-food restaurants didn't beckon from nearly every street corner.

The backbone of the diet was kernels—kernels of wheat and other grains growing in reassuring profusion. Families ate freshly cooked food and thick slices of home-baked bread around their own tables. They enjoyed hot cereals, corn bread, and biscuits. They ate rice, pasta, and corn, along with beans, potatoes, vegetables, and fruit. These nutritious high-fiber foods made up the larger percentage of their total daily calorie intake.

But times and tastes have changed dramatically. Freshly cooked breakfast cereals have largely been replaced by cold, presweetened flakes. Lunch typically consists of a salad soaked in oily dressing, or a hamburger, fries, and a soda, or perhaps a pizza. Dinner often comes frozen in a cardboard box or from the Colonel. Between meals there are sodas, chips, and doughnuts. Nutritious, high-fiber foods now represent only 22 percent of our daily calories, while fat consumption has nearly doubled and sugar intake has increased 240 percent.

The choice is yours. You can have the same freedom from heart disease, stroke, and cancer that our ancestors enjoyed simply by changing your habits of diet and exercise.

Hans Diehl and Aileen Ludington, *Dynamic Health* (Lake Mary, FL: Siloam, 2003), 10–12.

DECEPTION HAS THREE *PS*

by Gregory L. Jantz, PhD, with Ann McMurray

YOU MAY THINK that *deception* has only one *p* in the middle of the word. Actually, the kind of deception I'm talking about has three *ps*. They stand for packaging, processing, and portioning. Who is responsible for these three *ps*? Well, think of the food industry as a little like the serpent in that it is deceptive and does not have your best interests at heart.

The first *p* of deception—packaging

The packaging isn't about delivering information; it's about image. Image is all about highlighting even the obvious in order to sell the product. Packaging is not merely the vehicle for transporting and storing the food product; packaging is the vehicle to sell it. So they make every effort to produce packaging that makes food look good. This makes us buy food for the wrong reason, only because of the way it's packaged.

The second *p* of deception—processing

Food processing has allowed us to obtain whatever type of food we want without having to bother to make it ourselves. Food processing has allowed us to merge food with convenience. Without a great deal of time or effort, we are able to eat pretty much what we want.

All of this processed food is generally high in calories, sugar, fat, and often sodium. The flour used in baking these goodies is usually highly processed. It is generally referred to as white or processed flour. With white flour, components of the grain fiber are removed to make it lighter. If they used whole-wheat flour, why, they'd have to use more flour to achieve the same loaf dimension, and it would cost more to ship because it would weigh more.

Are you getting the idea here that there's a lot more that goes into the processing of your food than what's going to be the best food for you?

Because much of the fiber has been milled out, your body converts the carbohydrates in the flour into sugar.

The third *p* of deception—portioning

Portioning works in two ways when it comes to food. The first way is the oversized portion, usually provided at restaurants, fast-food outlets, and your Aunt Minnie's house at Thanksgiving. It's the fourth of pie that masquerades as "one slice." It's the two cups of mashed potatoes and gravy that parade as a "single helping," allowing you to go back for seconds when the first was really first, second, and third helpings all rolled into one. It's the salad-plate-sized cookie that only counts as "one cookie."

The second deception when it comes to portioning is the itsy, bitsy portion, usually hidden away on—you guessed it—food packaging. It's finding out by reading the fine print that the salad-plate-sized cookie really represents four servings at 150 calories a piece.

The smaller they can make the "portion," the fewer calories they have to list on the package. They can say, "Just 50 calories per serving!" Of course, normal people will eat four servings without even blinking and still reach for more. Be warned. Watch both the calories and the serving size. Only by adding them together can you get past this deception and on to the truth of what you're actually consuming.

Gregory L. Jantz with Ann McMurray, *The Body God Designed* (Lake Mary, FL: Siloam, 2007), 58–64.

WHY WHOLE GRAINS ARE BETTER THAN PROCESSED FOODS

by Don Colbert, MD

WHOLE-GRAIN PRODUCTS ARE nutrient-dense and pass on lots of vitamins and minerals to your body. Whole grains also contain lots of fiber, which is a fabulous toxin-trapper.

There's no USDA seal of approval for whole grains as there is for organic food. However, an organization called the Whole Grains Council created an official packaging stamp in 2005. The Whole Grain Stamp helps you to know how much whole grain content is included in various products.

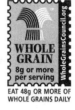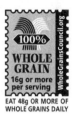

Finding a grain described as 100 percent whole grain in the ingredients list is more important than finding the words "whole grain" used loosely on the front of the package. If the first ingredient includes the word *whole*, it's more likely that the product contains whole grain, although it's not guaranteed.

SIMPLE WAYS TO "HIDE" WHOLE GRAINS IN YOUR DIET

- Add brown rice or rolled oats to recipes for meatballs, meatloaf, or hamburgers. A general rule of thumb: add ¾ cup of uncooked grains to every pound of meat.
- The next time you make cookies or muffins, try substituting half of the white flour with whole-wheat flour.
- Add ½ cup of cooked brown rice, wild rice, sorghum, or barley to your next batch of homemade or canned soup.
- Add ½ cup of cooked wild rice to your next batch of dressing or stuffing.
- Replace white rice with brown rice, basmati rice, or quinoa the next time you make risotto or rice pilaf.
- Sprinkle a handful of rolled oats on salad, yogurt, or ice cream.
- Use whole-grain pasta for your favorite pasta dishes.
- Blend your favorite ready-to-eat cereal with whole grains such as spelt or buckwheat.[1]

SPROUTED BREADS

I also encourage you to eat sprouted breads and flat breads. Ezekiel 4:9 bread and manna bread are both terrific flourless breads made from live, sprouted grains.

When you buy grain products, look for the word *sprouted* on the ingredient list.

Sprouted-grain products do go bad quicker, especially if you leave them on the counter, but there's nothing wrong with that. It means they aren't loaded with preservatives. The food God gave the Israelites during their sojourn in the wilderness—manna—bred worms after one day. It's characteristic of live food. You should learn to be suspicious of foods that don't go bad quickly.

WATCH OUT FOR CORN

Because so many people who visit me in the office discover that they have a sensitivity to corn, I recommend that you limit your consumption of whole-grain products that contain corn. Corn also typically contains a lot of mycotoxins, which are mold-associated toxins.[2]

Don Colbert, *Eat This and Live!* (Lake Mary, FL: Siloam, 2009), 56–57.

THE TEN COMMANDMENTS OF HEALTHY EATING AND DRINKING

by David B. Biebel, DMin, and Harold Koenig, MD

IT DOESN'T TAKE a degree in nutrition to know what the "right foods" are for you to eat—fruits, vegetables, lean meats, less sugar, and less processed foods. Most importantly, these foods should be eaten in smaller, healthier amounts.

Here are what we like to call "The Ten Commandments of a Healthy Diet." These are practical suggestions to show you where to begin:

1. Go "back to the garden" (as in the Garden of Eden), and consume a variety of healthy foods daily from all of the food groups (including adequate amounts of fiber).
2. Eat a healthy breakfast every day. Breakfast eaters perform better at work or school and find it easier to control their weight, since a good breakfast jump-starts your metabolism after your overnight fast.
3. Drink about one-half ounce of pure water per pound of your weight per day, 15 percent more when you exercise.
4. Eat at least nine servings of vegetables, fruits, and whole grains—whole, pesticide- and herbicide-free—daily. Variety is essential.
5. Consume several small amounts of lean protein daily as opposed to consuming large amounts at one sitting. Vegetarians should be careful to consume enough high-quality protein, including leucine, an amino acid essential to developing lean muscle and regulating hormones related to appetite and metabolism.
6. If you drink alcohol, stick to red wine, and no more than two servings per day. If you're pregnant, do not drink alcohol at all.[1]
7. Keep healthy snacks handy. Almonds, cashews, pecans, or walnuts provide fiber, vitamin E, and monounsaturated fats. They are "heart healthy" but high in calories, so use moderation. Note for chocolate lovers: a small amount of dark chocolate can be a health-enhancing reward, due to the type of flavonoids in it.[2]
8. Avoid most processed foods, especially those containing refined sugar or flour, excess salts, unnecessary fats, MSG, trans fats, and other additives.
9. Ban sugar-loaded soft drinks, candy, and other calorie-dense but nutrition-deficient foods from your house. Nobody can snack on what is not available. Forget "fast food" and "TV dinners," and stick to "slow" food that you can enjoy with your family around your dining room table as often as possible. This fellowship will build quality relationships and enhance spiritual connections with each other.
10. Become an informed consumer. Know what you are eating and where it came from. Read the labels. This is one of the most important factors.

David B. Biebel and Harold G. Koenig, *Simple Health* (Lake Mary, FL: Siloam, 2005), 68–71.

EAT MORE FIBER

by Don Colbert, MD

I FREQUENTLY TREAT PEOPLE in my practice who tell me they have only one bowel movement a week and think that's normal. They're shocked when I tell them a healthy person should have a bowel movement after every meal. Every time you eat food, the colon should experience peristalsis, which is the gastrocolic reflex that propels food through your digestive system.

There are two types of fiber: insoluble and soluble. Insoluble fiber increases the frequency of our bowel movements and the weight of our stool, and it helps prevent constipation, irritable bowel syndrome, hemorrhoids, diverticulosis, and other intestinal disorders. Bran (from any grain) is a good source of insoluble fiber. Most people can tolerate rice bran very well, so I often recommend this over the more popular wheat bran. Other good sources are high-fiber cereals and the skins of vegetables and fruits.

Soluble fiber lowers cholesterol, stabilizes blood sugar, slows digestion, and helps your body bind and eliminate toxins. Good sources of soluble fiber include fruits, beans, legumes, lentils, carrots, oats, and seeds such as psyllium seed and flaxseed.

It's important to get both types of fiber in your diet. Generally speaking, the higher the fiber content of your foods, the better. But I recommend that you increase your fiber intake slowly to avoid bloating, cramping, and excessive gas.

MORE FIBER MEANS MORE WATER

Fiber and water work together to stimulate the colon. As you increase the amount of fiber in your diet, you should increase the amount of water you drink.

QUICK WAYS TO ADD MORE FIBER TO YOUR DIET

- Add berries, almonds, or walnuts to your bowl of high-fiber cereal in the morning.
- Eat an orange or grapefruit instead of drinking a glass of juice. If you prefer drinking juice, squeeze your own and add the pulp back into the juice before drinking it.
- Sprinkle some pinto beans, garbanzo beans (chickpeas), or almonds on your salad.

Don Colbert, *Eat This and Live!* (Lake Mary, FL: Siloam, 2009), 58–59.

THE SCOOP ON FAT

by Terry Dorian, PhD

MOST AMERICANS ARE aware of the controversy surrounding our culture's low-fat diet scenario that promotes weight loss and protection against certain diseases.

But it is the *type* of fat that is the most significant factor in reversing chronic degenerative disease. Cells' membranes require omega-3 fatty acid derivatives (EPA and DHA) for fluidity. Monounsaturated fats found in nuts and extra-virgin olive oil balance the fluidity in the cells' membranes. Too much omega-3 would have an oxidizing (disease-causing) effect on the cell. Those healthy monounsaturated fats and vitamin E prevent that from happening.

Our bodies are able to manufacture these omega-3 derivatives from vegetarian sources, particularly green foods when we are healthy. The elderly and people on drugs or in a weakened state may not be able to make enough omega-3 derivatives. In those cases, we must consume the omega-3 fatty acids directly from animal sources by eating cold-water fish such as salmon, mackerel, tuna, and sardines, as well as grass-fed beef.

When we store excess fat in our bodies, we store mostly saturated fat. Grain-fed beef that dominates the beef market in the United States is high in saturated fat. The organic grass-fed beef that is now available in some markets has not been injected with hormones, does not contain pesticides, and is high in omega-3 fatty acids.

The Mediterranean diet of the 1960s, high in monounsaturated fats, offers enormous health benefits. And it convincingly proves, in comparison with the Chinese low-fat consumption, that it is the type of fats, rather than the quantity of fat, that is the distinguishing factor in healthy diets.

Poor fat sources

When we consume excessive amounts of carbohydrates (especially the processed, devitalized, no-fiber varieties), we end up with a diet that produces saturated fat. Even though we are consuming zero-saturated fat from animal sources and are following a low-fat diet, we are storing saturated fat from our high-carbohydrate intake.

Eating excessive amounts of "junk" carbohydrates is the single deadliest feature of the American diet. Everything from devitalized grains to sugary soda and candy, foods that are not real foods at all, are the products Americans crave most. Yet they are advertised as "fat-free" items in order to convince us that we should include them in our low-fat diets. This is one of the reasons we have become a nation of sick people who are getting sicker.

At the other extreme, a high-protein diet can be equally as harmful as a high-carbohydrate diet. We need adequate protein, but too much protein also makes us sick. Physical activity does have a bearing on the amount of protein the body requires. If we consume more protein than we require daily, it is converted to body fat when our energy requirements have already been met by other dietary components.

Terry Dorian, *Total Health and Restoration* (Lake Mary, FL: Siloam, 2002), 78–80.

WATER—HOW MUCH?

by Don Colbert, MD

O UR BODIES YEARN for pure, clean water. But one of the most common questions I hear is, "How much water should I drink?" I'm going to give you the answer to that question. To determine how much water your body needs, take your body weight (in pounds) and divide it by two. That's how many ounces of water you need every day.

_____ (weight in pounds) ÷ 2 = _____ (ounces per day)

Usually, that amounts to 2 or 3 quarts a day. Picture a gallon container of milk, and imagine it three-quarters full. If you are an average-sized person, that's about how much water your body needs daily. If you weigh 120 pounds, you will need 60 ounces of water; if 220 pounds, you'll need 110 ounces. Most people have no idea they require that much.

But you won't consume it all in liquid form. Simply by eating lots of fruits and vegetables—as you should—you will get about a quart a day. Foods such as bananas are 70 percent water; apples, 80 percent water; tomatoes and watermelons are more than 90 percent water; and lettuce is 95 percent water. If you eat an inordinate amount of starches, like breads or pastries, you will need more water, because these foods add little water to your body.

WHEN TO DRINK WATER

Most people wait until they are thirsty or until they have a dry mouth before they take a drink. By that time you are most likely already mildly dehydrated. A dry mouth is one of the last signs of dehydration.

Other people only drink during meals—another mistake. When you drink too much with a meal, it washes out the hydrochloric acid, digestive juices, and enzymes in your stomach and intestines, which delays digestion. Fluids, and iced drinks in particular, quench the digestive process similarly to pouring water on a fire.

You can drink some water with a meal. I usually drink room-temperature unsweetened tea or bottled water with a slice of lemon or lime squeezed into it. But don't go overboard. Meals are not the time to get most of your fluids. Stick to 4 to 8 ounces with a meal.

If you live in a warmer or drier climate, you will need more water. Most of us lose about a pint of water a day through perspiration. Our bodies also lose water through exhalation (about a pint a day) and through urination and stool (about 1 to 2 pints a day).[1] Two pints equal 1 quart, so our bodies lose about 1 ½–2 quarts a day. However, this doesn't account for excessive perspiration.

Don Colbert, *Eat This and Live!* (Lake Mary, FL: Siloam, 2009), 112–113.

IS BOTTLED WATER SAFE?

by Don Colbert, MD

MANY PEOPLE DRINK bottled water instead of tap water, making bottled water the second most popular beverage in the United States behind soft drinks.[1] People today consume twice as much bottled water as they did a decade ago, and the growth in the bottled water industry is "unparalleled," according to the Beverage Marketing Corporation.[2]

But is bottled water healthier for you? Does that attractive bottle with the pictures of snowy mountains and crystalline streams really mean the water inside is pure?

Bottled water is actually *less regulated than tap water.* Bottled water is considered a "food," and so it is regulated by the FDA. Tap water is regulated by the EPA.[3] The only requirement placed on bottled water is that it be as safe as tap water. But while the EPA makes cities test public drinking water daily, the FDA requires only yearly testing for bottled water.[4] The EPA forbids the presence of bacteria, which indicate the presence of fecal material, but the FDA has no such rule, meaning bottled water can contain fecal bacteria and still be legal.[5]

WHERE BOTTLED WATER REALLY COMES FROM

Brace yourself for this one. Dasani and Aquafina waters, two of the biggest brands in America, are reprocessed tap water from cities around the country. One of Aquafina's sources is the Detroit River![6] In fact, about one-fourth of bottled water is tap water, according to government and industry estimates.[7]

DR. COLBERT APPROVED: GLASS OR STAINLESS STEEL BOTTLES

Because studies continue to show that some forms of plastic are not as safe as people believe, I prefer drinking water from glass bottles or from stainless steel bottles.

The topic and debate over which plastics are safest will continue, and so will the recommendations. As for now, the safest plastics to use are HDPE (#2), LDPE (#4), and PP (#5). The rest—PET (#1), PVC (#3), PS (#6), and polycarbonate (#7) are not safe.

Don Colbert, *Eat This and Live!* (Lake Mary, FL: Siloam, 2009), 114–115.

PHYTONUTRIENTS: A RAINBOW OF HEALTH

by Don Colbert, MD

THE PHYTONUTRIENTS IN fruits and vegetables can be grouped according to color. Each group has its own set of unique protective benefits. You need to try to consume all seven colors of the phytonutrient rainbow every day to receive the protection you need. To do this, you need to eat a variety of foods. Think of phytonutrients as a "rainbow of health," God's promise to you to keep you healthy. Let's look at each group.

1. Red—tomatoes, watermelon, guava, and red grapefruit contain a powerful carotenoid called *lycopene,* which is about twice as powerful as beta-carotene. Lycopene is the main pigment responsible for the red color. Lycopene is linked to prevention of heart disease and prostate cancer.

2. Red/purple—blueberries, blackberries, hawthorn berries, raspberries, grapes, eggplants, red cabbage, and red wine contain a powerful flavonoid called *anthocyanidin*, which contains approximately fifty times the antioxidant activity of vitamin C and is twenty times more powerful than vitamin E.

3. Orange—carrots, mangoes, cantaloupes, pumpkin, sweet potatoes, yams, squash, and apricots, have high amounts of carotenoids, which help prevent cancer and heart disease. Typically, the more orange the fruit or vegetable is, the higher the concentration of *provitamin A carotenoids.*

4. Orange/yellow—oranges, tangerines, lemons, limes, yellow grapefruit, papaya, pineapple, and nectarines are rich in vitamin C and *citrus bioflavonoids* and protect us against free-radical damage. They prevent allergies and inflammation and have also been used to prevent and treat bruising, hemorrhoids, varicose veins, and spider veins.

5. Yellow/green—spinach, kale, collard greens, mustard greens, turnip greens, romaine lettuce, leeks, and peas are typically rich in *lutein* and *zeaxanthin*. Lutein is able to reduce the risk of macular degeneration, which is the leading cause of blindness in older adults.

6. Green—broccoli, cabbage, brussels sprouts, cauliflower, watercress, bok choy, kale, collard greens, and mustard greens are considered cruciferous vegetables. Broccoli sprouts have some of the highest concentrations of protective phytonutrients. Young broccoli sprouts that are about three days old contain twenty to fifty times more phytonutrients than mature broccoli.

7. White/green—onions contain the flavonoid *quercetin*, which has anti-inflammatory, antiviral, and anticancer properties. Quercetin is often recommended by nutritionists to treat both allergies and asthma. Apples, red wine, and black tea also contain quercetin.

   Garlic inhibits the formation of *nitrosamines*, which are cancer-causing compounds formed during digestion. Garlic has significant antimicrobial activity against bacteria, viruses, fungi, and even parasites. It also has cholesterol-lowering activities and can even lower blood pressure as well as help prevent blood clots.

   Green tea's active constituents are *polyphenols*, which have been shown to reduce the risk of cancers of the stomach, small intestines, colon, and pancreas, as well as lung and breast cancers. As an antioxidant, green tea is two hundred times more powerful than vitamin E and five hundred times more powerful than vitamin C.

Don Colbert, *Eat This and Live!* (Lake Mary, FL: Siloam, 2009), 68–71.

VARIETY IS THE SPICE OF LIFE

by Pamela M. Smith, RD

T HE BEAUTIFUL THING about good, balanced nutrition is this: everything fits together in such a perfect way that just focusing on eating (early, often, balanced, and lean) will give you a blessing of nutrients. You don't have to analyze your intake continually to be sure you've had your zinc today.

What you are responsible to do is to choose healthy foods with a sense of balance and variety—the cornerstones of good nutrition.

Your health doesn't depend on a single food or a single meal. No one food is perfect; no one food contains all the nutrients you need.

Healthy variety occurs when you make good food choices over a period of time.

Be sure to provide whole grain, low-fat meals that are full of a variety of brightly colored fruits and vegetables. The bright coloring is a sign of the nutritional content of a vegetable or fruit; generally the more vivid the coloring, the more essential nutrients it holds. That deep orange or red coloring in carrots, sweet potatoes, cantaloupes, peaches, and strawberries signals their vitamin A content. Dark green leafy vegetables such as turnip or mustard greens, spinach, romaine lettuce, brussels sprouts, and broccoli are loaded with vitamin A as well as folic acid. Vitamin C is found in more than just citrus; it is also power-packed into strawberries, cantaloupes, tomatoes, green peppers, and broccoli. Remember: you may not be able to tell a book by its cover, but you can tell the power of a fruit or veggie by its color!

Are you still saying yuck to the same veggies you didn't like when you were young? Open your mind, your taste buds, your likes and dislikes, your schedule, and your menu to these storehouses of nutritional power—they are worth it.

BREAKING THE RUT

Healthy eating doesn't need to be anything less than enjoyable, tasty, and full of variety. Yet for many people, healthy eating means eating in a rut, a boring rut.

We settle into a limited variety of dishes with which we feel safe and don't have to think about much. We don't want to have to make decisions; it's just easier to have the same bowl of cereal for breakfast, a "ditto" turkey sandwich at lunch, and a piece of baked chicken for dinner.

Why such a rut? It's easier for us to trust the rut than to trust ourselves to make healthy choices. Some people are subconsciously trying to work wonders, thinking that just the right (or only one) combination of food will work and be safe. Some people seem to punish themselves with the same old, boring foods, thinking they are paying some kind of penance for their last binge. Others, who don't care enough about themselves to do anything differently, feed themselves with as much fore-thought and effort as they feed their pets.

So what's the problem with ruts? Time and again I see people set up to overindulge as soon as they get the taste of anything more exciting. Then once they get off track, it becomes very difficult to get back on track—since, to them, "on track" means returning to the same old, boring rut.

Eating a variety of foods in their whole form provides you with a gamut of vitamins and minerals, including as yet hidden benefits.

Pamela M. Smith, *Food for Life* (Lake Mary, FL: Siloam, 1994, 1997), 89–91.

THE TOP TEN HEART-HEALTHY FOODS

by Francisco Contreras, MD

THE FOODS WE eat are the most important single factor in determining whether or not we develop heart disease. Let's look at the heart-healthy foods we want in our pantries and refrigerators.

1. Fruits and vegetables don't contain cholesterol, and they are naturally low in fat, saturated fat, calories, and sodium. They are also rich in protein, potassium, fiber, folic acid, vitamin C, and phytochemicals.

2. Olive oil contains phenols that increase the production of substances that help open arteries, which in turn reduces artery resistance to the blood flow, and blood pressure is decreased.

3. Nuts—no other food has been so consistently associated with a marked reduction in heart disease risk in people of all habits, races, and health profiles.[1] A 50-gram serving of nuts exceeds the recommended daily allowance for vitamin E, which has been shown to reduce the risk of coronary heart disease.[2]

4. Grape juice—drinking an average of about 2 cups (450 ml) of purple grape juice a day for one week vastly reduced the "stickiness" of blood platelets. It also contributes to increasing the opening of the arteries.

5. Red wine contains abundant polyphenols that have been shown to inhibit LDL cholesterol oxidation, help prevent atherosclerosis, increase antioxidant capacity, and raise plasma levels of HDL ("good") cholesterol.[3] Drinking two servings (240–280 ml) of red wine per day will provide approximately 40 percent of the total antioxidant polyphenols present in a healthy diet, as well as polyphenols like resveratrol that are virtually absent from fruit and vegetables.

6. Green tea—a single cup of green tea usually contains about 200–400 mg of polyphenols. Studies have indicated that drinking tea protects against heart disease.[4]

7. Coffee—the Scottish Heart Study found the prevalence of heart disease to be the highest among those who abstain from coffee drinking.[5] However, coffee should be consumed in moderation.

8. Chocolate—40 grams of milk chocolate contain almost as many polyphenols as a standard serving of red wine, which prevents hardening of the arteries, reduces the risk of atherosclerosis, and decreases morbidity and mortality from heart disease.[6]

9. Fiber—soluble, viscous fibers like psyllium, oat bran, guar, and pectin decrease serum cholesterol and LDL cholesterol serum levels, which may contribute to their protective role against heart disease.

10. Fish—omega-3 (n-3) fatty acids from fish and plant sources protect against heart disease and prevent deaths from heart disease and heart attack by preventing fatal cardiac arrhythmias, preventing the formation of blood clots, widening the arteries, inhibiting plaque formation, reducing high blood pressure, and preventing arteries from becoming inflamed.[7]

Francisco Contreras, *A Healthy Heart* (Lake Mary, FL: Siloam, 2001), 79–99.

THE PERFECT "COMFORT FOOD"

by Janet Maccaro, PhD, CNC

ARE YOU LOOKING for the perfect "comfort food"? Do you need something that will improve your mood within minutes and maybe keep you feeling good for some time?

Eat carbs.

Carbohydrates—if they are complex carbohydrates—boost your brain's serotonin levels, and serotonin is known as the "good mood" chemical. Avoid carbohydrates such as candy, sweet baked goods, and junk foods, even if they are the only things available in the vending machine at work. Those are simple carbohydrates, and their sugar content alone will give you a temporary "buzz," only to let you down badly later. Instead, try some air-popped popcorn, fresh fruit, or whole-grain crackers.

Eat foods that provide folic acid.

Many people who suffer from low moods have been shown to have a folic-acid deficiency. Choose foods such as asparagus; avocados; garbanzos, soybeans, and other beans; lentils and other legumes; oranges; broccoli; and spinach and its dark leafy cousins.

Eat foods that provide magnesium.

Magnesium relaxes your tense muscles. Here again, avocados and spinach can help. You can also get magnesium from dark chocolate (in small servings, please), almonds, and pumpkin or sunflower seeds.

Eat foods that provide niacin.

Some experts believe that niacin can help alleviate depression, anxiety, or panic. It is found in dairy products, poultry, fish, lean meats, brown rice, nuts, and eggs.

Eat foods that provide zinc.

If you lack zinc in your diet, you will have a very short "fuse." You will be irritable and easily angered. See if you can improve your bad mood with some zinc-containing whole-grain bread, a glass of milk, an egg or two, or even some oysters.

Eat foods that are low in sodium.

The average American adult consumes more than twice as much sodium in a day than is recommended. This has the negative effect of making a person retain water, which makes him or her feel sluggish. It also causes blood pressure to rise, which is hard on every part of a person's body.

Eat foods in moderation.

Even mood-enhancing foods should not be eaten in large quantities, or you will have too much of a good thing. Don't let your low mood drive you to overeat. If you do, you will undo many of the effects of the good nutrition by raising your blood sugar and consequent insulin and cortisone levels. You want your food to *enhance* your mood, not swing it wildly back and forth.

Janet Maccaro, *Change Your Food, Change Your Mood* (Lake Mary, FL: Siloam, 2008), 89–91.

HAVE A CHOCOLATE PEPPER!

by Francisco Contreras, MD, and Daniel E. Kennedy

ENDORPHIN SECRETION MAY also be triggered by the consumption of certain foods, such as chocolate and chili peppers.

Indeed, the characteristic increase in bodily endorphin levels caused by chocolate could explain why we often turn to it as a comfort food in times of stress. Chocolate is by far the most popular endorphin-producing food on the earth.

Known by the Aztecs as the "food of the gods," chocolate is derived from cacao beans that were revered by the Aztecs, who believed that eating chocolate would confer wisdom and vitality. Chocolate contains more than three hundred different compounds, including anandamide, a chemical that mimics marijuana's soothing effects on the brain. It also contains chemical compounds such as flavonoids (which are also found in wine) that have antioxidant properties and reduce serum cholesterol.

Although the combined psychochemical effects of these compounds on the central nervous system are poorly understood, the production of endorphins is believed to contribute to the renowned "inner glow" experienced by chocolate lovers. But as with red wine, moderation is the key. More than 50 g a day are not recommended.

Many popular ethnic foods, including Tex-Mex, Mexican, Cajun, Indian, Chinese (especially Szechuan), and Thai, are renowned for their spiciness. The resulting endorphin rush keeps diners coming back for more. Chili peppers provide a stimulating heat and "bite" that increases the body's production of endorphins.

Chili peppers are not all created equal: red peppers are generally more pungent than green ones, and hotter chilies grow at higher attitudes and warmer temperatures. Chilies also release their heat differently; some are experienced as "hot" immediately, or their pungency is released over time; some chilies cause a burning sensation in the back of the throat, while others affect the tongue or the lips.

And while chili peppers vary as to flavor, texture, and color, they all provide important vitamins and minerals, including vitamin A, calcium, and vitamin C. Moreover, due to the endorphin release associated with chili peppers, they have been utilized in various kinds of medical treatments, especially as part of therapy for chronic pain, and are sometimes considered an aphrodisiac.

I'm sure this is one of the reasons why Mexicans have such a low incidence of cancer and are so warm and happy.

Francisco Contreras and Daniel E. Kennedy, *Fighting Cancer 20 Different Ways* (Lake Mary, FL: Siloam, 2005), 119–120.

HIGH-FRUCTOSE CORN SYRUP

by Kara Davis, MD

HIGH-FRUCTOSE CORN SYRUP (HFCS) is a sweetener made from corn, not the plants we typically associate with "sweetness" like sugar cane and sugar beets, which give us table sugar (sucrose). It is made by milling corn into corn starch, then processing the corn starch into corn syrup, which is almost entirely composed of the sugar known as glucose. Enzymes are added to the corn syrup, changing the glucose into fructose. The end result is a sweetener—HFCS 90—that is almost 90 percent fructose, although there are other ratios as well (HFCS 55 and HFCS 42).

Since its introduction in the 1970s, HFCS use has increased, completely replacing table sugar in many foods and beverages. From a business standpoint, HFCS has clear advantages over sugar. In the United States, corn is abundant and inexpensive compared to sugar, making HFCS much cheaper to use. Because it is a liquid, it is easier to transport than sugar, and this also affects pricing. Foods containing HFCS have a longer shelf life and less freezer burn than foods made with sugar. So these factors have made HFCS the ideal sweetener for food manufacturers. Their preference is reflected in our consumption of HFCS, which now exceeds that of table sugar. In 2005 the average American consumed about 28.4 kilograms of HFCS compared with 26.7 kilograms of sucrose sugar.[1]

But what's good for business is not always good for our health. From the start, there have been health concerns relating to HFCS, with animal studies showing a connection to liver damage and obesity. Food manufacturers have dismissed such studies and maintain the effects on the body from HFCS are essentially the same as those of table sugar. Animal studies aside, we cannot ignore the parallel trends between obesity and the consumption of soft drinks sweetened with HFCS.

Some countries, including Mexico and Canada, still use sucrose in their soft drinks, but in the United States, the major soda manufacturers use HFCS. Between 1970 and 1990, HFCS consumption increased by more than 1,000 percent, in large part because of the switch from sucrose to HFCS in soft drinks. Our consumption of soft drinks increased by 135 percent between 1977 and 2001, and soft drinks are now the largest source of added sugars in the American diet. During this same interval, the incidence and prevalence of obesity have skyrocketed.[2]

A recent study presented at the 2007 Scientific Session of the American Diabetes Association involved human (not rodent) subjects. In it, volunteers who were overweight or obese consumed drinks sweetened with either fructose or glucose. At the end of the study, the fructose group had a 212 percent increase in the level of triglycerides, while the glucose group's triglycerides dropped by 30 percent. In addition, the LDL cholesterol and other "bad" fats—i.e., substances that accelerate atherosclerosis— were all significantly increased in the fructose group but remained unchanged in the glucose group.[3]

While the final report is not yet available, the investigators concluded that their preliminary data strongly suggest a connection between HFCS and not only weight gain but also weight-related disease. They advised that people at risk for diabetes or cardiovascular disease limit their consumption of fructose-sweetened beverages.

It seems this would be reason enough to just eliminate high-calorie beverages from the menu altogether. To me, that's just common sense.

Kara Davis, *Spiritual Secrets to Weight Loss* (Lake Mary, FL: Siloam, 2002, 2008), 179–181.

CAUTIONS ABOUT DAIRY

by Don Colbert, MD

MANY PEOPLE EAT dairy products with great abandon because they associate milk with health, robustness, and wholesomeness. But from a physician's point of view, I'm highly aware of the problems caused by dairy products. Most children I see in my practice with chronic ear infections and sinus infections have dairy sensitivities. I know of other doctors who say that eliminating dairy products is often the only thing they need to do to stop recurrent ear problems in children. One doctor reported that, of all the children he saw who required tubes to be put into their eardrums for drainage purposes, three out of four did not need the tubes when they stopped eating dairy products.[1]

Dairy products, and cow's milk in particular, are also linked to all kinds of allergies and sensitivities, including skin rashes, eczema, fatigue, spastic colon, excessive mucus production, nasal allergies, and chronic sinus infections. Some people even have diarrhea due to lactose intolerance. If you (or especially children) have any of these, stop all dairy products—including skim milk, butter, and even yogurt—for a week or so, and watch the improvement. Small wonder that man is the only species in the animal kingdom to drink cow's milk as an adult.

Another problem with milk is that it is pasteurized by heating it at 161 degrees for fifteen seconds, which denatures milk enzymes and changes its protein structure, making it difficult for our bodies to assimilate and digest.[2] However, I do not recommend raw milk since it may contain toxic bacteria such as *Brucella*, which is associated with brucellosis.[3]

Finally, dairy products tend to have lots of saturated fat, which is associated with high cholesterol and heart disease. Butter is 81 percent saturated fat. Cheese is 75 percent fat. Regular milk is 4 percent saturated fat, which means that 48 percent of its calories come from fat—way too high for a healthy diet. And toxins are concentrated in those dairy fats. High amounts of pesticide residues are usually found in butter and cheese.

Here are tips to eating healthy dairy products.

- Consider goat's milk. Goat's-milk products generally cause fewer allergies and sensitivities than cow's milk. Make sure the goat's milk is from grass-fed goats.
- Consider organic coconut milk.
- Choose organic skim dairy products. They have no saturated fat, and they are much lower in calories. Use small amounts of organic butter or ghee, which is clarified butter. It's best to avoid ice cream and frozen yogurt since they are high in sugar.
- Eat kefir and yogurt from time to time if you are not sensitive to dairy. The best dairy product for you is low-fat organic kefir or yogurt, which contains good bacteria that help maintain a healthy GI tract. Buy plain low-fat organic yogurt or organic goat's-milk yogurt, and add your own fresh fruit. Or try goat's-milk kefir or coconut-milk kefir.

Don Colbert, *Eat This and Live!* (Lake Mary, FL: Siloam, 2009), 104–105, 126–127.

CAUTIONS ABOUT MEAT

by Don Colbert, MD

You can enjoy meat by taking some precautions. Here are my recommendations:

- Try to choose organic, free-range, or grass-fed meat, and always look for the leanest cuts—chicken breast, turkey breast, or very lean cuts of filet mignon or tenderloin. This will help you avoid potential toxins in the fat. Free-range meats are healthiest because the animals were not fed antibiotics. The breasts of free-range chickens contain some of the lowest amounts of animal fat. Organic and free-range animals feed on grasses and have more omega-3 fats in the meat than grain-fed cattle. Grain-fed cattle are usually much fatter and contain more omega-6 fat as well as saturated fats.[1] The fat content of wild game is about 4 percent, whereas grain-fed beef typically contains 30 percent or more fat.

- If you cannot afford organic or free-range meat or poultry, get the leanest cuts, trim off any visible fat, and remove any skin. Make sure the meat has not been irradiated.

- Turkey is one of the best choices of meats. Turkey breast is one of the leanest meats and contains the least amount of pesticides and toxins. Other relatively safe meats include the leanest cuts of lamb, venison (U.S.), rabbit, and buffalo.

- Some people worry about giving up meat because they wrongly believe they won't get enough protein in their diet. But a balanced diet that includes small amounts of lean meats and generous portions of beans and whole grains can give you the protein you need. For example, whole-grain bread and hummus make a complete protein when eaten together. Remember, only about 1 percent of a gorilla's diet is derived from animal meat.

- If you choose to eat red meats, limit them to only 4 to 6 ounces, once or twice a week. A diet high in red meat is associated with an increased risk of breast[2] and prostate[3] cancers.

- When preparing poultry, trim off the skin and any visible fat before it is cooked. If you leave the fat and skin on, the pesticides collected in these parts of the animal may seep into the meat. Bake, broil, grill, or lightly stir-fry your meat. (Don't deep-fry your chickens or turkeys, as some people have begun doing.) Scrape off charred portions, because char contains benzopyrenes, which are carcinogens and are associated with colorectal cancer.

- Cook meats thoroughly since most poultry contains dangerous bacteria such as salmonella, campylobacteria, and staphylococcus, which are associated with food poisoning.

Once you start buying the right kinds of meats and preparing them in a healthy way, you can fully enjoy them as part of your regular diet.

Don Colbert, *Eat This and Live!* (Lake Mary, FL: Siloam, 2009), 100–101.

CAUTIONS ABOUT FISH

by Don Colbert, MD

I USED TO RECOMMEND fish much more heartily than I do now, but new studies keep emerging about the high mercury content of fish, even fish formerly considered safe. For that reason I'm much more cautious now about fish.

Because the oceans, lakes, and rivers have suffered from the toxic onslaught of chemicals along with the rest of the environment, fish are no longer free of toxins. But if you are careful about which fish you eat, they can be your best source of healthy omega-3 oils, which study after study has shown is one of the best oils on the planet. Here are my recommendations:

- Fish with the highest concentrations of omega-3 oils are Pacific herring, king salmon, wild Pacific salmon, anchovies, and lake trout. Wild Pacific salmon contains higher omega-3 fat than farm-raised Atlantic salmon.
- Look into buying tongol tuna, which is much lower in mercury and comes from much smaller tuna. Most store-bought tuna comes from larger tunas, which contain much higher mercury content. Tongol tuna is generally found in health food stores.
- Other good fish are tilapia, flounder, haddock, mackerel, and sole.
- Avoid shark and swordfish. They have some of the highest levels of mercury and pesticides of any fish in the sea. Sharks will eat anything, and they eat a lot of pesticides. In many areas trout have also been subjected to contamination through industrialization. Use caution, and select fish taken from fresh, pure-water areas.

If you purchase your fish from a grocery store, use wisdom. Nearly 40 percent of your grocer's fish may have already begun to spoil. Ensure the quality of your purchases by using this brief checklist:

- Look for fish that is shiny, bright, and bulging. If the scales are shiny, the fish is good.
- If the flesh doesn't spring back when you touch it, don't buy it.
- If it smells fishy, don't buy it.
- If the fish has not been kept on ice at 32 degrees, don't buy it. It is likely that it has already begun to spoil.
- Certain ocean waters are known for their purity. Fish from Australia, Chile, New Zealand, and Greece are extremely clean and should be safe to eat.
- Shrimp contains higher levels of cholesterol than other seafood, but it is usually free from contamination from pesticides, though it usually contains the heavy metal cadmium, which is associated with hypertension. Most shellfish contain cadmium, so if you choose to eat shellfish, do so infrequently and eat those from less-industrialized areas where the waters remain uncontaminated.

Don Colbert, *Eat This and Live!* (Lake Mary, FL: Siloam, 2009), 102–103.

TIPS FOR HEALTHY SHOPPING

by David B. Biebel, DMin, and Harold Koenig, MD

FOR MANY FOOD products, multiple choices are available in most grocery stores. Health-conscious consumers make healthier shopping choices. Some brands listed below may not be available where you shop, but the key is to read the labels and compare ingredients in order to identify the healthier brands. Be wary of the following terms: enriched, refined, or fortified. The basic principles include: choose whole foods free of herbicides or pesticides, hormones or antibiotics, additives, preservatives, refined sugars, salts, artificial sweetening, caffeine, coloring or flavoring, hydrogenated or partially hydrogenated oils (trans fats), hodrolyzed vegetable protein, nitrates, nitrites, and MSG.[1]

Our friend Toni Olson is a health educator whose passion is helping parents understand how to provide optimal nutrition for their families. This is Toni's guide to buying healthy groceries:

SHOPPER'S GUIDE

FOOD	BRAND	COMMENTS
Applesauce	Leroux Creek	Organic, gluten free with delicious berry blends
	Mott's Natural	Contains only apples, water, and ascorbic acid
	Santa Cruz Organic	Certified organic, variety of blends
Bars	Larabars	Better than most
	Nature Valley	No trans fats
Bread	Alvarado St. Bakery	No pesticides/herbicides, chemical fertilizers, genetically modified organisms (GMOs), artificial ingredients, preservatives, or trans fats. Buy 100 percent whole-grain breads or try sprouted grains.
	French Meadows Bakery	
	Rudi's Organic	
	Nature's Own Whole Wheat	Also good. More choices are available in the health food section.
Cereal	Mother's Peace Cereal	There are many brands of great-tasting cereals that contain organic ingredients, natural sweeteners (no refined sugar, aspartame, Splenda), no hydrogenated oils, and minimal flavorings, preservatives, etc.
	Nature Valley	
	Kashi	
	Nature's Path Instant Oatmeal	
Dairy	Nest Fresh Eggs	Organic, free-range chicken eggs that contain more nutrition with no hormones, antibiotics, toxic pesticides
	Horizon milk, cheese, and butter	Organic milk with no hormones, antibiotics
	Royal Crest Delivery	Also good quality
Deli Meats	Applegate Farms	Their meats and cheeses contain no colorings, flavorings, etc.
	Boar's Head	You can also get nitrate-free oven-roasted turkey from most deli counters.

Flour	Whole grain	Try whole wheat, spelt, rice, oat bran, amaranth, etc.
Fruits and Vegetables	Organic	Buy organic fruits and vegetables when they are available. When they aren't available, soak soft-skinned fruits and veggies in a mix of 1 gallon water and 1 tablespoon sea salt or vinegar for five minutes to remove pesticide residue.
Juice	Northland, Hansen	100 percent real fruit juice without added sugars
	Juicy Juice	
	R.W. Knudsen	
Macaroni and Cheese	Annie's Organic	
	Simply Organic	Just five ingredients of real food. Organic without added artificial flavorings, colorings, preservatives, and chemicals.
Meats	Maverick Farms	We buy only organic meat. Smaller portions of leaner, healthier meats without the hormones, antibiotics, and poor animal conditions are very important for a healthy diet.
Nut Butters	Adam's	
	Arrowhead Mills	Just real peanuts. Turn jar upside down in your pantry to keep the oil off the top. Have the kids grind their own at the store (Vitamin, Maranatha, Cottage, Wild Oats, Whole Foods).
Popcorn	Your own!	You can pop popcorn in a paper bag in the microwave with canola oil. Or use an air popper. Sprinkle some Herbamare seasonings or coconut flakes on it.
Potato Chips	Boulder Chips	Contain no preservatives, additives, artificial colors, or hydrogenated oils. Read the ingredients on "flavored" chips as these may contain some questionable flavorings, including MSG.
	Guiltless Gourmet	
	Lay's Natural	
Potstickers	Ling Lings	No harmful ingredients. Easy, pretty healthy, and kids love them.
Salt	Sea salt	Salt in its natural form is much better for you!
Sugar	Sucanat	Great replacement for refined sugar; hasn't gone through as much processing. Can be used as a 1:1 substitute for white sugar in baking.
Sweeteners	Stevia	Concentrated natural sweetener. Great in coffee, tea, etc. Stevia is a slow-release sweetener and helps maintain even blood sugar levels. Please avoid artificial sweeteners, as their safety is open to question.
Waffles	Vans	Delicious without the artificial ingredients, hydrogenated oils, and preservatives.
	Lifestream	
Yogurt	Stoneyfield Farms	Organic yogurt that contains natural sweeteners. Sugar content of this yogurt is much less than others.
	Mountain High	
	Redwood Hills	
	Goat yogurt	

David B. Biebel and Harold G. Koenig, *Simple Health* (Lake Mary, FL: Siloam, 2005), 63–67.

HEALTHY GROCERY LIST

by Pamela M. Smith, RD

GRAINS

Brown rice: ☐ Instant ☐ Long grain
☐ Short grain
☐ Wild rice
☐ Cornmeal
☐ Whole-wheat bagels
☐ Whole-wheat bread *(100 percent: first word of ingredients: "whole")*
☐ Whole-wheat English muffins
☐ Whole-wheat hamburger buns
Whole-wheat pasta: ☐ Elbows ☐ Flat
☐ Lasagna ☐ Spaghetti ☐ Spirals
☐ Whole-wheat pastry flour
☐ Whole-wheat pita bread
☐ _____
☐ _____

CEREALS *(whole grain and less than 5 grams of added sugar)*:

☐ Cheerios
☐ Grape-Nuts
☐ Grits
☐ Muesli
Oats: ☐ Old-fashioned ☐ Quick-cooking
Puffed cereals: ☐ Rice ☐ Wheat
☐ Raisin Squares
☐ Shredded Wheat
☐ Shredded Wheat'n Bran
Unprocessed bran: ☐ Oat ☐ Wheat
☐ Wheatena
☐ _____
☐ _____

CRACKERS

Crispbread: ☐ Kavli ☐ Wasa
☐ Crispy cakes
☐ Harvest Crisps 5-Grain *(not all whole grain, but good for variety)*

☐ Rice cakes
☐ Ry-Krisp
☐ _____

DAIRY

☐ Butter
Cheese *(low fat; less than 5 grams of fat per ounce)*:
Cheddar: ☐ Kraft Light Naturals
☐ Weight Watchers Natural
☐ Cottage cheese, 1 percent
☐ Farmer's
☐ Jarlsberg Lite
Cream cheese: ☐ Philadelphia Light *(tub)*
☐ Philadelphia Fat-free
Mozzarella: ☐ Nonfat ☐ Part-skim
☐ String cheese
☐ Laughing Cow Light *(nonrefrigerated)*
☐ Parmesan
Ricotta: ☐ Nonfat ☐ Part skim
☐ Egg substitute
☐ Eggs
☐ Fleischmann's Squeeze Spread
☐ Milk *(skim or 1 percent)*
☐ Nonfat plain yogurt
☐ Stonyfield Farm Yogurt
☐ _____
☐ _____

CANNED GOODS

☐ Swanson's Natural Goodness chicken broth
Soups: ☐ Pritikin ☐ Progresso Black Bean
☐ Progresso Lentil
Tomatoes: ☐ Paste ☐ Sauce ☐ Stewed
☐ Whole
☐ _____
☐ _____
☐ _____

FRUITS

☐ Apples ☐ Apricots ☐ Bananas ☐ Berries
☐ Citrus ☐ Cherries ☐ Dates *(unsweetened,*
pitted) ☐ Grapes ☐ Kiwi ☐ Lemons ☐ Limes
☐ Melon ☐ Nectarines ☐ Peaches ☐ Pears
☐ Pineapple ☐ Plums ☐ Raisins
☐ _____
☐ _____
☐ _____

VEGETABLES

☐ Asparagus ☐ Broccoli ☐ Cabbage ☐ Carrots
☐ Cauliflower ☐ Celery ☐ Corn ☐ Cucumbers
☐ Green beans ☐ Greens ☐ Kale
☐ Mushrooms ☐ Onions ☐ Peas ☐ Peppers
☐ Red potatoes ☐ Romaine lettuce ☐ Spinach
☐ Squash ☐ Sweet potatoes ☐ Tomatoes
☐ White potatoes ☐ Zucchini
☐ _____
☐ _____
☐ _____

BEANS AND MEATS

Beans and peas: ☐ Black ☐ Chickpeas/
   garbanzo beans ☐ Kidney ☐ Lentils
   ☐ Navy ☐ Pinto ☐ Split peas
   ☐ _____
Beef (lean): ☐ Deli sliced ☐ Ground round
   ☐ Round steak
   ☐ _____
Chicken: ☐ Boneless breasts ☐ Parts
   ☐ Whole fryer
   ☐ _____
Fish and seafood: ☐ Fresh ☐ Frozen
Lamb: ☐ Leg ☐ Loin chops
Turkey: ☐ Breast ☐ Ground ☐ Sliced ☐ Whole
   ☐ _____
Veal: ☐ Chuck ☐ Leg chops ☐ Loin chops
   ☐ Round ☐ Rump ☐ Shoulder chops
Water-packed cans: ☐ Chicken ☐ Salmon
☐ Tuna ☐ Charlie's Lunch Kit
☐ _____
☐ _____

MISCELLANEOUS

All-fruit jam and pourable syrup: ☐ Knudsen
   ☐ Polaner's ☐ Smucker's Simply Fruit
Bean dips: ☐ Guiltless Gourmet
Boullion cubes: ☐ Beef ☐ Chicken
Cooking oils: ☐ Canola ☐ Olive
☐ Cornstarch
Fruit juices (unsweetened): ☐ Apple ☐ Apple-
   cranberry ☐ White grape ☐ Orange
Garlic: ☐ Cloves ☐ Minced
☐ Honey
Mayonnaise: ☐ Light ☐ Miracle Whip Light
☐ Mustard
☐ Nonstick cooking spray
Nuts/seeds (dry roasted, unsalted): ☐ Peanuts
   ☐ Sunflower kernels
Pasta sauce: ☐ Pritikin ☐ Ragu's Chunky
   Gardenstyle
☐ Peanut butter *(natural)*
Popcorn: ☐ Orville Redenbacher's Light
   Natural Microwave ☐ Plain kernels
Salad dressing: ☐ Bernstein's Low-Calorie
   ☐ Good Seasons ☐ Kraft-Free ☐ Pritikin
☐ Soy sauce *(low sodium)*
Spices and herbs: ☐ Allspice ☐ Basil ☐ Black
   pepper ☐ Cayenne pepper ☐ Celery seed
   ☐ Chili powder ☐ Cinnamon ☐ Curry
   ☐ Dill weed ☐ Garlic powder ☐ Ginger
   ☐ Mustard ☐ Nutmeg ☐ Oregano
   ☐ Onion powder ☐ Paprika ☐ Parsley
   ☐ Rosemary
Tortilla chips: ☐ Baked Tostitos
   ☐ Guiltless Gourmet
☐ Vanilla extract
Vinegars: ☐ Balsamic ☐ Cider ☐ Red wine
   ☐ Tarragon
☐ White Wine Worcestershire Sauce
☐ _____
☐ _____
☐ _____

Pamela M. Smith, *Food for Life* (Lake Mary, FL: Siloam, 1994, 1997), 121–123.

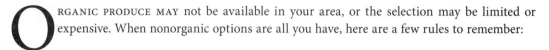

WHEN ORGANIC PRODUCE IS NOT AVAILABLE

by Don Colbert, MD

ORGANIC PRODUCE MAY not be available in your area, or the selection may be limited or expensive. When nonorganic options are all you have, here are a few rules to remember:

- **Look for thicker peels.** Generally, the thicker the peel or rind, the safer the fruit. For example, bananas have a thick peel; therefore, it is less likely that pesticides are absorbed deeply enough to reach the fruit inside. Oranges, tangerines, lemons, grapefruit, pineapples, watermelons, and figs also have thick peels. You can feel pretty safe purchasing nonorganic selections of these fruits because you remove the peel—and, therefore, the toxins—before eating them.
- **Watch thin peels.** The following produce have thin peels and have been known to carry much higher levels of pesticide residue: apples, bell peppers, celery, cherries, imported grapes, nectarines, peaches, pears, potatoes, red raspberries, spinach, and strawberries.[1] Since it is difficult to peel this produce, I strongly recommend organic.
- **Be careful if there's no peel.** And what about produce that has no peel, such as lettuce and broccoli? Enjoy your salad, but peel off the first two or three layers of lettuce leaves to remove any pesticide-tainted leaves if you do not purchase organic lettuce. Some broccoli can contain higher levels of pesticides, so if you are eating a lot of broccoli, you may want to purchase an organically grown variety or wash it well.
- **Wash your produce.** You can purchase a natural, biodegradable cleanser from most health food stores, or simply wash the wax off of your produce with a mild detergent such as pure castille soap. Wait until you are ready to eat the produce before you wash it.
- **Soak your produce.** Another good way to remove waxes and pesticides is to soak fruits and vegetables in a sink of cold water to which you have added 1 tablespoon of 35 percent, food-grade hydrogen peroxide for five to fifteen minutes. Then rinse thoroughly with fresh water. Another option is to soak produce in a sink half full of cold water with 1 teaspoon of Clorox bleach for five to fifteen minutes. Again, rinse the produce thoroughly after soaking.

Don Colbert, *Eat This and Live!* (Lake Mary, FL: Siloam, 2009), 57.

COMBATING EXCUSES FOR NOT LIVING HEALTHY

by Ron Kardashian, NSCA-CPT

AS A PROFESSIONAL trainer, I have heard a multitude of "exceptions" that clients try to use to exempt themselves from responsibility for healthy living. Some are listed below with cautions or suggestions as to how to handle *your* pet "need."

"But I'm a vegan or vegetarian."

This lifestyle can be very healthy if you learn how to supplement your eating habits with protein, vitamins, and minerals you need for optimal health to avoid deficiencies of nutrients found in other eating patterns.

"But I am dying for a burger and fries!" (Stop saying "I'm dying.")

Purchase grass-fed, organic beef, and make your burger with good bread and natural condiments. Try sweet potato fries. (They are available in more restaurants now.)

"What about my coffee?"

Coffee is best if it is organic and is consumed fresh. Decaffeinated coffee is highly processed and removes some of the antioxidant benefits contained in the natural coffee beans.

"But I need my soda."

Try a sparking bottle of water. Pellegrino with fresh lime or lemon is wonderful.

"But I need a 'cheat' day."

Then have one. Just make sure you are not giving in to an addiction to your favorite food or drink or bingeing because of emotional eating. Emotional eating will lead to an addiction. When you feel a "cheat" coming on, make sure it is worth it to lose sight of your goals for even one day.

"But we're going to a birthday party—mine!"

Before going to the party, declare to yourself, "God is strong in me. I am not going to eat everything I see. I am going to have a small portion of cake." You'll be the one who comes out dancing the night away.

"But I need a drink."

Addiction to alcohol consumption is no different from any other addiction. As you embrace the goals you have set for living a healthy life, your tastes will change, and your "need" for alcohol will diminish. And don't be afraid to get some professional help. God will be with you.

"But my grandfather smoked for years and lived to be eighty!"

Smoking has a greater negative effect on health in our world because our general health is more at risk, and it is a fact that smoking causes cancer. I encourage you to meditate on the reality that your body is the temple of God. This revelation will strengthen your resolve to respect the presence of God in your body. As you do, smoking will be gone forever.

"But I need my bedtime snack."

To meet your fitness goals, especially regarding losing weight, you must avoid late-night eating. When you eat late at night, the food has nowhere to go, except to a storage compartment in your body to be stored as fat—even if it is fat-free.

Ron Kardashian, *Getting in Shape God's Way* (Lake Mary, FL: Siloam, 2009), 253–255.

DINING OUT GUIDE

by Ed and Elisa McClure

WHICHEVER TYPE OF restaurant you choose, you must learn to speak up for yourself. Ask your server questions, and don't hesitate to make special requests. Some chefs are willing to leave off certain ingredients or to adapt a recipe. More and more restaurants now have a gluten-free section of the menu, and servers and kitchen staff are becoming more knowledgeable about food issues. Here are some quick guidelines to help you eat healthy when dining out.

MENU GUIDELINES BY CUISINE TYPE

Steak houses

Steak houses have plenty of protein choices, which can usually be broiled or grilled, and some reliable side dishes, such as steamed or grilled vegetables and sweet potatoes. Skip the baked potato, pass on the Hollandaise or Béarnaise sauces, and ask them to leave off the honey butter or sweetened topping that sometimes comes with the sweet potato. If anything, use a little butter—not margarine. Although butter is saturated fat, it is much healthier for you than margarine.

Mexican

Some items in typical Mexican food restaurants are problematic—for instance, fried tortillas. Some restaurants still use lard. You have to be careful about ingredients. When in doubt, ask your server.

Almost every Mexican restaurant will have homemade charro beans, which are a good choice. Fresh salsas and guacamole are full of good ingredients. Fajita meats are grilled and served with peppers and onions; just avoid the cheese and sour cream toppings.

Diners and coffee shops

Avoid bacon, often cured in sugar, and sausage, as both are filled with nitrates and other ingredients you don't want. Try steak and eggs, because the steak doesn't have additives like other breakfast meats and eggs are a good, whole food. Also try oatmeal topped with berries.

For lunch and dinner, stick with a grilled pork chop, grilled chicken, or steak with green beans or a steamed vegetable mix. You can always ask for a grilled hamburger patty with lettuce and tomato.

Asian/Chinese

Ask for brown rice, which is now a staple in most Asian restaurants, rather than white rice or noodles. Try some of the broth soups, especially in Thai cuisine. Many Asian restaurants have great fresh vegetables and a different approach to preparation. Avoid adding extra soy sauce to your dishes as it is very high in sodium. You can make good choices in these restaurants; it is just a matter of asking the questions and not doing the usual things.

Barbecue

You can get smoked chicken, brisket, and ribs—all kinds of meats. But watch the rubs. If the rubs have too many ingredients, we recommend avoiding them. But straightforward smoked meat is great. Most barbecue places either have pinto beans or green beans. If they are cooked with bacon, pick that out and just eat the beans. Balance the protein with some beans, and you will do fine.

Fast food

When it comes to the drive-through, we always say it's better to drive by—and keep going! But there are times when fast food may be the only available option. You can find salads and fresh fruit now, or you can order a hamburger patty or grilled chicken. Flexibility when ordering is going to be very limited.

Italian

We have found a way to eat at Italian restaurants and do it well. Because of food sensitivities to wheat, we usually skip the pasta when dining out. However, some establishments have gluten-free pasta as an option. Keep your pasta as a side dish rather than an entrée. If you choose a salad, ask for balsamic vinaigrette or olive oil and lemon. Try any number of fresh grilled items, including seafood, chicken, and veggies. As always, ask your server, and check online to see if your favorite Italian restaurant has ingredients posted.

Indian

Indian restaurants usually have pappadam, a crispy cracker-type bread made with pure lentil flour—it is wonderful! The tandoori chicken, baked in a traditional clay oven or pot, is another good choice. They will usually have grilled shrimp and some fresh vegetable items. Ask if they have brown rice.

Pit stops and airports

If you do any amount of traveling, you will always wind up stopping at a convenience store or an airport vendor for a snack or meal. These places offer few choices, but here are some tips for that inevitable quick stop. Stick with packaged nuts or seeds. Grab some bottled water and some fresh fruit.

There you go. Keep in mind the three basic rules—knowing your food plan, preplanning, and speaking up—and dining out can be an enjoyable experience that won't derail your weight-management program.

Ed and Elisa McClure, *Eat Your Way to a Healthy Life* (Lake Mary, FL: Siloam, 2006), 221–229.

RECONSTRUCT YOUR FAVORITE FOODS WITH HEALTHY INGREDIENTS

by Ed and Elisa McClure

ACH OF US has a unique and distinct heritage, which includes food preferences formed by our ethnicity, our regional foods, and our family traditions. As an example, the cuisine of New Orleans is much different from the cuisine of New York's Little Italy. Both are excellent and reflect the culture and heritage of the people of that region. Far be it from us to take the spice out of life! It is possible to enjoy your favorite traditional foods without compromising your health or weight.

That is where the deconstruction and reconstruction of recipes comes in. Almost any recipe can be deconstructed and reconstructed. The trick is to know the dos and don'ts when finding the alternative food products. Keep reading, and you will learn how to spot the harmful ingredients you need to replace as you "reconstruct" your favorite foods.

GROCERY STORE DETECTIVES

Food labels on packaging are divided into two parts: the list of ingredients and the Nutrition Facts panel. Both are important to know how to read and understand. Interpreting food labels is integral to your success because it helps you make informed food choices for a healthy new you. Ingredients are listed in descending order, so keep in mind that the predominant ingredient is listed first.

As a general guideline, look for labels with fewer ingredients. If there is a paragraph of ingredients full of words you can't pronounce, then don't buy that product. Put it back on the shelf and look for a better choice. There are better choices. Whole, fresh foods do not need ingredient panels: they are what they are. You don't need a list of ingredients for an orange, a blueberry, or a green pepper. When shopping, look for food products that have recognizable, clearly stated ingredients with no additives, preservatives, or artificial or altered ingredients.

The Nutrition Facts panel is also important to know how to read. The first item listed in the Nutrition Facts panel is the serving size, usually measured in gram weight. Do you know gram weight vs. ounce weight? Most of us don't. The rule of conversion is that 28 grams equal 1 ounce. If the serving size is 56 g (grams), then divide the serving size by 28, and you will know that the serving size is 2 ounces, or 168 g is 6 ounces, and so on.

Pay close attention to the serving size. Quite often the serving size listed on the label is a smaller portion than what we realistically consume. If the serving size is 2 ounces (56 g) and you actually consume 4 ounces, then that is two servings. So you must multiply the calories, fat, cholesterol, sodium, carbs, and protein listed on the label by two to get the real value of your consumption.

The best choices are always whole, fresh, unaltered, minimally packaged, colorful, naturally healthy foods. They will always be the most nutritious and lowest calorie choices you can make. Learning to read and understand the ingredients list and the Nutrition Facts panel will help you discern what naturally healthy ingredients are. You will become a better shopper and will find it easier to maintain a healthy lifestyle.

Ed and Elisa McClure, *Eat Your Way to a Healthy Life* (Lake Mary, FL: Siloam, 2006), 114–117.

RECIPES WITH SIMPLE INGREDIENT SWAPS

by Ed and Elisa McClure

H ERE ARE FOUR examples of foods that you could purchase premade at the grocery store— full of preservatives, additives, sugars, etc.—but why ruin your health that way? By simply taking a look at the ingredients (deconstruction) and swapping out the unhealthy items with whole foods (reconstruction), you can very easily create the foods you love right in your own kitchen. Almost all recipes can be made more health-friendly by following the principle of deconstruction and reconstruction. (See Secret #36.)

Scrambled Eggs Fiesta—*Serves 4*

1 Tbsp. unsalted butter	6 large eggs
½ cup red bell peppers, chopped	1 fresh avocado, sliced
½ cup green peppers, chopped	4 Tbsp. fresh salsa
1 Tbsp. jalapeño pepper, minced (about 1 pepper)	15-oz. can vegetarian refried beans
½ cup onion, chopped	4 spelt tortillas

Heat butter in a sauté pan and add peppers and onion; sauté until slightly soft. Beat eggs in a separate bowl and add to pan. Reduce heat and cook until eggs are scrambled. Serve with avocado slices, salsa, refried black beans, spelt tortilla, and pico de gallo (see recipe below).

Per serving (including tortilla and toppings): 400 calories, 21 g total fat (6 g sat fat), 420 mg cholesterol, 590 mg sodium, 39 g carbohydrate (8 g fiber, 6 g sugar), 20 g protein

Grilled Chicken Fajitas—*Serves 4*

2 lbs. boneless skinless chicken breasts and thighs	1 tsp. cracked black pepper
2 Tbsp. olive oil	1 tsp. cumin powder
1 tsp. granulated garlic	Spelt tortillas
½ tsp. sea salt	

Cut chicken into strips; place in bowl and add olive oil, garlic, sea salt, black pepper, and cumin powder. Marinate for 30 minutes. Heat broiler and cook chicken 4 inches from broiler for 15 minutes, turning as necessary. Serve on warmed spelt tortillas. Top with pico de gallo (see recipe below), guacamole, and sautéed onions and peppers.

Pico de Gallo (Fresh Salsa)—*Makes 3½ cups*

2½ cups fresh tomatoes, diced	½ cup Serrano peppers, minced
1 cup onion, diced	Pinch of sea salt
½ cup cilantro, chopped	Squeeze of lemon juice

Mix all ingredients in a bowl. Chill and serve as a condiment with beans, fajitas, or eggs.

Ed and Elisa McClure, *Eat Your Way to a Healthy Life* (Lake Mary, FL: Siloam, 2006), 188, 193, 195, 202.

EAT FOR YOUR BLOOD TYPE

by Joseph Christiano, ND, CNC

YOUR BLOOD TYPE can tell a lot about you. It is a great place to begin when you are trying to choose what to eat. Below is a *very* brief overview of some of the more beneficial foods for each blood type. For more details, please refer to my book *Bloodtypes, Bodytypes, and You* for menus and food lists that will help you with the balance to insure an anabolic state.

BLOOD TYPE A

The foods most harmful to As in the long run are meat and dairy. The elimination of these two food groups will allow type A individuals the greatest potential to avoid heart disease and cancer. Tofu, soy products, unsalted redskin peanuts, red wine, and green tea are especially good for type As because they help fight cancer.[1] Type As typically have lost the ability to make pepsin, a protein-digesting enzyme. Therefore, a more vegetarian diet or one of less-dense protein products such as chicken, turkey, and Cornish hens is more easily digestible for As. Whole grains such as quinoa, millet, brown rice, and wild rice are preferable over wheat products due to an oversensitivity to such products.[2]

BLOOD TYPE B

Type B individuals should eliminate all wheat, corn, tomatoes, peanuts, and especially chicken from their diets. Chicken contains a dangerous lectin that may clot the blood and can also lead to heart disease, cancer, diverticulitis, irritable bowel syndrome, spastic colon, and intestinal tract illnesses.[3] Blood type Bs share the diet of both types A and O, which means they can eat and happily digest a wide range of foods. Type Bs can tolerate dairy products in moderation. Fermented dairy products like yogurt, kefir, and cottage cheese would be the best for type Bs. Moderation is the key word for type Bs, who can handle a little bit of everything but should not go overboard on any single food.[4]

BLOOD TYPE AB

The single worst food for ABs is chicken. Chicken contains a dangerous lectin that may clot the blood and may also lead to heart disease, cancer, and/or a host of other digestive and intestinal tract illnesses. Tofu, soy products, salted redskin peanuts, red wine, and green tea are especially good for type AB because they help fight cancer and heart disease.[5] Most dairy products can be tolerated in moderation.

BLOOD TYPE O

For type O, both dairy and grains should be eaten sparingly.[6] Many Os are lactose intolerant. Soymilk and soy cheeses are the easiest and most tasty ways of replacing dairy products. Type Os have a greater predisposition to celiac/sprue disease, which is the inability to digest gluten. Therefore, try to stay away from the predominantly gluten-rich grains—wheat, rye, oats, and barley.[7] I also recommend that they eliminate most dairy, nuts, and grains. Type Os who eliminate dairy and grain products and stick to lean protein tend to have very low cholesterol levels and stay quite healthy.[8]

Joseph Christiano, *Bloodtypes, Bodytypes, and You* (Lake Mary, FL: Siloam, 2000, 2004, 2008), 116–118.

BREAKFAST ON THE GO

by Pamela M. Smith, RD

O NE SERVING OF a muffin and shake (both recipes below) gives 1 complex carbohydrate (the muffin), 1 ounce protein (the milk), and 2 simple carbohydrates (the juice and the raisins).

Shake-'em-up Shake

8 oz. (1 cup) skim or 1 percent milk	1 tsp. vanilla
½ cup fresh orange juice	4–5 ice cubes

Pour all of the ingredients in a large cup with a lid. Shake wildly and drink up!

Spiced Bran Muffins

¼ cup molasses	1½ tsp. baking powder
3 Tbsp. honey	1 tsp. ground ginger
2 large egg whites	1 tsp. ground cloves
¼ cup plain, nonfat yogurt	1 tsp. cinnamon
¼ cup 1 percent or skim milk	¼ cup chopped pecans
¼ cup wheat bran	¼ cup golden raisins
¼ cup oat bran	Nonstick cooking spray
1 cup whole-wheat pastry flour	

Preheat oven to 350 degrees. Warm the molasses and the honey in the microwave or in a saucepan until they just begin to steam (about 110 degrees). Let the mixture cool. Whisk the egg whites, yogurt, and milk together until blended. Add the molasses-honey mixture while whisking. Gently stir in the brans, flour, baking powder, and spices; then fold in the pecans and raisins.

Spray a 12-cup muffin tin with nonstick spray, and fill each cup two-thirds full with batter. Bake for 15 to 20 minutes or until a toothpick inserted into the center of a muffin comes out clean. Serve warm, or freeze individually in freezer bags to use later.

Baked Breakfast Apple

1 small Golden Delicious apple, cored	1 Tbsp. raisins
2 Tbsp. old-fashioned oats	2 Tbsp. apple juice
¼ tsp. cinnamon	½ cup nonfat ricotta cheese (or cottage cheese)

Place the apple in a microwaveable bowl. Mix together the oats, the cinnamon, and the raisins. Fill the cavity of the cored apple with the mixture. Pour the apple juice over the apple. Cover and microwave on high for 2 minutes, turning bowl halfway after 1 minute. Spoon the cheese onto a plate, and top it with the apple and juice mixture.

Makes 1 serving, giving 1 complex carbohydrate (the oats), 2 ounces protein (the cheese), and 1 simple carbohydrate (the apple, juice, and raisins).

Pamela M. Smith, *Food for Life* (Lake Mary, FL: Siloam, 1994, 1997), 93–97.

LUNCH EXPRESS

by Pamela M. Smith, RD

Pita Pizzas

1 whole-wheat pita, cut in half into rounds (like a saucer)

2 Tbsp. spaghetti sauce (or tomato sauce)

1½ oz. or ⅓ cup part-skim or nonfat mozzarella cheese, shredded

1 small apple, cut into wedges (optional)

Preheat oven to 375 degrees. Place the two pita circles on a baking sheet. Spread each one with half of the spaghetti sauce, and top each with half of the cheese. Bake for 8 to 10 minutes or until cheese is bubbly. Serve with apple wedges (optional).

Makes one serving, giving 2 complex carbohydrates (the pita bread), 2 ounces protein (the cheese), and 1 simple carbohydrate (the sauce).

Terrific Tuna Grill

2 cans (6½ oz. each) solid white tuna, water-packed, drained

½ cup carrots, shredded

1 stalk celery, diced

1 apple, diced (½ cup)

2 Tbsp. light mayonnaise

2 Tbsp. orange juice

3 Tbsp. plain, nonfat yogurt

1 tsp. Dijon mustard

½ tsp. Creole seasoning

2 plum tomatoes, sliced

8 slices 100 percent whole-wheat bread

Nonstick cooking spray

Combine the tuna, carrots, celery, and apple. In a separate bowl, stir together the mayonnaise, orange juice, yogurt, mustard, and creole seasoning until blended. Pour the mixture over the salad, stirring to coat it. Divide the salad into four portions, spreading each portion onto one slice of bread. Top each with 2 slices of tomato and the other slice of bread. Spray a nonstick skillet with cooking spray and heat on medium high. Grill the sandwiches until brown.

Makes 4 servings, each giving 2 complex carbohydrates (the bread), 3 ounces protein (the tuna), and 1 simple carbohydrate (veggies and fruit).

Grilled Turkey and Cheese Sandwich

2 tsp. Dijon mustard

2 slices 100 percent whole-wheat bread

1 oz. (¼ cup) grated light cheese (such as Laughing Cow Light)

1 plum tomato, sliced

2 oz. skinned turkey breast, fully cooked and sliced

Nonstick cooking spray

1 cup watermelon chunks

Spread the mustard on each slice of bread. Put half the cheese, the tomato, and turkey on one slice of bread. Top with remaining cheese and slice of bread. Grill the sandwich on a hot griddle or a nonstick skillet coated with cooking spray. Cook until bread is lightly toasted and the cheese melts. Serve with melon chunks.

Makes 1 serving, giving 2 complex carbohydrates (the bread), 3 ounces protein (the turkey and cheese), and 1 simple carbohydrate (the fruit).

Pamela M. Smith, *Food for Life* (Lake Mary, FL: Siloam, 1994, 1997), 100–105.

MAKE-IT-QUICK DINNER

by Pamela M. Smith, RD

Sicilian Chicken and Pasta (serve with Marinated Cucumbers)

4 boneless, skinless chicken breasts	2 Tbsp. cornstarch
½ tsp. Creole seasoning	¼ tsp. Tabasco sauce
½ tsp. dried basil	1 clove minced garlic
½ tsp. dried oregano	¼ cup grated Parmesan cheese
2 cans (15 oz. each) Italian-style stewed tomatoes	1 small package of angel hair pasta (8 oz.)

Preheat the oven to 425 degrees. Sprinkle the chicken with the seasoning, and pat it with the herbs. Place the chicken in a baking dish, and cover it with foil. Bake for 15 minutes.

While the chicken is baking, pour the canned tomatoes into a medium saucepan and add the cornstarch, the Tabasco sauce, and the garlic. Cook the mixture until it is thickened, about 5 minutes.

After 15 minutes, remove the chicken from the oven, pouring off any liquid from the pan. Pour the heated sauce over the chicken and sprinkle the grated cheese on top. Place the pan back in the oven and cook, uncovered, for 10 more minutes.

Cook the pasta according to the package directions. Drain and place it on a platter. Top the pasta with the chicken and the sauce.

Makes 4 servings, each giving 1 complex carbohydrate (the pasta), 3 ounces of protein (the chicken and the cheese), and 1 simple carbohydrate (the tomatoes).

Nutritional profile per serving

27 g carbohydrate, 25 g protein, 9 g fat, 20 percent calories from fat, 50 mg cholesterol, 878 mg sodium, 396 calories

Marinated Cucumbers

4 cucumbers	½ cup no-oil Italian dressing
1 small red onion, thinly sliced	4 romaine or green leaf lettuce leaves
1 tsp. dried dill weed	

Wash and peel the cucumbers; slice in rounds. Add the onion slices and toss with the dill weed. Pour in the dressing and refrigerate at least 2 hours to blend the flavors. Serve on a lettuce leaf. Makes 8 servings of a healthy munchie.

Nutritional profile per serving

9 g carbohydrate, 1 g protein, 0 g fat, 0 percent calories from fat, 0 mg cholesterol, 280 mg sodium, 40 calories

---

Pamela M. Smith, *Food for Life* (Lake Mary, FL: Siloam, 1994, 1997), 106–118.

SWEET ENDING

by Pamela M. Smith, RD

Chocolate Marble Cheesecake

1 cup yogurt cheese (see recipe below)
1½ cups reduced-fat chocolate graham cracker crumbs
3 Tbsp. apricot all-fruit spread, melted
1 cup skim milk ricotta cheese
4 egg whites
1 pkg. (8 oz.) light cream cheese

1 Tbsp. unbleached flour
1 tsp. vanilla

½ cup sugar
¼ cup unsweetened Dutch-process cocoa
1 tsp. almond extract

Preheat oven to 350 degrees.

Prepare yogurt cheese; set aside. Coat a 9-inch springform pan with cooking spray. In a bowl, mix graham cracker crumbs and all-fruit spread. Lightly press crumb mixture into bottom of pan. Bake for 8 minutes. Set aside. Increase oven temperature to 375 degrees.

Process ricotta cheese in a food processor until almost smooth. Add egg whites and process until smooth. Add yogurt cheese, cream cheese, flour, half of sugar, and the teaspoon of vanilla. Process until a smooth batter forms. Pour half of filling into a bowl. Add cocoa, remaining sugar, and the teaspoon of almond extract. Stir until well combined.

Alternately pour batters, half of each at a time, into crust. Gently swirl batters with a spatula.

Bake until a knife inserted into the center comes out clean, 35 to 40 minutes. Cool on wire rack for 15 minutes. Run a knife blade around the edge of pan. Cool for 30 minutes. Remove side from pan. Cool completely. Chill for at least 4 hours.

Cut into 12 slices.

Nutritional profile per serving

17 g carbohydrate, 6 g protein, 1 g fat, 9 percent calories from fat, 1 mg cholesterol, 69 mg sodium, 100 calories

Yogurt Cheese

Low-fat yogurt cheese is easy to make and has a rich, creamy consistency that's just right for making cheesecakes, dips, and spreads. To make yogurt cheese, simply line a strainer with cheesecloth and spoon in nonfat plain yogurt (with active cultures). Place the strainer over a deep bowl and refrigerate for 24 hours. Two cups of yogurt make 1½ cups of cheese.

Pamela M. Smith, *The Good Life* (Lake Mary, FL: Siloam, 1996), 160, 167.

POWER SNACK CHOICES

by Pamela M. Smith, RD

When most people think of snacks, they picture potato chips, candy, and sodas. These types of snacks are "empty calories," providing high amounts of fats, sugars, salt, and calories but little or no vitamins or minerals.

A healthy snack provides you with needed nutrition and will keep your blood sugar level from dropping too low, leaving you sleepy and craving sweets. The following gives some power snack suggestions that balance carbohydrates with protein.

- Baked Tostitos or Guiltless Gourmet tortilla chips with ⅓ cup fat-free bean dip and salsa
- One-half sandwich on whole-grain Kaiser roll or whole-wheat bread, made with turkey and mozzarella or ham and fat-free cheese
- Whole-grain cereal with skim milk
- Fat-free cream cheese spread and whole-grain crackers
- Tuna lunch kit or small pop-top can of tuna with whole-grain crackers
- Harvest Crisps crackers or Raisin Squares cereal with Laughing Cow Light cheese wedge or low-fat string cheese
- Health Valley Graham Crackers with 2 Tbsp. natural peanut butter
- Crispbread crackers with sliced turkey and Dijon mustard
- Light popcorn with 2 Tbsp. freshly grated Parmesan cheese
- Stonyfield Farm yogurt or plain, nonfat yogurt mixed with all-fruit spread
- 12 grapes or 10 fresh strawberries with low-fat string cheese or Armenian cheese
- 1 cup of gazpacho with low-fat string cheese
- Fruit shake (skim milk blended with frozen fruit and vanilla extract)
- Low-fat cheese tortellini salad in vinaigrette with carrots and celery
- Dill tortilla rolls: tortilla with fat-free cream cheese, lemon juice, fresh dill, and Creole seasoning
- Trail mix (1 cup unsalted, dry-roasted peanuts; 1 cup unsalted, dry-roasted, shelled sunflower seeds; and 2 cups raisins)—make in abundance and bag into ¼ cup portions
- Homemade low-fat bran muffin and skim milk

Pamela M. Smith, *Healthy Expectations* (Lake Mary, FL: Siloam, 1998), 17–19.

MORE HEALTHY RECIPES

by Ed and Elisa McClure

Mediterranean Pasta—*Serves 6*

2 Tbsp. extra-virgin olive oil
6 garlic cloves, chopped
28-oz. can whole peeled tomatoes, chopped in food processor (or crushed tomatoes)
½ cup sun-dried tomatoes, chopped with tomatoes in food processor
½ tsp. cracked black pepper
½ cup fresh basil, chopped slightly, loosely packed
¼ tsp. red pepper flakes (optional)

15-oz. can artichoke hearts, drained, quartered
15-oz. can black olives, drained, halved
¼ lb. fresh baby spinach

1 Tbsp. pine nuts

16-oz. package brown rice penne pasta
Grated Parmesan cheese

In a medium saucepan heat 1 Tbsp. olive oil; add chopped garlic and sauté lightly but do not brown. Add tomatoes and pepper, simmering for 10 minutes. Add basil, pepper flakes, artichoke hearts, olives, and spinach; simmer for 10 minutes. Add nuts and reduce heat to low. Cook pasta according to package directions and transfer to a large bowl. Pour sauce over pasta and top with grated Parmesan cheese if desired.

8-oz. serving: 230 calories, 7 g total fat (1 g sat fat), 0 cholesterol, 530 mg sodium, 41 g carbohydrate (6 g fiber, 4 g sugar), 5 g protein

Broccoli Italian Style—*Serves 4*

1 head broccoli
2 Tbsp. olive oil
¼ tsp. granulated garlic

¼ tsp. sea salt
¼ tsp. cracked black pepper
¼ tsp. sesame seeds

Separate broccoli florets and cut stems to about 1 ½ inches. Steam until cooked to desired tenderness. Remove from steamer and arrange on serving platter. While still hot, drizzle olive oil and sprinkle garlic, salt, black pepper, and sesame seeds over florets. Serve at room temperature.

6-oz. serving: 110 calories, 8 g total fat (1 g sat fat), 0 cholesterol, 100 mg sodium, 8 g carbohydrate (5 g fiber, 3 g sugar), 5 g protein

Garlic Bread—*Serves 8*

¼ tsp. granulated garlic
¼ tsp. cracked black pepper
¼ tsp. oregano

¼ tsp. crushed red pepper
16 slices spelt sourdough bread (or any gluten-free bread of your choice, thinly sliced (¼-inch thick)

Mix garlic, cracked black pepper, oregano, and crushed red pepper. Place bread slices on a baking sheet, spray with olive oil, and sprinkle with spice mixture. Place about 4 inches from broiler for about 3–4 minutes until browned.

1 ½-oz. serving: 120 calories, 2 g total fat (0 g sat fat), 0 cholesterol, 300 mg sodium, 22 g carbohydrate (1 g fiber, 1 g sugar), 4 g protein

---

Ed and Elisa McClure, *Eat Your Way to a Healthy Life* (Lake Mary, FL: Siloam, 2006), 195–196, 202–204.

WEIGHT LOSS

HOOKED ON FOOD?

by Pamela M. Smith, RD

Y ES, MILLIONS OF Americans are hooked—emotionally dependent—on food. What does that mean?

It has nothing to do with your present weight; you may be very overweight or very thin. Rather it has to do with an improper relationship with food in which food and eating have assumed an unnatural importance in your life. In this improper, love-hate relationship, food has an unnatural control over you. You may love the way it tastes and makes you feel, but you hate it for what it does to your body and how it controls your life. Like any unhealthy relationship, it results in a roller coaster of emotions: gratification and satisfaction, guilt and remorse, being "good" only to be "bad." The obsession fills your thoughts and actions, robs you of well-being, and affects your self-esteem; it holds you captive. It has life-damaging consequences.

Food is a trap when it is used as a substitute for love, friendship, or success, or when it's used to cover up more serious emotional issues. Unhealthy eating and overeating can become a way of life and a way of coping with life. And because we must eat for life, we obviously can't abstain from it as we can from other substances people abuse. Food is quite another story, even for people who have given up smoking.

Food is not inherently evil. Humans must have it to survive and thrive; we are physically dependent upon it. God created us to need food, and He created us to enjoy the taste of food. He also designed the eating of it to be pleasurable while we're benefiting from its nourishment.

The problems begin when we become emotionally dependent on food to cope with everyday life, when it becomes our source of joy. Food becomes an evil when we love eating more than we love ourselves, more than we love other people, and more than we love God.

People who never touch alcohol, drugs, or cigarettes often use food as their vice or real pleasure in life. How many church socials have I attended where people proudly declare they don't need liquor to have a good time—but don't dare take away their cake table!

Scripture is full of illustrations about food and gluttony, messages often ignored. Food—and finances—are two vulnerable issues for us because we can't live without them. Many do well in the abstinence issues; denominations are even formed around them. We find strength in abstinence. We can live without alcohol, nicotine, and narcotics—even though withdrawal can be deadly. But food and money are not objects we can abstain from; we must have them to survive.

We must apply the fruit of self-control to them, however, and keep them in their appropriate place—not loving them more than God or more than people. And that's why they become a trap. That's why the Bible calls the love of money the root of all sorts of evil (1 Tim. 6:10)—not because it is inherently evil, but because it can so easily become a lord over our lives. Neither is food inherently evil until it becomes our golden calf.

As Scripture records in Exodus 32, God, Moses, and the top of Mount Sinai seemed too far away for the Israelites waiting in the valley below. Anxious for a quick-fix god that they could see and touch, the Israelites molded a calf of gold.

We likewise turn to food because it's always at hand and gives immediate gratification.

Pamela M. Smith, *Food for Life* (Lake Mary, FL: Siloam, 1994, 1997), 186–187.

WE EAT TOO MUCH

by Kara Davis, MD

GOOD EATING HABITS are reflected in both the quality and the quantity of food. Weight gain results from too many calories, irrespective of the quality of the food. Put another way, it's altogether possible to have "too much of a good thing." Yes, overeating low-quality food leads to weight gain, but so does overeating high-quality food. In terms of weight gain, food quality is not as big an issue as is net calories. Don't fall into the erroneous mind-set that healthy foods are exempt from quantity restriction.

Below is a sample menu for breakfast, lunch, dinner, and a snack from a 1,600-calorie diet plan. Pay particular attention to the serving sizes (the *quantity* of food) and the relative absence of foods that are comprised of empty calories (the *quality* of food).

BREAKFAST	LUNCH	DINNER	SNACK
1 cup oatmeal	2 slices whole-wheat bread	5 oz. chicken leg, no skin, baked	1 cup cantaloupe
½ cup fruit	2 oz. turkey or ham and 1 oz. low-fat cheese	1 cup whole-wheat pasta	¼ cup 1 percent cottage cheese
1 cup plain, low-fat yogurt	¼ avocado sliced	4 Tbsp. low-fat vinaigrette (2 Tbsp. for marinade for chicken and 2 Tbsp. to toss with pasta)	
Black coffee or tea with lemon	Alfalfa sprouts	1 cup broccoli and 1 cup zucchini, steamed and tossed with pasta	
	1 tsp. mayonnaise	8 oz. skim milk	
	½ cup baby carrots		
	2 tablespoons nonfat dressing for dipping carrots		
	1 apple		
	Water or noncaloric beverage		

Most of my patients are amazed at the difference between the amount of food they *should* be eating and what they actually eat. Even the foods that are nutritionally sound are restricted in terms of quantity. Notice, for instance, the breakfast meal has *one* cup of oatmeal, not two. And the meat allowed with dinner is one small, skinless, baked chicken leg—not three large pieces fried extra crispy and drenched with barbeque sauce.

This sample diet also reveals how empty calories are a major problem. Where are the chips, candy, cookies, ice cream, and soft drinks in this 1,600-calorie menu? They aren't included because once the daily nutritional needs are met, there is not much room left to allow for empty calories.

The truth of the matter is that in order to live a life governed by self-control, we must be willing to hold ourselves accountable for our choices and accept responsibility for our actions.

Kara Davis, *Spiritual Secrets to Weight Loss* (Lake Mary, FL: Siloam, 2002, 2008), 153–156.

OBESITY AND DIABETES

by Kara Davis, MD

A S THE PREVALENCE of obesity and being overweight has increased over the past few decades, there has been a parallel increase in the prevalence of type 2 diabetes. These two conditions are so tightly linked that the term *diabesity* was coined to emphasize the connection between the two. Before examining some of the issues relating to type 2 diabetes, let's clarify terminology.

Diabetes exists in two forms—type 1 diabetes and type 2 diabetes. Type 1 diabetes was previously called insulin-dependent diabetes or juvenile-onset diabetes. This form is less common, constituting 5 to 10 percent of all cases of diabetes. In type 1 diabetes, the cells in the pancreas that make insulin are destroyed by an immune-mediated process. What triggers this process is not entirely clear, whether genetic, environmental, or an autoimmune disorder. It is usually diagnosed in children and youth, and there is no known way of preventing it. Type 1 diabetics always require insulin. They cannot be treated with oral medications. This form of diabetes is not connected to the obesity epidemic.

Type 2 diabetes constitutes 90 to 95 percent of all diabetes cases. In years past, it's been known as non–insulin dependent diabetes or adult-onset diabetes. Both of these terms are misleading since many type 2 diabetics require insulin, and not all cases are diagnosed in the adult years. Type 2 diabetes, unlike type 1, does not begin with insulin *deficiency* but rather insulin *resistance*. The cells of the body do not respond properly to the insulin produced by the pancreas (i.e., the body *resists* the insulin present in the bloodstream). To compensate, the pancreas of the type 2 diabetic will make more insulin. Over time, however, the pancreas loses its ability to produce insulin—it "burns out." At this point, the type 2 diabetic will require insulin, even though the diabetes may have been controlled with oral medications or lifestyle modification when the disease was initially diagnosed. Weight loss serves to reverse this insulin resistance, making the body more sensitive to it and preserving the function of the pancreas.

There are many risk factors for type 2 diabetes. Of course, obesity is a significant risk factor, as is a sedentary lifestyle, but there are other risks as well. Age, family history, and race play a major role. African Americans, Hispanics, Native Americans, some Asian Americans, and Native Hawaiians are all at increased risk.

Diabetes is a major risk factor for cardiovascular disease, the number one cause of death in the United States. In addition to heart disease, peripheral vascular disease, and stroke, there are other complications of diabetes, including kidney failure, hypertension, blindness, amputation, nerve damage, periodontal disease, depression, and difficulties during pregnancy.

Lifestyle modification with dietary changes, regular exercise, and weight loss can actually prevent diabetes from developing in people at risk. The same lifestyle changes will optimize the control of those already diagnosed with the disease and reduce the chance for complications.

Kara Davis, *Spiritual Secrets to Weight Loss* (Lake Mary, FL: Siloam, 2002, 2008), 194–195.

FAD DIETS

by Kara Davis, MD

THERE IS A quality in human nature that desires "something for nothing." It's this tendency that makes fad diets so appealing—they promise a quick and easy solution to a complex and difficult problem. The following are examples of just a few of the more popular fad diets.

The grapefruit diet

The specific instructions for this diet vary depending on the source, but in general, the plan requires that a whole or half of a grapefruit be eaten before each meal. The dieter is also encouraged to drink lots of coffee or tea. This diet is based on the premise that grapefruit contains an enzyme that burns fat. In reality, no such enzyme has ever been discovered. Grapefruit is a good source of vitamin C and folic acid and should be part of any healthy diet, but like any other food, it shouldn't be eaten exclusively or in excess. If you happen to lose weight on this diet, then it is because grapefruit is a low-calorie, low-fat food—not because of any mystery enzyme.

Everyone who drinks coffee knows that caffeine has a diuretic effect—it causes excessive urination. So "success" with the grapefruit diet may simply result from dehydration—losing water weight, which will reaccumulate once you replenish your body's fluids. The combination of large amounts of citric acid and caffeine may also exacerbate gastroesophageal reflux disease (GERD) in those who are susceptible.

The cabbage soup diet

This diet appeals to people who want to lose weight fast. It claims that up to ten pounds can be shed in a one-week period of time without ever feeling hungry. That claim alone should generate suspicion, but those who want a "quick fix" often lose sight of what makes (or doesn't make) common sense. This is also a single-food diet. Instead of grapefruit, the dieter is allowed to eat unlimited quantities of cabbage soup. The plan also recommends caffeine-containing beverages, so once again, any drop in the scale is likely to represent water weight.

High-protein diets

These diets are based on the premise that carbohydrates make us hungry, and this leads to overeating. The proposed solution is to eliminate carbohydrates from the diet and substitute them with large quantities of protein and fat.

One obvious problem with this approach is that it will lack many of the vitamins and nutrients that are found exclusively in carbohydrate foods. These diets may also generate ketones in the body, and high ketones can cause headaches, nausea, fatigue, and dizziness. There is some evidence to suggest that high-protein diets may adversely affect the kidney function. People with kidney diseases should never try these diets.

Weight loss occurs when the calories we consume are consistently less than the calories we utilize for an extended period of time. Don't get burned by fad diets. Accept the weight-loss process, and make permanent lifestyle changes for better health.

Kara Davis, *Spiritual Secrets to Weight Loss* (Lake Mary, FL: Siloam, 2002, 2008), 212–214.

BARIATRIC SURGERY

by Kara Davis, MD

BARIATRIC SURGERY ("WEIGHT-LOSS" surgery) has been around since the 1950s but has become more popular over the last decade as the prevalence of obesity has increased. The operation changes the anatomy of the stomach and intestinal tract, modifying either the stomach alone or the stomach and the small intestine combined.[1]

More than one type of bariatric procedure is available. They can be broadly categorized into those that restrict the amount of food you can eat and those that decrease the number of calories absorbed. The restrictive procedures include gastric stapling, the vertical (sleeve) gastrectomy, and the adjustable gastric band. The latter is so appealing because the band is fully adjustable and the procedure can be done laparoscopically. The thought of surgery may seem dramatic at first, but depending on the patient, the body weight, and the presence or absence of weight-related medical conditions, it could prove to be a totally reasonable option.

Obviously the patient should be well informed about the procedure and know what to expect after the operation is over. Bariatric surgery will not get you "off the hook" in terms of following a healthy lifestyle. All patients must be motivated to implement good eating and exercise habits. Most health plans require documentation that medically supervised weight-loss attempts have failed and a preoperative psychiatric assessment is in order. Depression is extremely common and would need to be treated prior to having any procedure.

Studies indicate the long-term success rate for bariatric surgery exceeds that for diet and exercise alone. Surgery is actually the treatment of choice for people with extreme obesity, defined as a body mass index (BMI) over 40, who have failed traditional approaches to weight loss (i.e., lifestyle modification and prescription medications).

The BMI is calculated using weight and the height. *Overweight* is defined as a BMI greater than 25; *obese* as a BMI greater than 30; and *extreme obesity* is any value over 40. It is estimated that about 5 percent of the total adult population has extreme obesity, but the percentage is higher in some subgroups. For instance, 16.5 percent of all African American women aged forty to fifty-nine have a BMI of 40 or more. Their prevalence of extreme obesity more than doubles that of white women (7 percent) and Mexican American women (7.8 percent) who are the same age.[2]

Another thing to consider in making a decision about bariatric surgery is whether there are medical conditions influenced by body weight, like type 2 diabetes, sleep apnea, and hypertension. In these instances, surgery is appropriate with a BMI of 35 or more. Diabetics in particular respond well to bariatric surgery with many patients experiencing full remission of the disease.

If you have been in the valley of decision over bariatric surgery, are in the extreme obesity category, or suffer from medical conditions caused by body weight, make it a point to talk things over with your family and your primary care physician. Ask your doctor to refer you to a surgeon who can give you even more information about the operation. This is not a decision to take lightly, and the Scriptures say that there is wisdom in a multitude of counselors. Seek God as you determine whether this procedure is right for you.

Kara Davis, *Spiritual Secrets to Weight Loss* (Lake Mary, FL: Siloam, 2002, 2008), 191–192.

WEIGHT-LOSS MEDICATIONS

by Kara Davis, MD

MUCH RESEARCH IS being devoted to the development of weight-loss medications. Some of these drugs have been approved for long-term use, others have not yet been approved in the United States, and still others have been withdrawn from the market because of safety concerns.

In 1992, the use of a combination of two drugs, fenfluramine and phentermine ("fen-phen"), gained widespread attention.[1] For a sizable fee, you could go to a weight-loss "clinic" and get a coveted fen-phen prescription, regardless of whether you needed it or not. Many "patients" who were prescribed fen-phen were *not* obese; some weren't even overweight. It was widely prescribed for cosmetic purposes in the absence of solid medical indications.

In 1996 the drug dexfenfluramine received approval for use as a weight-loss medication.[2] Until this time, the Food and Drug Administration had not approved any medications for weight loss for twenty-three years. Unlike fenfluramine, dexfenfluramine was authorized for continuous use up to a year. The drug was so popular that 3.3 million prescriptions were written from June 1996 to April 1997. In the spring of 1997, reports began to surface that people using fenfluramine and dexfenfluramine were developing abnormalities in their heart valves. Soon thereafter, the FDA withdrew both drugs from the market.[3]

Subsequent to the withdrawal of fenfluramine and dexfenfluramine, sibutramine and orlistat were released. Orlistat became available in an over-the-counter formula in February 2007.[4] A third drug, rimonabant, has been available in several countries in Europe and South America since 2006.[5] In 2007, however, the Advisory Committee of the FDA determined that more safety information was needed before the drug could be approved in the United States.[6]

Sibutramine works as an appetite suppressant. It alters the balance of chemicals in the brain such as norepinephrine, serotonin, and dopamine. Studies have shown that patients taking sibutramine were able to lose 7 to 8 percent of their initial body weight over the course of a year, compared to a 1 to 2 percent loss in patients taking a placebo.[7]

Some of the side effects of sibutramine include headache, dry mouth, constipation, insomnia, and elevations in blood pressure and pulse rate. People using sibutramine should have these monitored at regular intervals.

Orlistat works at the level of the intestine through preventing the absorption of dietary fat from the intestines into the bloodstream. Obviously, fat that never gets into your bloodstream cannot add inches to your waistline, but it has distressing side effects: oily stool, loose stool, flatulence, and (for some) a loss of bowel control. These effects are not universal, but they are fairly common.

Orlistat may impair the absorption of the four vitamins that require an oil-based medium to dissolve—vitamins A, D, E, and K. Because of this, patients are advised to take a multivitamin supplement containing these four vitamins. Patients who respond to prescription strength orlistat can expect to lose 8 to 10 percent of their initial body weight in six to twelve months.[8]

Neither sibutramine nor orlistat is approved for cosmetic weight reduction. These drugs should only be prescribed to patients who are obese or to patients who are overweight and have a weight-related medical condition.

Kara Davis, *Spiritual Secrets to Weight Loss* (Lake Mary, FL: Siloam, 2002, 2008), 188–190.

STRESS CAN MAKE YOU FAT

by Don Colbert, MD

Y OU CAN IMPROVE your lifestyle greatly by reducing the impact of stress on your body. The excessive stress that you are under on a daily basis can contribute to obesity. Let me explain. You see, when you are under stress, your body produces a hormone called cortisol, which is very similar to cortisone. If you've ever taken cortisone, you are well aware of the side effects. Cortisone causes you to gain weight. Well, cortisol can have the same effect.

When your adrenal glands produce cortisol during periods of high anxiety and stress, it can actually cause your body to gain weight. Because when cortisol levels are raised—as a result of a mental or physical stress reaction—a person craves sugar as well as carbohydrate-rich foods, such as breads, pasta, potatoes, corn chips, crackers, and so forth. These foods calm the emotions temporarily by increasing blood sugar levels and serotonin levels in the brain. Two or three hours after eating these foods, however, a person's insulin level skyrockets, causing blood sugar to drop. If insulin levels remain elevated, the body continues to store fat for energy. In other words, chronically elevated insulin levels from eating excessive amounts of sugar or carbohydrates on a frequent basis literally program the body to be in a fat storage mode and unable to burn stored fat for energy.

Most obese people can't break out of this cycle because they are constantly craving sugars and carbohydrates throughout the day, and they mindlessly seek to satisfy those cravings with readily available "snack" foods.

Elevated cortisol causes the release of stored sugar or glycogen from the liver and muscles. Muscle cells may begin to break down their proteins to amino acids to eventually convert them into sugar. The net effect is that blood sugar levels rise again. Elevated cortisol may stimulate the appetite by causing neurotransmitter imbalances, especially with serotonin and dopamine. These imbalances may cause cravings for sugars and carbohydrates; low dopamine and serotonin levels are also linked to depression. With the eating of sugars and carbohydrates, blood sugars rise, insulin production soars, blood sugar levels may plunge, and the entire cycle is repeated.

Several major research studies have demonstrated that excessive stress, obesity, and elevated cortisol go hand in hand.[1] Therefore, reducing your level of stress can help you lose weight and keep it off.

Don Colbert, *The Bible Cure for Weight Loss and Muscle Gain* (Lake Mary, FL: Siloam, 2000), 77; Don Colbert, *Stress Less* (Lake Mary, FL: Siloam, 2005), 174–175.

DRINKING ON THE POUNDS

by Dino Nowak

W HILE I WAS finishing up my book *The Final Makeover*, I spent quite a bit of time in Starbucks. When I say quite a bit of time, I mean from noon until closing time. I understand why people go to write there: it is more conducive to getting work done. At home there are too many distractions, and at the library you go crazy with fluorescent lighting and lack of natural light (plus, it's too quiet).

I am amazed at the size of the drinks people get at Starbucks (and other places like Starbucks). I am also amazed at what people get in their drinks. People must think that drinks do not count toward their total energy intake, because when you look at the calories in these drinks it is no wonder people gain fat.

One of the heavyweights is a Starbucks Java Chip Frappuccino (20 ounces) with whipped cream, coming in at a whopping 650 calories. A 16-ounce Caffe Mocha: 400 calories. A 16-ounce Mocha Frappuccino blended coffee: 420 calories. A 16-ounce White Chocolate Mocha: 490 calories.[1] There are, of course, smaller sizes, and Starbucks is even testing out the waters with lower-calorie versions of their drinks. But the point remains that what you drink does impact body fat.

Drinking on the pounds is not limited to the coffees listed above. One of the bigger source of calories is, of course, soda. In 2001 Americans spent more than $61 billion on soft drinks.[2] It's also the single biggest source of refined sugars in the American diet.[3] Check your soda label next time: every 4 grams of sugar is like swallowing a teaspoon of it. (Yet we keep blaming carbs—where is the soda diet?) Let's look quickly at the calories in an average soft drink:

- A 12-ounce can will give you 140 calories.
- A 20-ounce bottle supplies 250 calories.
- Then you have the 32-ounce Big Gulp at 400 calories.

You may say you would never order one of those humongous sizes, but how many cans or bottles do you drink a day? Possibly close to three of them. Well, that is worse than drinking a Big Gulp because with three 20-ounce bottles you just took in 750 calories. You could have just had water and eaten a whole chocolate cake by yourself.

Watch for smoothies and juices. Smoothies can have as many as 1,000 calories in them. And some juices are just water "juiced up" on sugar. Look to make sure they are 100 percent fruit juice.

So here is what we are going to do (and hopefully it will develop into a lifelong habit for you): no more regular sodas. But for every diet soda you have, the next drink in line for the day is either a glass of milk or a glass of water (or zero to low-calorie flavored water). Once you finish that, your next drink can be another diet soda if you want. Of course, if you want to stick with water or flavored water, that is fine; you do not *have* to have a diet soda in between.

We have to stop drinking on the pounds.

Dino Nowak, *The Final Makeover* (Lake Mary, FL: Siloam, 2005), 84–84.

BODY FAT DISTRIBUTION

by Kara Davis, MD

BODY FAT DISTRIBUTION plays such an important role in health that many clinicians advocate using the waist circumference (which reflects the distribution of fat) in combination with the BMI (which reflects the absolute weight) when assessing a person's risk for cardiovascular disease and type 2 diabetes. This is because abdominal fat, also called "central obesity," "upper body obesity," or "truncal obesity," has metabolic consequences that are more striking than when the fat is located peripherally—predominantly on the hips and thighs.

In other words, if two people weigh exactly the same amount, the person with the "apple" shape will have a higher risk for cardiovascular disease than the person with the "pear" shape.

Body fat distribution is assessed most easily in an office setting by measuring the waist circumference, or the waist-to-hip ratio (the waist measurement divided by the hip measurement). Some studies show the waist measurement alone is better at predicting the risk for cardiovascular disease than the waist-to-hip ratio; however, a recent study showed a parallel association between the waist-to-hip ratio and mortality in middle-aged women.[1]

The waist measurement is included in the criteria for metabolic syndrome, which is a set of health risk factors that are associated with an increased chance for developing such conditions as heart disease, peripheral vascular disease, stroke, and diabetes. The syndrome is confirmed if three or more of the following five criteria are met:

CRITERIA	DEFINING LEVEL
Abdominal obesity, waist circumference in inches	Men > 40 in
	Women > 35 in
Triglycerides	> 150 mg/dl
HDL cholesterol	Men < 40 mg/dl
	Women < 50 mg/dl
Blood pressure	> 130/85
Fasting glucose	> 100 mg/dl

Three of the criteria (triglycerides, HDL cholesterol, and fasting glucose) are determined by blood tests; the other two are determined by simple measurements that can be taken in or outside your doctor's office.

It is currently estimated that fifty million American adults have metabolic syndrome. Several factors contribute to the development of metabolic syndrome, including genetics, being overweight, and being physically inactive. Recent studies also link the quality of the diet to the development of the syndrome. The typical Western diet—one high in meat, refined grains, fried foods, and soda (including diet soda)—increases the chance of developing the metabolic syndrome,[2] while a Mediterranean diet is likely protective. Both quality and quantity are important for our total health.

Kara Davis, *Spiritual Secrets to Weight Loss* (Lake Mary, FL: Siloam, 2002, 2008), 173–174.

THE RIGHT WEIGHT DEBATE

by Hans Diehl, DrHSc, and Aileen Ludington, MD

A PERSON'S WEIGHT IS a highly individual issue, but here are some guidelines. By definition, obese means being 20 percent or more above one's ideal weight. A person with an ideal weight of 120 pounds would be obese at 144 pounds or more. Overweight, on the other hand, means being 10–19 percent above one's ideal weight. Our hypothetical person with an ideal weight of 120 pounds would be overweight at 132–143 pounds.

Ideal weight can be set in several different ways. One way is to look at the records of large life insurance companies that are interested in finding predictors of longevity. They have discovered that certain ideal weight-to-height relationships correlate well with optimum life expectancy. The massive actuarial data of the Metropolitan Life Insurance Company formed the basis of its gender-specific Table of Desirable Weight, based on height and bone size.

Although most people have a pretty good idea of their frame size, wrist and sometimes ankle measurements provide a more reliable method. In general, a wrist measurement for women of 5 ¼ inches or less is considered small-boned, between 5 ¼ to 6 inches is medium, and over 6 inches is large. For men, anything under 6 inches is small and anything over 7 inches is large.

Here is a time-honored rule of thumb:

- For men—allow 100 pounds for 5 feet of height. For each additional inch, add 6 pounds. The ideal weight for a man 5 feet 10 inches tall would therefore be 160 pounds.
- For women—allow 106 pounds for 5 feet of height, but add 5 pounds for each additional inch. For a woman who is 5 feet 5 inches tall, that comes to 131 pounds.
  Large-boned men and women should add 5 percent to these figures.

A simpler, more practical test is the pinch test. Trained health professionals use calipers to measure the thickness of skin folds at different places on the body. With the proper tables, they can then calculate body fat percentages with fair accuracy.

You can do a simplified pinch test yourself. Reach over to your left side, just below the last rib, and pull the skin and fat away from the underlying muscle. Hold it between your thumb and index finger and squeeze. If the space between your thumb and finger is more than three-fourths of an inch, you're in trouble!

Knowing your ideal weight is important. Studies show that people who remain near their target live longer, healthier lives. Find out how close (or far) you are from your ideal weight.

Hans Diehl and Aileen Ludington, *Dynamic Health* (Lake Mary, FL: Siloam, 2003), 87–89.

BASIC NUTRITION AND EXERCISE GUIDELINES

by Kara Davis, MD

BELIEVE IT OR not, lifestyle modification is not rocket science! We can't allow ourselves to become intimidated at the thought of learning and implementing a few changes for better health. Yes, there is a natural fear of the unknown, and there is comfort with the familiar, but if "familiar" habits are destroying your health and the health of your children, then it is time to learn some new things and not be apprehensive about it. With that in mind and with a desire to keep things uncomplicated, our approach will begin with seven very simple pieces of advice.

1. Your diet should be comprised primarily of plant-based foods. Reduce your intake of meat, especially meats that are processed, smoked, dried, and salted. Plant-based foods such as whole grains, vegetables, legumes, seeds, nuts, and fruits should constitute the majority of your diet.

2. Spend more time in your kitchen. In other words, cook more often so that you eat out less often. It is extremely hard to maintain control of what you eat if you do not prepare it yourself.

3. Watch your beverages. If you aren't careful, you can accumulate hundreds of empty calories each day through what you choose to drink. A recent study found that even diet soda was associated with the development of metabolic syndrome, a finding that clearly warrants further study.[1]

4. Limit, LIMIT, *LIMIT* the amount of sugary and salty snacks you eat or allow your children to eat. Since these types of foods are heavily advertised, you will need to make a habit of turning off the television—a practice that promotes good health in and of itself. Snacks have their role; just make sure what you choose is beneficial and not detrimental.

5. Stop going for seconds. Enough said.

6. Stop putting enough food for seconds on your first plate. Enough said.

7. Exercise regularly (aim for sixty minutes, most days of the week), but also look for other opportunities to move—and be diligent about it. For instance, unless you are physically disabled, there is really no need to hunt for a parking space close to the entrance of the store. In doing so, you are denying yourself a much-needed opportunity to move.

Seven rules, with seven being the number of completion. If you carefully adhere to these seven pieces of advice, you will see results.

Kara Davis, *Spiritual Secrets to Weight Loss* (Lake Mary, FL: Siloam, 2002, 2008), 11–13.

FOUR STRATEGIES FOR CONTROLLING YOUR IMPULSES

by Kara Davis, MD

WHEN WE CONSIDER self-control, one way to gauge ourselves is to examine how we handle impulses. Keep in mind, the biblical precepts about self-control may not be specific to eating and exercise habits but should be applied to all areas of our lives.

1. Stewardship

Everything belongs to God; we are just His stewards, which is another term for "manager." The Bible tells us our bodies are not our own, but they belong to God: "Do you not know that your body is a temple of the Holy Spirit, who is in you, whom you have received from God? *You are not your own; you were bought at a price.* Therefore honor God with your body" (1 Cor. 6:19–20, NIV, emphasis added).

A faithful steward understands that *personal* desires are not part of the plan. The good manager will diligently seek and adhere to whatever it is that the *owner* desires. If his or her personal desires fail to line up with the owner's desires, then it is the *personal* desires that are relinquished.

2. Discerning needs vs. wants

The sad truth is that many people refuse to accept that *needs* take precedence over *wants*. What frequently happens is that their "needs" are compromised because they have misappropriated their resources toward satisfying "wants." We *want* so many foods that we ought to restrict or avoid, and then we avoid the kinds of foods our bodies truly *need*. Clearly, if our impulses are left unchecked, we set ourselves up for becoming sick.

3. Proper planning

In the area of finances, planning requires a budget. In the area of weight control, planning requires a meal plan. If we don't have a budget, we are prone to lose control and spend money impulsively.

Likewise, a menu is crucial to good eating habits. But I find that many people who are overweight or obese or who have medical conditions influenced by diet do surprisingly little meal planning. Trying to manage money is difficult without a budget, and trying to eat a nutritionally sound, calorie-appropriate diet is difficult without a meal plan. When we fail to plan, we are prone to eat whatever is available, and that often means fast food, junk food, or highly processed meals that are high in sodium and calories.

4. Discipline

Discipline is vitally important both to temple stewardship and capital stewardship. Without discipline, both our spending habits and our eating habits tend to become erratic and excessive. And without discipline, both the practice of saving and investing and the practice of regular exercise fall by the wayside.

Believers are indwelt by the Holy Spirit, whose very character is that of self-control. If yielding to impulses has prevented you from making lifestyle changes to improve your health (or your finances), then please understand that God has equipped you through the power of the Holy Spirit to lead a self-controlled life. Reflect on this truth, and manifest it in your daily living. Don't, as the apostle Paul warned, become "disqualified for the prize" because of uncontrolled impulses.

Kara Davis, *Spiritual Secrets to Weight Loss* (Lake Mary, FL: Siloam, 2002, 2008), 157–159.

EATING TIPS

by Don Colbert, MD

1. Eat the protein portion of your meal first since this stimulates glucagon, which will depress insulin secretion and cause the release of carbohydrates that have been stored in the liver and muscles, which will help prevent low blood sugar.
2. Chew each bite at least twenty to thirty times, and eat slowly.
3. Never rush through a meal. Rushing will cause hydrochloric acid to be suppressed, making digestion difficult.
4. Never eat when you are upset, angry, or bickering. Eating should be a time of relaxation.
5. Limit your starches to only one serving per meal, and eliminate them entirely after 6:00 p.m. Never eat bread, pasta, potatoes, corn, and different starches together at one meal. This elevates insulin levels. If you do go back for seconds, choose fruits, vegetables, and salads, but not starches.
6. If you are craving a dessert, simply eliminate the starch or the bread, pasta, potatoes, and corn and have a small dessert. Or better yet, have it for lunch. However, be sure to have your protein and fat to balance out the sugar in the dessert. Also, don't eat desserts regularly. Only do this on special occasions such as birthdays, holidays, and anniversaries. Take 10 grams of fiber to help bind and eliminate toxins and fats. Remember, fiber covers a multitude of dietary sins.
7. Avoid alcoholic beverages, not only because alcohol is toxic to our bodies, but also because it triggers a tremendous insulin release and promotes storage of fat.
8. Try to eat 10 grams of fiber with each meal, or take two fiber capsules (such as PGX Fiber) with 16 ounces of water at the beginning of a meal to prefill your stomach.
9. Eat three well-balanced meals each day, with 3–5 ounces of protein, 1–2 tablespoons of good fats, starch the size of a tennis ball, and all the salad and green veggies you want.
10. Eat breakfast like a king, lunch like a prince, and dinner like a pauper.

Note: The information in this secret has been updated from its original text to include the latest medical and nutritional breakthroughs.

Don Colbert, *The Bible Cure for Weight Loss and Muscle Gain* (Lake Mary, FL: Siloam, 2000).

YOUR DAILY CALORIE BANK

by Gregory L. Jantz, PhD, with Ann McMurray

Y OU HAVE A certain number of calories per day in the "bank." Your goal is twofold: (1) You don't want to spend more calories than you have in your bank. (2) You want to invest your calories in the right mix of nutrients in order to enjoy a health dividend.

For example, my pyramid says I have 2,400 daily calories a day in the "bank," figured for my gender, age, and activity level. Here's how I could be spending that on any given day:

- In the morning, I make a Starbucks run and get a venti caffé mocha with whipped cream and nonfat milk and a blueberry scone. I have just deducted 870 calories, or 36.25 percent, of my daily total.
- For lunch, I go to McDonald's and get a grilled chicken sandwich, small fries, and low-fat milk. Lunch is 770 calories of my 2,400 per day, or 32 percent.
- For dinner, it's vegetable lasagna! Now, the package says the serving size is 1 cup, but I have 2 cups, a multigrain English muffin with butter, a small green salad with dressing, and a glass of water. That's 810 calories of my 2,400, or 33.75 percent.

I've eaten 2,450 calories. Not bad. Of course, I didn't factor in the candy bar in the afternoon (250 calories) or the ice cream I had after dinner (350 calories), but who's counting? Oh, yeah, we are. I've now eaten 650 calories more than my daily guidelines tell me, or about 25 percent more calories than I should have had for the day.

Oh, I failed to mention that in order to have this level of caloric intake, I'm supposed to get in at least 30–60 minutes of physical exercise each day. But it just didn't happen. So, actually, I really should deduct 200 calories, according to my tracking sheet, which means I'm now at 850 calories over for the day.

Are you getting the idea how quickly that bank of daily calories can be taken up? If I only have 2,400 calories per day to fuel my body and give it the vitamins, minerals, and amino acids it requires to perform, I need to do a better job and choose food wisely.

- Instead of Starbucks, I could have had a cup and a half of cooked oatmeal, peanut butter, a medium orange, and a cup of nonfat milk for a total of 515 calories. That's 355 calories less than the Starbucks run and a lot cheaper.
- I still have McDonald's for lunch, but instead I choose their Asian salad with grilled chicken, a package of apple slices, and low-fat milk. That's only 505 calories, 265 calories less than my other trip to McDonald's. Plus, I would have had both fruits and vegetables.
- For dinner, I eat a cup and a half of veggie lasagna, add to the salad broccoli heads and orange and red pepper strips. My dinner is 700 calories.
- For snacks, I have a protein bar at 200 calories and low-fat yogurt at 250 calories.

Now I've made some fairly simple-to-do, real-world changes and I'm still under my 2,400-day by over 200 calories. I chose whole grains with the oatmeal, ate several different types of vegetables, had my two cups of fruit, got my protein from the grilled chicken in the salad, the dairy products, and the peanut butter. I've still had three meals with an afternoon snack and dessert after dinner, and today I consumed almost 900 fewer calories, and I came much closer to my goals.

Gregory L. Jantz with Ann McMurray, *The Body God Designed* (Lake Mary, FL: Siloam, 2007), 78–83.

EAT MORE, WEIGH LESS

by Hans Diehl, DrHSc, and Aileen Ludington, MD

TODAY'S WORLD IS full of contradictions. Popular magazines and TV screens brim with beautiful, slender people—and with full-color ads of rich, fattening foods. Supermarkets offer 25,000 slickly packaged, calorie-dense products, along with magazines touting the latest quickie diet. Fast-food restaurants tempt from nearly every street corner with *takeout* service—while nutrition is what they take out!

Modern food technology has turned inexpensive, low-calorie, high-volume foods into expensive, high-calorie, low-volume *caloric bombs*. It's now possible to eat a whole meal's worth of calories with only a few bites of food. No wonder people feel hungry and dissatisfied—and overeat!

How does it happen? *Processing* strips seven pounds of sugar beets of their bulk, fiber, and nutrients, producing one pound of *pure sugar*. Sugar and other refined sweeteners now account for about 20 percent of daily calories eaten.

Almost 50 percent of the modern Western diet consists of processed and concentrated calories devoid of vital nutrients and valuable fiber—a sure-fire formula for being overweight.

SO HOW DO I GO ABOUT LOSING WEIGHT?

If you love food but want to lose weight, then follow these food selection principles:

Eat freely from the following:

- Fruits—all fresh fruit (avocado and olives sparingly)
- Vegetables—all vegetables, greens, squash, tomatoes
- Legumes—all beans, peas, lentils, garbanzos
- Tubers—potatoes, yams, sweet potatoes
- Grains—all whole grains, breads, pastas

Eat sparingly from the following:

- Nuts
- Flesh foods, if you insist—small amounts (3 ounces no more than three times a week) of skinless fowl, fish, fillet, lean beef

Optional:

- Dairy—nonfat milk, plain yogurt, skim-milk cheeses, buttermilk, and low-fat cottage cheese in moderation
- Eggs—whites only; substitute two egg whites for one egg in recipes.

Hans Diehl and Aileen Ludington, *Dynamic Health* (Lake Mary, FL: Siloam, 2003), 91, 93.

THREE-DAY MEAL PLAN

by Don Colbert, MD

I WOULD LIKE TO help you plan three days of menus to jump-start your weight-loss plan, but please refer to my book *The Bible Cure for Weight Loss and Muscle Gain* for a full seven-day meal plan. Be sure to drink spring or filtered water with a squeeze of lemon or lime with each meal.

DAY ONE

BREAKFAST	
Men	Women
1 cup old-fashioned oatmeal with ¼ cup blueberries	½ cup old-fashioned oatmeal with ¼ cup blueberries
½ cup skim milk	⅓ cup low-fat cottage cheese
2 tsp. walnuts	2 tsp. walnuts
1 tsp. agave nectar	¾ tsp. agave nectar
½ cup low-fat cottage cheese	

LUNCH	
Men	Women
4–5 oz. chicken breast	3–4 oz. chicken breast
1 tsp. grapeseed mayonnaise	1 tsp. grapeseed mayonnaise
Lettuce	Lettuce
Tomato slice	Tomato slice
2 slices toasted Ezekiel bread	1 ½ slice toasted Ezekiel bread
A spinach salad with 10–20 sprays of salad spritzer	A spinach salad with 10–20 sprays of salad spritzer

MIDAFTERNOON SNACK	
Men	Women
A snack bar (Jay Robb Jaybar or Go Free Dark Chocolate Crunch)	A snack bar (Jay Robb Jaybar or Go Free Dark Chocolate Crunch)

DINNER	
Men	Women
4 oz. salmon	3 oz. salmon
Salad with peppers, onions, mushrooms, celery, cucumber, and sprouts	Salad with peppers, onions, mushrooms, celery, cucumber, and sprouts
10–20 sprays of salad spritzer	10–20 sprays of salad spritzer
½ cup fruit cocktail	⅓ cup fruit cocktail

DAY TWO

BREAKFAST	
Men	Women
¾ cup low-fat cottage cheese	½ cup low-fat cottage cheese
2 cups peaches	1 ½ cup peaches
1 Tbsp. slivered almonds	½ Tbsp. slivered almonds

LUNCH	
Men	Women
4 oz. water-packed tuna, preferably tongol tuna (lowest in mercury)	3 oz. water-packed tuna, preferably tongol tuna (lowest in mercury)
1 tsp. grapeseed mayonnaise	1 tsp. grapeseed mayonnaise
Chopped celery, chopped onions, lettuce, tomato	Chopped celery, chopped onions, lettuce, tomato
2 slices double-fiber or Ezekiel bread	1 ½ slice double-fiber or Ezekiel bread

MIDAFTERNOON SNACK	
Men	Women
Protein shake or supplement such as whey protein or Life's Basic Plant Protein	Protein shake or supplement such as whey protein or Life's Basic Plant Protein
DINNER	
Men	Women
4 oz. turkey	3 oz. turkey
1 cup steamed broccoli spears	1 cup steamed broccoli spears
1 small baked potato or sweet potato (size of tennis ball) with pat of organic butter	1 small baked potato or sweet potato (size of tennis ball) with pat of organic butter

DAY THREE

BREAKFAST	
Men	Women
1 whole egg and 2 egg whites, scrambled with onions and chopped tomatoes	1 whole egg and 1 egg white, scrambled with onions and chopped tomatoes
1 oz. low-fat cheddar cheese	1 oz. low-fat cheddar cheese
2 slices Ezekiel or double-fiber toast with pat of butter	1 slice Ezekiel or double-fiber toast with pat of butter
1 orange	1 orange
LUNCH	
Men	Women
Chicken fajitas with 4–5 oz. chicken strips	Chicken fajitas with 3–4 oz. chicken strips
2 8-inch spelt tortillas	1-½ 8-inch spelt tortillas
2 Tbsp. guacamole	2 Tbsp. guacamole
½ cup salsa	½ cup salsa
Chopped lettuce	Chopped lettuce
MIDAFTERNOON SNACK	
Men	Women
4 oz. low-fat cottage cheese	4 oz. low-fat cottage cheese
1 cup strawberries	¾ cup strawberries
DINNER	
Men	Women
4–5 oz. lean filet mignon, preferably free-range meat	3–4 oz. lean filet mignon, preferably free-range meat
1 small baked potato with a pat of butter	1 small baked potato with pat of butter
1 cup steamed asparagus	1 cup steamed asparagus
Large salad with 10–20 sprays of salad spritzer	Large salad with 10–20 sprays of salad spritzer

Note: The information in this secret has been updated from its original text to include the latest medical and nutritional breakthroughs.

Don Colbert, *The Bible Cure for Weight Loss and Muscle Gain* (Lake Mary, FL: Siloam, 2000).

KEEP A JOURNAL OF YOUR EATING HABITS

by Ed and Elisa McClure

ONE OF THE most important things I did in the process of losing 200 pounds was to keep a daily journal. Each day I recorded everything I ate and drank, my weight, and the amount and type of activity or exercise I did. It was eye opening, to say the least.

The primary purpose of keeping a food log is to create awareness of what, when, and how much or how little you eat. And if you will record your emotional state before and after eating, you will also begin to learn more about why you eat—reasons besides the primal instinct of true hunger, that is. I can't stress enough how important it is to be completely truthful with yourself as you are taking inventory, setting goals, and keeping your food log.

Keeping a daily journal is a proven principle of weight-loss success. Participants in the National Weight Control Registry listed journaling as one of the top five components of their success at losing weight and keeping it off. A daily journal not only helps you plan what to eat, but it also provides structure and discipline to other areas of your life as well. If you start feeling overwhelmed at how far you still have to go to reach your destination, just look back at your journal and rejoice at the progress you have made so far. If you feel stuck and don't see the scale moving in the right direction, the answer will be in the pages of your daily journal.

The format of your journal is not that important. While I was at Structure House, I used logbooks provided for me. They were very detailed, with hour-by-hour entries and spaces for recording emotional reflections. Lately I have used a very inexpensive record book with blank ruled pages. The important thing is to simply develop the habit of writing everything down.

Ed and Elisa McClure, *Eat Your Way to a Healthy Life* (Lake Mary, FL: Siloam, 2006), 127–128.

THE GLYCEMIC INDEX

by Don Colbert, MD

In 2005 the USDA updated its recommendations for eating fresh foods. It used to recommend five to seven servings of fruits and vegetables every day. Now it recommends five to thirteen servings a day—almost double the previous recommendation.

It's hard to go wrong with fresh, organic fruits and vegetables. They should be the major part of your diet. One note of caution, however: fruits and vegetables can be low glycemic or high glycemic. The glycemic index (GI) is a numerical system of measuring how fast a carbohydrate triggers a rise in your blood sugar. The higher the number, the greater the blood sugar response. A low-glycemic food will cause a small rise, while a high-glycemic food will trigger a dramatic spike.

- Low-glycemic foods are 55 or less.
- Medium-glycemic foods are 56–69.
- High-glycemic foods are 70 and above.

I recommend eating produce with a glycemic index of 50 or less. For people trying to lose weight, the chart below will give you glycemic values for some fruits and vegetables:[1]

GLYCEMIC INDEX VALUE	FOOD	
< 15	Artichoke	Green beans
	Asparagus	Lettuce, all varieties
	Avocado	Peppers, all varieties
	Broccoli	Snow peas
	Cauliflower	Spinach
	Celery	Young summer squash
	Cucumber	Zucchini
	Eggplant	
15	Tomatoes	
22	Cherries	Peas, dried
24	Plum	
25	Grapefruit	
28	Peach	
31	Dried apricots	
32	Baby lima beans, frozen	
36	Apple	Pear
52	Orange juice, not from concentrate	
53	Banana	
54	Sweet potato	
55	Sweet corn	
64	Beets	Raisins
66	Pineapple	
72	Watermelon	
97	Parsnips	
103	Dates	

Don Colbert, *Eat This and Live!* (Lake Mary, FL: Siloam, 2009), 54–55.

SUPPORTING YOUR WEIGHT LOSS WITH SUPPLEMENTS

by Don Colbert, MD

L ET'S EXPLORE SOME of these natural substances that can promote health and vitality as you defeat obesity in your life. We will also look at some of the supplements available that you should avoid as you take the necessary steps to reach your ideal weight.

A good multivitamin. When you purchase a vitamin supplement, be sure that it contains vitamin K_1. You may want to choose a multivitamin you can take two to three times a day.

A good multimineral. Find a mineral supplement that is chelated rather than one that contains mineral salts. Chelation is a process of wrapping a mineral with an organic molecule such as an amino acid that increases absorption dramatically.

Many colloidal minerals have extremely high amounts of aluminum in them. They may also contain mercury, arsenic, and other toxic materials. Therefore, avoid colloidal mineral supplements.

B-complex vitamins. To prevent our adrenal glands from becoming exhausted, we need to supplement our diets daily with a comprehensive multivitamin and mineral formula with adequate amounts of B-complex vitamins, especially B_5 or pantothenic acid.

Ginseng. Taking 200 mg of ginseng two to three times per day will help support the adrenal glands, thus allowing you to handle stress.

DSF Formula is an adrenal glandular supplement by Nutri-West. It is an important aid in helping your body to cope with the effects of stress, which can actually cause you to gain weight. Take ½ to 1 tablet at breakfast and at lunch.

5-HTP. Many overweight individuals are depressed, and I have found that supplements of 5-HTP (5-hydroxytrptophan) in a dose of 50 to 100 mg three times a day with meals will not only help depression but will also promote satiety, thus fewer calories are consumed at meal times. You should not take 5-HTP if you are taking any other antidepressant.

Fiber. Very effective in promoting weight loss and stabilizing insulin levels, fiber also helps control blood sugar and lowers insulin levels. Two to four capsules of PGX fiber with 16 ounces of water taken before a meal will prefill your stomach.

Green tea. Consumption of green tea can reduce body weight, abdominal fat, and increase fat oxidation and energy expenditure. It also reduces cholesterol, free fatty acids, and triglycerides. Take two high-potency green tea capsules, or drink several cups of green tea each day to maximize weight loss.

Irvingia. Leptin is a hormone that tells our bodies when they have consumed enough calories, but as we get older, our bodies become resistant to this hormone. Irvingia helps to counteract that by reversing leptin resistance and reducing the amount of glucose that is converted to fat in the body. A dose of 150 mg of irvingia should be taken twice a day.

Note: The information in this secret has been updated from its original text to include the latest medical and nutritional breakthroughs.

Don Colbert, *The Bible Cure for Weight Loss and Muscle Gain* (Lake Mary, FL: Siloam, 2000).

UNDERSTANDING VOLUMETRICS

by Ed and Elisa McClure

Now, I LIKE to eat—make no mistake about that! I have learned that not only are you what you eat, but also you need to eat for who you are. Let me explain that by helping you understand something called volumetrics.

The weight-management principles of volumetrics center around the fact that people tend to eat about the same volume (or weight) of food every day. An excellent resource on the topic is the book *Volumetrics* by Dr. Barbara Rolls.

Restricting the amount you eat, which is what most diet programs recommend, is counterproductive. Your brain is programmed to be satisfied with a certain amount of food, and eating less than that will result in feelings of deprivation that will eventually cause powerful cravings. However, eating the same volume of food but switching to lower-glycemic, less energy-dense foods will help you lose weight while still feeling full.

Which would make a better snack: a garden-fresh tomato or fat-free pretzel sticks? If you guessed the tomato, you are right. The entire tomato provides only 25 calories, the equivalent of no more than four or five of the tiny pretzel sticks. Now, be honest. Would you be satisfied with only a few bites of the dry, fat-free pretzel sticks? Not likely. You would probably wind up eating far more than the 25-calorie portion size. Obviously, you will feel more satisfied by eating the greater volume of the tomato for the same number of calories.

So the first point to understand about volumetrics is that it is important to eat enough. If you do not eat the volume of food your body is accustomed to, it will backfire on you, stalling your weight loss.

There is a qualitative aspect to volumetrics. Not only do you want to choose less energy-dense foods, but you also want to consider what a food is doing for your body nutritionally. What is the sodium content? What about antioxidants and vitamins? How much fat are you getting in an average serving, and what kind of fat is it—saturated fat or one of the more beneficial fats?

There is also a quantitative aspect to volumetrics; you can factor in food cost in addition to volume and calories. Being a "numbers guy," I quickly realized that you don't have to spend a significant amount of money. Take a look at A Tale of Two Meals.

A TALE OF TWO MEALS			
STIR-FRY			
AMOUNT	ITEM	COST	CALORIES
5 oz.	Chicken breast	$1.10	225
1 Tbsp.	Sesame oil	$0.40	100
½ cup	Broccoli	$0.30	15
¾ cup	Brown rice	$0.10	200
½ cup	Cabbage	$0.20	10
½ cup	Carrots	$0.30	20
Total amount: 21.5 oz. Total cost per person: $2.40 Total calories per person: 570		Total cost per oz.: $0.11 Total calories per oz.: 26.5	

A TALE OF TWO MEALS			
PRIME RIB			
AMOUNT	ITEM	COST	CALORIES
9 oz.	Prime rib	$5.04	630
6 oz.	Baked potato	$0.30	190
1 oz.	Butter	$0.16	200
3 oz.	Spinach	$0.10	20
½ oz.	Cream	$0.40	50
1 oz.	Sour cream	$0.20	50
1 oz.	Cheese	$0.20	115
Total amount: 21.5 oz. Total cost per person: $6.40 Total calories per person: 1,255		Total cost per oz.: $0.30 Total calories per oz.: 58.5	

Both meals contain the same amount of food, 21.5 ounces. But one meal contains more than twice as many calories and costs almost three times as much. Put the principle of volumetrics to work in your food plan, and you can achieve your weight-loss goals without breaking your food budget.

Ed and Elisa McClure, *Eat Your Way to a Healthy Life* (Lake Mary, FL: Siloam, 2006), 128, 130–132.

IDENTIFY YOUR ROADBLOCKS TO WEIGHT LOSS

by Ed and Elisa McClure

MOST PEOPLE SEEM to face the same roadblocks over and over. Once you identify your roadblocks, you can blast right through them to reach your goals.

Roadblock #1: Prescription medications

Many medications such as antidepressants, antibiotics, and blood pressure reduction drugs either cause weight gain or can hinder you from losing weight. However, you should never stop taking a prescription drug without consulting your doctor.

Roadblock #2: Candida

Candida albicans is a type of yeast, a single-celled organism abundant in our intestinal environment. A number of things—antibiotics, prednisone, hormones, stress, diabetes, or eating too much sugar and processed foods—can change the intestinal balance and cause overgrowth of yeast.

Roadblock # 3: Stress

Cortisol is a hormone released in response to stress, and it plays an important role in fat storage, especially around the abdomen. When you do not manage stress well, you are literally expanding your waistline!

Roadblock #4: Lack of sleep

One effect of a chronic lack of sleep is an increased appetite due to interference with the appetite-regulating hormones leptin and ghrelin. Leptin signals your brain when it is time to eat as well as when satiety, or fullness, has been reached. Ghrelin stimulates appetite and is elevated significantly when sleep is inadequate.

Roadblock #5: Hormones

Too much estrogen leads to increased fat storage and interference with insulin regulation; too much insulin leads to more fat storage, insulin resistance, and blood sugar irregularities; too little testosterone makes it extremely difficult to build muscle mass and metabolize fat.

Roadblock #6: Food sensitivities and intolerances

Common foods that might be a hindrance to your health and weight are corn, yeast, wheat, sugar and sweeteners, dairy products, wheat, peanuts, fish, shellfish, and soy.

Roadblock #7: Sabotage

Sabotage is real, and it can be present in one or more of the following three ways: (1) self-sabotage—people knowingly or unknowingly sabotaging their own efforts through self-destructive behaviors; (2) family—they will not change with you; (3) co-workers and friends.

Roadblock #8: Compartmentalization

I implore you not to compartmentalize yourself. Don't try to eat the right foods and not increase your activity. Don't become a marathon runner and remain a hostage to emotional issues that should be in your past. Recognize and treat yourself as a whole, marvelous creation deserving of abundant health, peace, joy, and happiness.

Ed and Elisa McClure, *Eat Your Way to a Healthy Life* (Lake Mary, FL: Siloam, 2006), 87–109.

THE POWER OF POSITIVE WORDS

by Ed and Elisa McClure

Positive thinking plus positive words can revolutionize your life. Thoughts produce corresponding feelings and emotions. It is not the other way around. What you think about will determine your feelings, so it is absolutely crucial to change old, negative thought patterns to new, positive thought patterns, which will produce positive feelings and emotions.

One of the best ways to change your thoughts is to hear yourself say aloud the positive principles you want to establish in your mind. Not only are you what you eat, but you are also what you think and speak.

The following affirmations will help reprogram your "internal software" with life-changing attitudes based on God's Word. Repeat these statements aloud daily.

- I am beautiful, capable, and lovable. I am valuable. I love myself unconditionally and nurture myself in every way. I am unique, the apple of God's eye.
- I am a child of God. I love people and show love, warmth, and friendship to all. I am healed of all my childhood wounds, and I hold no account of wrong done to me. I can be intimate with others and with myself. All of my relationships are based on integrity and respect.
- I am intelligent and have great creativity. I can concentrate easily. I can analyze and solve problems. I learn quickly and have an excellent memory. I have the mind of Christ. I make decisions with confidence.
- I am diligent and faithful, and I have a spirit of excellence. Whatever I put my hand to will prosper. God always causes me to triumph in Christ.
- I let go of things I cannot control. I have the courage to change things I should change, the serenity to accept the things I cannot change, and the wisdom to know the difference. I have no need to control people or situations. I am controlled by the Holy Spirit.
- I am a success. I can do anything I put my mind to. I can do all things through Christ, who strengthens me. I see each day as a new and positive adventure. I give thanks in all things.
- I express my potential more and more each day. I see problems as exciting challenges that cause me to grow stronger and stronger in my faith. I visualize myself as the person God wants me to be. I see myself achieving my goals and fulfilling God's purpose for my life.
- I live every day with passion and power. I feel strong, excited, passionate, and powerful. I feel tremendous confidence. I have all the abilities I need to succeed.
- Every cell in my body vibrates with health, healing, vitality, and love. I am healthy and strong and filled with vitality. Jesus took every sickness and every disease away from me.[1]

Ed and Elisa McClure, *Eat Your Way to a Healthy Life* (Lake Mary, FL: Siloam, 2006), 139–142.

STEPS TO GET YOU MOVING

by Dino Nowak

1. **Ask God for help.** Ask God to give you the right motives, perseverance, lifelong perspective, and a sound mind that does not succumb to the images and messages of the culture. Ask God to remove the fear so that you can make this change. Ask Him for His power to act upon and not just your own. (See 2 Timothy 1:7.)

2. **Take inventory.** What is it you want to change exactly? Why do you want to change? Why now? What brought you to this decision? What role models are you looking to? Do you have an accountability or fitness partner? What is your meeting schedule?

3. **Goal setting and direction.** Start first with how you want to *feel*, and then what would you like to be able to *do* better or learn new altogether. Finally, list your physical goals. What would you like to change in your *appearance*? I have a saying: wrong motives lead to wrong goals, giving us wrong strategies, which lead to wrong methods and outcomes. Set yourself up for success by establishing *right* motives.

4. **What are your stumbling blocks?** Be specific and very detailed. Brainstorm how you plan to overcome each one. Do not filter your thoughts; just write them down as they come to you.

5. **Wipe the slate clean.** Forget everything you have ever tried or have ever been told in the past.

6. **Recognize that change is needed.** Do you need to make healthy changes? Look at others who have followed the same path for years. It happens gradually over time but is destined to the same result. What would be even better is to find some photos of your family or friends who are now overweight or obese who were not earlier in their life to show how the behaviors and habits you develop now *will* catch up to you in the future.

7. **Decide to make the change.** You need to make a personal decision and do so with conviction and for the right reasons. Make the commitment. Are you committed to the point it costs you something? Expect sacrifices (especially in your old thinking) to be made. They will benefit you far greater than what it is you are giving up.

8. **Accept in your heart and mind that the images you see in the media are not reality.** Until you accept this truth, you will continue to compare yourself and others to those false standards. Do you believe the images are not an accurate reflection of reality?

9. **Stop comparing yourself to others.** Get it in your mind that God made you special. (See Psalm 139.) There is no one else like you in the world, so stop comparing yourself to doctored pictures of supermodels.

10. **Once you start, commit to finish.** If you are not ready to see it through to the end, then do not start. We are looking to make a change once and for all. Make sure you are 100 percent fully committed to the process.

Dino Nowak, *The Final Makeover* (Lake Mary, FL: Siloam, 2005), 110–114.

SLIMMING RECIPES

by Joseph Christiano, ND, CNC

White Bean and Escarole (or Swiss Chard) Soup

2 Tbsp. olive oil
1 small diced onion
2–3 cloves smashed garlic
1 16-oz. can cannellini beans (or other appropriate
    white bean)
4–5 cups water

2 Tbsp. mellow white miso
½ Tbsp. rosemary, fresh or dried
Salt to taste
½ lb. escarole or Swiss chard, trimmed and coarsely
    chopped

Heat olive oil in large soup pot. Sauté onion and garlic for 3–5 minutes. Add beans and cook until warm.

Heat 1 cup water. Dilute miso in warm water. Set aside.

Puree ⅔ of onions and beans in food processor. Slowly add miso water to thin beans. The consistency should be somewhat loose. Add more water if necessary.

Add pureed beans to soup pot with whole beans and onion. Add balance of water, rosemary, and salt to taste. Bring to simmer. (Note: Miso should never be boiled. It breaks down easily under high temperatures.) Add escarole or Swiss chard. Cook for 10 minutes more. Serve immediately.

Makes 4–6 servings.

Tofu Burgers

1 lb. extra-firm tofu, drained well
½ cup cooked brown rice
½ cup dry bread crumbs
½ cup chopped scallions
2 egg whites

¼ cup grated carrots
½ cup low-fat mozzarella or soy cheese
2 tsp. soy sauce
2 tsp. ground walnuts (optional)

Mash tofu. Mix all ingredients thoroughly. Form burgers. Heat nonstick skillet to medium with spray of olive oil. Cook burgers until golden.

Makes 6 servings.

Marinated Tuna Steaks

⅓ cup olive oil
¼ cup tamari, shoyu, or light soy sauce
Lemon juice from half a lemon
2 cloves smashed garlic

2 Tbsp. fresh chopped coriander (cilantro)
1 dollop honey
4 tuna steaks (6 oz. each)

Combine all ingredients except tuna in large Ziploc bag or shallow bowl. Mix ingredients well. Add tuna to marinade. Cover tuna completely with mixture. Place in refrigerator for 15–30 minutes. Use this time to prepare other parts of your dinner.

Grill or broil tuna steaks on medium heat to desired doneness, 3–4 minutes per side for rare, 5 minutes for medium well. Let fish sit for 5 minutes before serving.

Makes 3–4 servings.

Joseph Christiano, *Bloodtypes, Bodytypes, and You* (Lake Mary, FL: Siloam, 2000, 2004, 2008), 215, 218, 226.

DETOXING

TOXIC ONSLAUGHT

by Don Colbert, MD

MOST PEOPLE ARE toxic to some degree—and I don't mean their personalities, but their physical bodies. Everyone has toxins stored in his or her body. Your body has waste management systems that keep you healthy when they function properly. But, like a city that neglects its trash removal, your body can eventually become overwhelmed with toxins. That's what it means to be toxic.

CAN TOXICITY BE AVOIDED?

I'm convinced that toxicity cannot be avoided entirely. We live in a toxic world. There are about eighty thousand chemicals registered for use in the United States, and we add about two thousand more every year. These chemicals are used in food, prescription drugs, supplements, household products, personal products, and lawn care products.[1]

Some of the air we breathe is toxic—more than 80,000 metric tons of carcinogens are released in the air annually in North America.[2] But we can clean our air inside our home and workplace. A significant amount of our water is polluted, with more than 2,100 chemicals in most municipal water supplies.[3] However, we can learn to choose clean, pure water. Much of the food supply also contains toxins. However, we can learn to choose living, organic foods instead of pesticide-laden foods.

Because of the way Americans eat and drink, and because of the toxicity of our environment—everything from manufacturing to agriculture—many people's bodies are backed up with microscopic garbage. It is as if their body's waste management department has gone on strike.

Thankfully, there is an answer: detoxification. There are simple things that you can start doing today to rid your body of toxins and to help your waste management systems keep them out. Decrease your exposure to toxins by:

1. Choosing more living, organic foods (especially veggies), free-range lean meats, and low-fat organic dairy. Consume 30 grams of fiber daily.
2. Choose clean, pure spring or filtered water instead of tap water.
3. Breathe clean air, and do not stroll, walk, or jog along busy roads or highways. Don't wait outside airport terminals, inhaling diesel exhaust. Avoid secondhand smoke in restaurants and public buildings.
4. Wear rubber gloves if you use chemicals for cleaning. Better yet, check for natural cleaning alternatives and natural personal care products.
5. Work with your doctor to try to get yourself off of as much medication as possible. This will give your liver a break and will allow it to rid your body of built-up toxins. Avoid even Tylenol; it has the potential to stress the liver if it is overused and can be the main cause of acute liver failure.[4]

Don Colbert, *The Seven Pillars of Health* (Lake Mary, FL: Siloam, 2007), 147–149.

WHEN BREATHING MAY BE HAZARDOUS

by Hans Diehl, DrHSc, and Aileen Ludington, MD

MANY MODERN HOMES and office buildings are tightly sealed to save energy costs. But this advantage may be offset by poor ventilation and potential accumulation of indoor air pollutants.

Tobacco smoke, of course, is the most dangerous pollutant, but there are others. Formaldehyde, for example, seeps from certain wood products, and other chemical fumes come from carpeting, copy machines, upholstery, cleaning products, and freshly dry-cleaned clothes. Carbon monoxide and nitrogen dioxide, two poisonous gases, may come from gas, oil, and coal furnaces; gas ranges; fireplaces; and kerosene heaters.

Other problems occur from dust, air mites, molds and fungi, ozone, lead, asbestos, pesticide residues, and, in some areas, radon gas.

These pollutants affect people with symptoms ranging from burning eyes, sore throats, coughing, and itching to headaches, sluggishness, nausea, dizziness, feelings of exhaustion, and depression. This cluster of symptoms is sometimes referred to as "sick building syndrome."

Here are some ways we can protect ourselves and improve indoor ventilation:

- Ban smoking indoors. Even secondhand smoke contains hundreds of chemicals.
- Make sure all gas, oil, and kerosene and coal-burning heaters and appliances are properly vented to the outdoors.
- Keep heating and air conditioning units well maintained. Clean air ducts and filters regularly.
- Keep chimneys open and in good repair.
- Use air fresheners, moth crystals, etc. sparingly.
- Avoid idling a vehicle in an attached garage or near an open window.
- Set air conditioners and heating systems to bring in 20–30 percent (or more) fresh air. Energy costs will be somewhat higher, but health benefits will more than compensate for this.
- Air out your house at least once a day. On smoggy days, air out the house at night or in the early mornings. In most areas, smog drops considerably once the sun has set.
- Sleep with an open window. Set up cross ventilation in your bedroom if possible. You'll wake up feeling refreshed.

People with allergies and certain lung ailments may find air purifiers helpful.

How does air relate to personal health?

Air is composed of about 20 percent oxygen, the rest being nitrogen along with a few other gases. Since the human body operates on oxygen, each one of its one hundred trillion cells must receive steady, fresh supplies, or die. Oxygen is picked up in the lungs from the air we breathe and delivered to our bodies via the red blood cells. Well-oxygenated cells are healthy and contribute to overall well-being. Anything that diminishes oxygen supplies to the lungs or its delivery to body cells is detrimental.

Hans Diehl and Aileen Ludington, *Dynamic Health* (Lake Mary, FL: Siloam, 2003), 222–225.

THE COLON: YOUR "INVIRONMENT"

by Joseph Christiano, ND, CNC

COLON HEALTH IS all about functionality, and the function of your colon is directly related to proper elimination, or bowel movements. Improving your health and ridding your body of poisonous toxins that contribute to poor health, disease, and sluggish metabolism start with what I call your "INvironment."

The colon's major functions are to absorb water and nutrients from partially digested food that enters from the small intestine and to send waste out of the body. It's a garbage bag that holds all the waste products of the foods that we've consumed, cellular debris, and so forth. These things need to be dumped out of our bodies, and the colon acts like a trash can that temporarily holds all of the garbage until it's time to take out the trash for good.

THE MALFUNCTIONING COLON

Most people who come to me for help with this problem ask me how the elimination process in their bodies got so bogged down. The answer is simple: when we ingest foods that are refined white flour products, a pasty mucus forms in our digestive tract. This gooey mucus builds up in the colon.

You see, when the digestive process of the colon is slowed down too much because of the refined sugar and flour that are plastering the walls of the colon and narrowing the passage, the fecal matter and mucus can become impacted. The fecal matter itself is now impacting all of that toxic waste into the colon. Instead of helping your body eliminate those toxins, your colon is actually storing them.

The little pouch or bulge developing below your navel may not be fat. This little bulge is often the result of the colon getting so impacted with fecal matter that it's getting larger and larger.

If you are experiencing any of the following symptoms, it may be a sign that you have a malfunctioning colon: headaches, skin problems, foul breath, lack of energy, stomach pain, and constipation.

Here are my recommendations for repairing and maintaining optimum colon function:

1. Keep a dietary record.
2. Avoid refined sugar, white flour, and fried foods.
3. Eat 30 grams of fiber each day from natural sources such as bran, psyllium, flaxseed, oatmeal, and fruit.
4. Drink alkaline water daily.
5. Minimize stress as much as possible in your life.
6. Exercise three to five times weekly.
7. Conduct a colon cleanse and detoxification program twice a year.

Joseph Christiano, *Bloodtypes, Bodytypes, and You* (Lake Mary, FL: Siloam, 2000, 2004, 2008), 49–52.

DETOXING 101

by Scott Hannen, DC

M ANY PEOPLE ARE not aware that the body has its own filters, so they have no idea that we must be responsible to help the body cleanse the filters. For the sake of discussion, let me list your body's five main filtration systems for you.

1. Your liver is your chemical filter.
2. Your kidneys are your fluid filters.
3. Your lungs and airways are your air filters.
4. Your spleen is your blood cell filter.
5. Your lymphatic system is your intercellular filter.

These five filtration systems dump many of their toxins into the colon. That is why cleansing these filters as well as the colon is vital for our health.

When food is digested, and the body breaks it down into tiny elements to be used by the body for energy, repair, and other processes, there are elements of debris collected as well. All of these unwanted leftovers, cellular debris, antigens, and other circulating waste are recycled through the liver, kidneys, spleen, and lymphatic system, where they can be properly discarded from the body, usually through the bowel and urinary tract.

If one of these filtering organs or systems is not functioning properly, the entire body may begin to suffer an accumulation of toxins. This can lead to extensive cell damage, symptoms, sickness, and disease. It can also prevent the body from absorbing nutrients, thus depriving the cells of proper nutrition. This nutrient deprivation can also lead to deficiencies that produce cell damage, symptoms, sickness, and disease. When you understand these fundamental workings of the body, you can see how providing adequate nutrients (such as vitamins, minerals, essential fatty acids, and enzymes) and maintaining proper filtration would lead to optimal health, thus greatly diminishing sickness and disease. This is what I call *primary health care.*

When we detect a problem with one of our body's filtration systems, we need to find a way to cleanse it. We read in Genesis 1:29 that God created herbs to be used by humans to sustain them.

There are specific herbs that cleanse every filtering organ of the body safely and effectively. Some bitter herbs can safely detoxify the liver, and then there are certain grasses that do the same for the kidneys, when used in moderation. Besides cleansing the body, herbs also offer wonderful healing and repairing potential.

Other herbs also have a protective effect as well.

Scott Hannen, *Healing by Design* (Lake Mary, FL: Siloam, 2003, 2007), 88–89.

SOUPS FOR DETOXIFICATION

by Janet Maccaro, PhD, CNC

S OUP IS A great way to sneak high-nutrient, high-fiber foods into your meals. Eating homemade nutritious soup that is low in salt will not only nourish you but will also flush waste from your body. This simple dietary change can cut your risk of premature death from heart disease, stroke, cancer, etc. Adding soup to the beginning of your meals not only boosts your nutrition but also curbs your appetite.

The key is to stick to a serving of low-calorie, high-fiber soup like vegetable soup or minestrone, which only has around 75 to 125 calories. For optimal nutrition and weight loss, try eating at least two homemade "soup meals" a day. And for the best results, try my favorite health-building Slimming Soup!

To get you started, I have included one of my all-time favorite vegetable-based, high-fiber soups that will fill you up—not out!

Dr. Janet's Very Veggie Slimming Soup

2 Tbsp. olive oil	1 zucchini, chopped
1 large onion, chopped	1 yellow squash, chopped
2 green and/or red bell peppers, chopped	1 can (14 ½ oz.) low-sodium stewed tomatoes
4 garlic cloves, minced	1 bottle (46 oz.) vegetable juice
½ tsp. ground cumin	½ tsp. ground black pepper
½ small head cabbage, sliced	¼ tsp. crushed red pepper flakes
2 large carrots, sliced	

Warm oil in a large saucepan over medium heat. Add onion and bell peppers. Cook five minutes or until tender. Add garlic and cumin. Cook one minute. Add cabbage, carrots, zucchini, squash, tomatoes (with juice), vegetable juice, black pepper, and red pepper flakes. Heat to boiling. Reduce heat to low, cover, and simmer one hour.

Makes six wonderful servings! It will be easy for you to get your five servings of vegetables today with this soup, and that is just "souper"!

Janet Maccaro, *100 Answers to 100 Questions About How to Live Longer* (Lake Mary, FL: Siloam, 2009), 74–75.

BATHS FOR PURIFICATION

by Janet Maccaro, PhD, CNC

YOU MAY EXPERIENCE flu-like symptoms during the detoxification because your body is ridding itself of poisons. You can get relief from these symptoms by taking baths using sea salt (1 to 2 cups) and baking soda (1 cup) in a tub of water and soaking for twenty minutes (more than twenty minutes may exhaust you). This bath also counteracts the effects of radiation, whether from x-rays, cancer treatment radiation, fallout from the atmosphere, or television radiation. On off days, you can put 1 cup of apple cider vinegar in the tub and soak. Here are some other baths you can use:

- Clorox bath: This will help to remove heavy metals from the body and add oxygen. Add ½ cup Clorox brand bleach, use ONLY this brand, to a tub of warm water. Soak for twenty-five minutes. You can shower off with soap and fresh water afterward, but it is not necessary. If you skin feels a bit itchy, this will relieve it.
- Epsom salts and ginger: This bath opens pores and eliminates toxins and relieves pain. Stir in 1 cup of Epsom salts and 2 tablespoons of ginger to cup of water first, then add it to the bath. Do not remain in the tub for more than thirty minutes.
- Epsom-sea-oil: This bath helps with dry skin and stress. Put 1 cup Epsom salts, 1 cup sea salt (from health food store), and 1 cup sesame oil into a warm to hot tub of water, and then soak for twenty minutes. Pat yourself dry.
- Vinegar bath: This is used when the body is too acidic and is a quick way of restoring the acid-alkaline balance. Mix 1 cup to 2 quarts of 100 percent apple cider vinegar to a bathtub of warm water. Soak forty to forty-five minutes. This is excellent for excess uric acid in the body and for the joints, arthritis, bursitis, tendonitis, and gout.
- Betonite bath: This is a fast detoxification method. Soak 2 to 4 pounds of betonite clay in a flat container overnight to dissolve it. Then add the dissolved clay to a tub of water. With 2 pounds of betonite, soak one hour; with 4 pounds, soak only about thirty minutes. The more betonite used, the faster the detoxification.

Janet Maccaro, *90-Day Immune System Makeover* (Lake Mary, FL: Siloam, 2000, 2006), 23–25.

GO AHEAD—SWEAT IT!

by Don Colbert, MD

I OFTEN SAY THAT summer was created by God to be our "sweat season," when our bodies expel toxins through the skin. God actually told Adam he would work by the sweat of his brow. The skin has been called "the third kidney" by some in the medical field because it is able to release so many toxins such as pesticides, solvents, heavy metals, urea, and lactic acid from the body. It is also called the third kidney because the consistency of the sweat is similar to our urine.[1] Approximately 99 percent of perspiration is water; the remaining 1 percent is toxic waste.[2] But because of air conditioners, antiperspirants, and a general bias against sweating, much of the U.S. population never really sweats.

Don't be afraid to perspire when you exercise; it means you are healthy! Exercise also improves circulation to the skin, which brings nutrients to the skin and removes cellular waste.

Here are some other suggestions for detoxifying your body through the skin.

HOP IN THE SAUNA

If you don't work outdoors in the heat, or if for some reason you cannot exercise, consider sauna therapy.

An infrared sauna is especially effective. Infrared saunas use an infrared radiant heat source that causes your body to eliminate up to three times more toxins in the perspiration than do conventional saunas. An infrared sauna stimulates the cellular metabolism and breaks up water molecules that hold toxins within the body, thus allowing the body to sweat out these toxins. This natural process may also burn up to 300 calories during a twenty- to thirty-minute session.

BRUSH YOUR SKIN

You are now aware that your body excretes toxins and waste through your skin every day. Therefore, taking proper care of your skin is extremely important. If the pores of your skin become clogged with dead skin cells, the toxins may remain locked inside your body, putting more stress on your liver and kidneys.

Dry-skin brushing is an excellent way to keep the pores of your skin open and clear so that your skin is allowed to breathe and excrete the toxins.

I strongly recommend investing in a loofah sponge or a natural soft-bristle brush. To brush your skin, start with the soles of your feet, working up your legs, torso, and arms until you have brushed the majority of your body, avoiding only your face. Use firm, hard strokes, brushing toward your heart to increase blood flow. The entire process should take about five minutes. It usually makes your skin feel warm due to increased circulation. I recommend dry-skin brushing prior to taking a shower.

In short, sweating, brushing your skin, and sauna therapy can help you detoxify through your skin.

Don Colbert, *The Seven Pillars of Health* (Lake Mary, FL: Siloam, 2007), 173–175.

GUIDELINES FOR YOUR DETOXING JUICE FAST

by Don Colbert, MD

I<small>F YOU DECIDE</small> to go on a juice fast, you will want to prepare yourself by eating only fruits and vegetables the day before you begin your juice fast.

I strongly recommend that you begin your juice fast on the weekend. By doing so, you will be able to spend more time resting. If you experience any side effects such as fatigue, light-headedness, or a headache, it will probably not interfere with your job (since it is the weekend).

It's very important that you juice raw, fresh fruits and vegetables (preferably organic). Prepared juices are simply not the same. Fresh juice contains the living enzymes, phytonutrients, antioxidants, vitamins, and minerals. Bottled, canned, and processed juices have been pasteurized. Many of the phytonutrients and enzymes have been lost in the process.

Don't drink alcohol or soft drinks. During your fast, drink only juices and herbal teas. You may also sip gently warmed vegetable juice or vegetable broth. (Avoid microwaves since they destroy most of the phytonutrients, antioxidants, and enzymes.) Good teas include organic black, green, and herbal teas. Also, drink plenty of clean, pure water, about two quarts a day.

When drinking your specially prepared juices, sip them slowly to mix the juice with saliva. Don't gulp them down.

Peel oranges and grapefruits, but be sure to leave on the white, pithy part of the peel. That is the part that contains the important bioflavonoids. Leave the skins on all other organic fruits and vegetables. Remove the green top portion from carrots, since they may contain a toxic substance. Slice the fruits and vegetables so that they fit nicely into your juicer.

Drink the juices immediately after juicing—do not store them. As soon as a fruit or vegetable is sliced, it begins to lose nutritional value.

Transfer your juice from the juicer to the blender and add crushed ice to create delicious smoothies from any juice recipe.

If your juicer spits out the fiber (pulp) from your fruits and veggies, which most juicers do, add 1 to 2 teaspoons of the fiber back into the juice before you drink it. The fiber helps to regulate your blood sugar, lowers cholesterol, prevents gallstones, and binds toxins.

When you create your own juices, there are four main fruits and vegetables that usually should form the base of each juice. These include carrots, celery, apples, and tomatoes. One of these, or a combination of them, should make up the greatest portion of your juice. You will find that they taste good and combine well with other fruits and vegetables. In addition, they are able to disguise the taste of veggies you may not like, such as cabbage and greens.

Don Colbert, *Get Healthy Through Detox and Fasting* (Lake Mary, FL: Siloam, 2006), 114–117.

DIETING VS. FASTING

by Lisa Bevere

GOD TOLD ME *not to diet*, then He told me *to fast*. This would seem a contradiction; both are a restriction of food. The difference lies in the purpose or motive that inspires them. A diet is designed to help you lose or gain weight. A change of diet may also be initiated to improve or correct health problems. Dieting is a natural physical application that alters our physical well-being, weight, or health. It changes the way we *look* or *feel*.

Fasting is not for weight gain or loss. Nor is it limited to natural healing. It is not designed to change the way we look and feel but to change the way we *perceive and live. A diet may change the way you look, but a fast will change the way you live.* A diet may change your appearance, but a fast will change the way you see it; it will alter your inner perspective. The world has perverted and reduced the fast, diminishing it to a diet. As such, it is not a spiritual renewal but a physical one. But the deepest transformations are wrought from the inside out.

Fasting changed my perception by changing my focus, causing me to change the way I lived. I didn't live for food or weight—I lived for God. Even on a natural fast you will experience an increase in eyesight clarity. On a spiritual fast you will have your spiritual eyes stripped of scales that have blinded them. When we lay aside the daily routine of food, drink, pleasures, and leisure, we are able to reevaluate our priorities.

Fasting is not about food; it is about separation. It represents a consecration to the Lord, a change in our relationship with Him. Whenever Israel truly fasted and turned to God for His assistance, He heard them. He responded with protection, provision, direction, and healing. There is not one of us who in our own strength could provide all this.

Fasting brings many benefits into our lives. Here are just a few of the benefits:

- Fasting creates a new hunger. (See Ezra 8:32.)
- Fasting increases sensitivity to God. (See Luke 2:36–38.)
- Fasting works humility. (See Psalm 35:13.)
- Fasting chastens or disciplines. (See Psalm 69:10.)
- Fasting changes our appetite. (See Acts 13:2.)
- Fasting increases our capacity. (See Esther 4:16.)
- Fasting brings answers to prayer. (See Isaiah 58:9.)
- Fasting leads to quick healing. (See Isaiah 58:8.)
- Fasting opens the door to God's protection and provision. (See Isaiah 58:8.)
- Fasting looses the chains of injustice. (See Isaiah 58:6.)
- Fasting frees the oppressed and breaks every yoke. (See Isaiah 58:6.)
- Fasting motivates us to provide food for the needy. (See Isaiah 58:7.)

Lisa Bevere, *You Are Not What You Weigh* (Lake Mary, FL: Siloam, 1998, 2007), 98, 100–102, 106, 114–121.

JUICE RECIPES

by Don Colbert, MD

BREAKFAST JUICES

½ small lemon or lime, peeled
1 cup berries
3 oranges, peeled
1 scoop phytonutrient powder

1 pink grapefruit, peeled
½ small lemon or lime, peeled
1 apple, cored and seeded
1 scoop phytonutrient powder

Handful of parsley
2 apples, cored and seeded
1 scoop phytonutrient powder

SNACK JUICES

2 celery stalks
2 apples, cored and seeded
2 carrots

Cut watermelon in sections and remove seeds. Juice enough melon for 8–12 ounces of juice.

3-inch slice pineapple with skin
¼-inch ginger root
Handful of parsley

LUNCH JUICES

1 beet
2 carrots
2 celery stalks
½ sweet potato, raw

½ head cabbage
Handful collard greens
2 carrots
1 apple, cored and seeded

Handful of parsley
1 tomato
2 celery stalks
1 garlic clove (optional)

DINNER JUICES

4 medium tomatoes
2 celery stalks
½ cucumber
Handful of bean or
    broccoli sprouts
1 clove garlic (optional)

2 carrots
1 beet
½ cucumber
2 celery stalks

3 carrots
Handful of collard greens, spinach,
    or beet greens
1 garlic clove
Handful of parsley

Don Colbert, *Get Healthy Through Detox and Fasting* (Lake Mary, FL: Siloam, 2006), 122–135.

FITNESS

PUTTING YOUR FIT INTO FITNESS

by Lorraine Bossé-Smith

W E'RE ALL DIFFERENT! A one-size-fits-all approach to fitness (or to anything, for that matter) will not work, and in my book *Finally FIT!* I have come up with a very unique way to customize your fitness program based on your specific personality traits. While I am going to give a brief overview below of those personality types or temperaments, you will do best by going to the book *Finally FIT!* to take the FIT Assessment to determine what category you fit into and how to achieve the best workout plan possible to achieve long-lasting results.

A customized approach to fitness will be that perfect FIT for you. It will be one you enjoy and that motivates you to stick with it. It's the program that will make *the* difference you have been hoping for. So now let's take a brief look at these FIT, or Fitness Individuality Trait, formulas.

The first category is the FAST FIT. If you're a FAST FIT person (like me), you prefer deciding for yourself. You assess things quickly without getting a lot of input from others. You are driven and goal oriented as well. You can be demanding on yourself and others. Can you see how this information will impact what type of exercise program you select? A FAST person, for instance, hates to wait in lines at the gym and may give up on fitness altogether rather than finding a faster way to work out. You need a program that is active, varied, and challenging. Understanding how you're wired will help you find success in fitness—and everything else, for that matter.

The next category is the FUN FIT category, and you like to interact with people. You blend or mingle well. You appreciate high-energy groups and a variety of options. You are an influencer, but you can also be easily influenced by others. You typically like large social or public gatherings. Can you imagine how you might approach fitness differently than the other styles? If you were to try to exercise alone all the time, you might get bored. It might not be very much fun, so you could end up quitting. You need to have a fitness program that is fun, full of variety, and allows you to interact with others.

In the FRIENDLY FIT category, you prefer a slow pace. You would much rather be in a small group setting than a large social event. You do not like a lot of change, preferring a routine. Your steady pace can lead to stubbornness if not monitored. You need a unique fitness program that "fits" you. Don't try to go it alone. Work out with a friend.

The final FIT category is the FACTUAL FIT category. If this is you, you like details and structure. You have a calculating and analytical mind that prefers working on tasks rather than engaging with people. Because of your attention to facts and figures, you may at times come across as cold. You approach fitness differently than others…more structured. One way for you to ensure success in fitness is to make sure you have a workout plan that helps you be consistent.

We are all uniquely wired, and while I have given you just a quick glimpse into the FIT categories, there is so much more you can uncover about yourself and how you relate to others. Be sure to read my book *Finally FIT!* to reap the full benefits of understanding how to customize a lifetime of healthy, active living specifically made for you.

Lorraine Bossé-Smith, *Finally FIT!* (Lake Mary, FL: Siloam, 2004), 26–27.

FOUR KEYS TO MAKE ANY DIET OR FITNESS PROGRAM WORK

by Ron Kardashian, NSCA-CPT

THERE IS A progression in understanding the keys to getting in shape God's way. You must begin with key #1, revelation, which unlocks the divine power of God's love into your life. Revelation makes it possible for you to know the truth and change your motivation and core beliefs that have contributed to your destructive mind-set and behavior patterns.

Once you have a vision of what is real, you are able to write power vision and mission statements to help you refine your vision and reach for your dreams.

Then you take key #2, declaration, in your hand and begin to unlock the power of your words to change your atmosphere and your life situation. As you learn to agree with the truth of God's Word for your life, your words begin to embrace your purpose and destiny that He wants to reveal to you.

Of course, that means you must embrace the necessity of change through key #3, application. You need to become a doer of God's Word, not just a hearer (James 1:22), in order to reap the wonderful harvest that you will plant through speaking and acting as the beautiful person God made you to be.

As you embrace the first three keys to getting in shape God's way, you will begin to experience key #4, manifestation, in your life—spirit, soul, and body. When you are manifesting the reality of keys one through three, it simply means that your healthy lifestyle is evident to all; it is easily perceived by the senses and especially by the sight.

Manifestation involves more than simply arriving at your stated fitness goals; it involves your entire life journey. And at every stage in life, there will be new challenges to face to maintain your goals for health and manifest your destiny in every area of your life—spirit, soul, and body.

God's intention is that love becomes the greatest source of power on Earth for you to unlock your destiny. As you learn to love God, love yourself, and love others, your lifestyle will be transformed. When love becomes your motivation, one of your main objectives will automatically become to honor your temple. That will include manifesting to the world that your lifestyle is one that establishes fitness for your body. You will take care for the health of your body, as well as your spirit and soul, as a gift of greatest worth.

Ron Kardashian, *Getting in Shape God's Way* (Lake Mary, FL: Siloam, 2008), 205–206.

FIVE COMPONENTS OF A WELL-ROUNDED EXERCISE PROGRAM

by Dino Nowak

HERE ARE THE components of a well-rounded physical activity program. Most likely you will recognize three of them, but the final two are key to keeping this going throughout the course of your life.

1. Strength

This is often referred to as resistance training where your body weight (such as with push-ups, sit-ups, or squats) or exterior weights (such as dumbbells, elastic bands, bungy cords, or weight machines) provide added resistance against muscles as they contract during a specific movement. Strength training allows our daily tasks to be completed more easily, reduces the risk of injury, and alleviates many aches and pains in conjunction with flexibility work.

Another reason this is so important is because lean muscle tissue boosts our metabolism and helps us burn more calories, even while resting.

2. Cardio

Cardiovascular training includes activities like walking, swimming, cycling, jumping on a trampoline, jogging, and any other activity that focuses on making your heart and lungs stronger and healthier.

3. Flexibility

This is the stretching routine after your workout and on your no-movement days. This helps with your posture, relieves stress, increases blood flow and circulation, and keeps you in the habit of doing something physical each day. Stretching after a workout is critical.

4. Reality

I call this the not-if-but-when principle. It means there will always be days you do not feel like going for that walk, or you will eat something you know you should not. That does not mean you are any less of a person and you blew everything. Shake it off, and move on to the next meal or the next workout. If you think you are going to start a fitness program and achieve perfection every minute of the day for the rest of your life, you need to let go of that mentality right now. The key is that what you do most often in your life is what will shape your outcome.

5. Plateau

Most people starting a physical activity program will plateau in one or two months. After a period of losing body fat, your body will stabilize for a while, making it more difficult as your body adjusts and tries to hold on to its fat stores. Remember, it has no idea that you are just trying to shed some body fat. This is why you need to change the activities and intensities. So look for consistent progress over time. There may be plateaus with a setback or two, but look at the big picture. Most people get frustrated or depressed by a setback and give up altogether. So let's get our attitudes correct from the beginning and remember to switch activities and increase intensity.

Dino Nowak, *The Final Makeover* (Lake Mary, FL: Siloam, 2005), 143–147.

KNOW YOUR HEART RATE TRAINING ZONE

by Ron Kardashian, NSCA-CPT

O NE OF THE biggest mistakes people make when they work out is that they don't exercise in a specific training zone. There are three percentages that are important to your overall knowledge of a cardiovascular workout regimen. They are 60 percent, 75 percent, and 85 percent—which represent the low-end, middle-range, and high-end heart rate targets, respectively.

In preparation for your participation in a fitness plan, please fill in the charts below, which will help you determine your safe training and your fat-burning zones. As with any fitness program, please see your physician before starting.

CALCULATE YOUR SAFE HEART RATE TRAINING ZONE

Calculate your safe training zone by completing the following equation.[1]

From the number 220 subtract your age:	
220 – _____ (your age) = _____ (maximal heart rate)	My maximal heart rate is _____.
Multiply your maximal heart rate by 60 to know your low-end training zone:	
(Maximal heart rate) _____ x .60 = _____ (low end)	My low-end training zone is _____.
Multiply your maximal heart rate by 85 to know your high-end training zone:	
(Maximal heart rate) _____ x .85 = _____ (high end)	My high-end training zone is _____.
Say this: "My safe heart rate training zone lies between _____ (low end) and _____ (high end)."	

FAT-BURNING ZONE

When you exercise, you always want to try to stay between your low-end and high-end heart rate training zones, which you calculated in the chart above. Don't be afraid to push yourself a little harder each time you exercise. The body responds well in a controlled stress environment.

Maintaining a heart rate target of 75 percent of your *maximal* heart rate during your workout will allow you to burn fat continually.

FAT-BURNING HEART RATE

Calculate your fat-burning heart rate by completing the following equation:[2]

Find your resting pulse. It is best taken in the morning before exertion or after sitting quietly for five minutes. Place two fingers on your neck to find your pulse. Count the beats for six seconds.

Multiply that number by 10 to get your resting pulse. (For example: if you counted seven beats in six seconds, 7 x 10 = 70, which would give you 70 beats per minute [bpm]).
My resting pulse is _____.
Now subtract your resting pulse from your maximal heart rate, which you determined from the chart above, to get your heart rate range:
_____ (maximal heart rate) - _____ (resting pulse) = _____ (heart rate range)
Now multiply that number (heart rate range) by .75 (which is your fat-burning intensity), and then add your resting pulse to get your personalized target fat-buring heart rate:
_____ (heart rate range) x .75 (fat-burning intensity) + _____ (resting pulse) = _____ (fat-burning heart rate)
Say this: "My personalized target fat-buring heart rate is _____."

Ron Kardashian, *Getting in Shape God's Way* (Lake Mary, FL: Siloam, 2009), 192–195.

EXERCISE STRATEGIES THAT WORK

by Don Colbert, MD

THINK ABOUT ALL the unused exercise equipment lying under beds, under sheets in guest bedrooms, and in garages across America. Big chains like Play-It-Again Sports thrive on good intentions that never take hold.

Your body will not do the right thing without some prodding. It doesn't like being exercised at first, but after about three weeks, your body will change its mind: it will desire and expect to exercise. Here are the best tips I know to bulletproof your exercise routine.

Build exercise into your schedule. Schedule it like an important doctor's appointment. Choose a time you won't waver from, and put yourself on automatic so you don't give yourself an "out."

A workout before breakfast, before lunch, or before dinner is great. Just don't exercise late at night, since you may be too charged up to sleep. Also, avoid exercise immediately after a meal. It will pull the blood from your stomach and intestines (where it's needed to help digestion) to your muscles. You are likely to start belching and have heartburn and other digestive problems. Exercise before you eat or two hours after you eat. However, a light snack before exercising is fine.

Choose an exercise you enjoy. The best exercise is the one you'll do. If you have arthritis and walking hurts your knees, choose biking, elliptical machines, pool exercise, yoga, or Tai Chi instead. Tailor your routine to your physical condition.

Have an exercise partner. Partners keep you accountable to do the exercise and should make the exercise time more enjoyable.

Choose a location you enjoy. Walk in malls, parks, mountains, on the beach, or near a lake. Make exercise a complete sensory experience.

Change it up. Change your routine, either by location, time of day, or by the exercise you do. Make it fun.

Do occupational/transportation exercises. Seize every opportunity to increase your activity level. Park at the far end of the parking lot and walk to the store. Use stairs when you can. Default to the active options.

Take cues from your body. On days when you are exhausted, or after nights in which you have not slept well, don't push yourself to exercise. Listen to your body, and learn when to take a day off. I say this from experience. For years I pushed my body very hard until I had a heat stroke and almost died. I had not allowed my body to stop when it needed to stop. Now older and wiser, I have slowed my pace, and I listen to what my body is saying.

Overtraining can suppress your immune system, increase your risk of injury, increase your body fat by raising cortisol levels, and interfere with your emotional and mental health. It can cause as much stress to the body as trauma, surgery, infections, and anxiety.

Don Colbert, *The Seven Pillars of Health* (Siloam, Lake Mary, FL, 2007), 141–144.

EXERCISING FOR YOUR BODY TYPE

by Joseph Christiano, ND, CNC

THE PEAR BODY TYPE

When the pear gains weight, the weight mostly goes to the hips, thighs, and buttocks. Pears can be considered bottom heavy and can have a shallow bust line, narrow shoulders, and a straight waist.

To redesign the pear body type, perform exercises designed to:

- Fill out the chest/bust
- Broaden back and add width to the shoulders
- Firm and tone the arms (biceps and trideps)
- Firm the abdominal muscles
- Isolate hips, thighs, and buttocks
- Elongate, firm, and tone
- Reduce lower body major muscles

Avoid any exercises or physical activities that would tend to stimulate the lower body to grow. Concentrate on building muscle mass for the upper body while reducing the lower body.

THE APPLE BODY TYPE

When the apple gains weight, the weight mostly goes to the upper body. The apple lacks upper body/lower body symmetry or balance. They are generally leaner but lagging in size in comparison to the upper body. Most of their body fat is around the waist, upper back, and arms.

To redesign the apple body type, perform exercises designed to:

- Shape and tone only the upper body
- Isolate abdominal muscles
- Build the upper and lower leg muscles
- Build, firm, and tone the buttocks

Avoid exercises that tend to build mass on the upper body. Exercises for the upper body should be done for the sole purpose of firming and toning each muscle group. Concentrate on the abdominal muscles for strengthening and flattening. Incorporate exercises that will stimulate lower body muscles. Using dumbbells will help develop a symmetrical hourglass shape.

THE BANANA BODY TYPE

When the banana gains weight, the weight goes equally to the upper and lower body. The banana mainly lacks curve or shapeliness and tends to have a straight-line figure or physique.

To redesign the banana body type, perform exercises designed to:

- Firm, tone, and build muscles in the upper body
- Strengthen and tone the abdominal muscles
- Elongate the thighs
- Firm and tone the buttocks

Incorporate exercises that will even out the shape and add curves and lines. Because the upper and lower are relatively balanced, or symmetrical, the fuller banana will want to add additional cardiovascular workouts to the body redesigning program.

Joseph Christiano, *Bloodtypes, Bodytypes and You* (Lake Mary, FL: Siloam, 2000, 2004, 2008), 290–292.

THERE'S NO MIRACLE IN A BOTTLE FOR INSTANT FITNESS

by Dino Nowak

HAVE YOU EVER seen the commercials that show those drastic before and after pictures? The ones that say you go from *this* to *this*—all by just taking a simple pill? I know of a woman who was actually a model for one of those.

Now, this woman had been active all her life. She always exercised and was in great shape. She also did some fitness modeling. When she and her husband were expecting a baby, a guy she knew who worked for this company approached her and said they would pay her quite well to have her pictures taken after she had the baby. This would be the "before" picture. He highly recommended she put on some more weight before the photo.

She took the offer and did just that. But once the picture was captured, man, did she go to work exercising. It didn't take too long for her to trim down. Since her body was so used to being fit and active all those years, it just bounced back when she returned to her workout routine. In just a few weeks she was ready for the "after" picture. She looked amazing (though she shared with me the photo was touched up too).

But guess what? Even though she was given a supply of the pills she was advertising, she took only a few in the beginning and stopped! You and I, however, and the rest of America are led to believe that all she had to do was take the magic little pill and her body went from before to after.

I wish I could say this is one of the exceptions.

Folks, this is why you don't hear much of the truth behind those advertisements you are exposed to: the contracts the models sign keep them from speaking the truth for fear of being sued. So take this one to heart as you are unlikely to hear many more.

You need to be aware of the strategies marketers use to separate you from your money. This is a multibillion-dollar-a-year business! That did not happen by accident. If all this stuff really worked, you would be fit already, and they would have put themselves out of business. Think about it.

Jesus said, "You shall know the truth, and the truth shall make you free" (John 8:32, NKJV). The truth is what frees us.

Here's a truth to get you started: there is no shortcut when it comes to losing fat or getting in better health. You have to eat with purpose and move. No supplement, gadget, or miracle gizmo is going to get you to that destination without traveling those paths.

Dino Nowak, *The Final Makeover* (Lake Mary, FL: Siloam, 2005), 2–6.

FIVE THINGS BEGINNERS NEED TO KNOW

by Ron Kardashian, NSCA-CPT

IF YOU HAVE never exercised or don't know much about it, please consider the following important information before you begin your workout. Again, remember to see your physician before beginning any exercise program.

Learning correct form

Take time and effort to learn the correct form for your workout so that it can become a natural part of your lifestyle. It is easier to learn to do something correctly the first time than to have to unlearn what you have practiced incorrectly when you realize it is not working for you.

Preventing injury

The key to preventing injury during your workout, after learning to exercise correctly, is to proceed slowly and with caution.

Muscle recruitment/isolation

Muscle recruitment does not mean that you are asking for volunteers to beef up your muscle mass. It is a term that refers to learning how to isolate or flex every muscle separately. For example, if I asked you to flex your calf muscle, you most likely could isolate it and do that. But if I asked you to flex your infraspinatus, you might ask me to repeat the question. Your infraspinatus is a muscle in your back near your underarm. It is possible to mentally locate and flex muscles you may not know that you have. These isolation techniques are vital to burning fat and increasing your lean muscle tissue in those hard-to-lose areas of the body. I encourage you to adopt the practice of recruiting your muscles—learn where they are and practice flexing and isolating them.

Cardiovascular work/breathing practice

You may be aware that it is possible to live without food for weeks. You can live without water for several days. But you can only live without oxygen for a few minutes. During your workout, make sure that anytime you are feeling pressure, you breathe out. For example, if you are doing a squat, when you begin to stand up, breathe out. As you are lifting up in a bicep curl, breathe out. As you reach and throw, breathe out. As you coordinate your breathing with your movement, it will create a wonderful oxygen flow—voluntary exchange—to all parts of your body.

Adaptation

It is important to understand the principle of adaptation working in your body. For example, when you stress your muscles through resistance training, the bones to which they are connected are also slightly stressed. This stress will actually improve your bone function and cause the bones to adapt to your new muscular fitness. The more resistance you apply in your workout, the better your muscles will work for you.

As God's highest creation, you were designed to grow under times of stress. Physical adaptation simply involves the improvement in your body's ability to function in strength and freedom because of your fitness training.

Ron Kardashian, *Getting in Shape God's Way* (Lake Mary, FL: Siloam, 2008), 197–199.

FIT OVER FIFTY

by Lorraine Bossé-Smith

JUST BECAUSE YOU are retired or nearing retirement doesn't mean you walk away from principles you learned in your youth. Some retirees take not having to work to an extreme and stop working on everything, including their health. I believe it is even more critical at the fifty-plus mark to monitor one's health and work on improving it.

Take a look around you, and you will see many retired folks spending their "free" days at the doctor's office or in line at the pharmacy. Is that how you want to spend your time? I wish more than that for you. I would like to see you enjoy a healthy lifestyle that allows you to do the things you have always dreamed of.

My father never had that chance. He died of cancer at the very young age of fifty-two. I remember him speaking of the day when he would get to travel and see the United States, but his day never came. His premature death is a very good reminder that we do not know how much time we have here on earth.

IT'S NEVER TOO LATE

Our bodies are amazing. We can abuse them by doing all the wrong things, but once we stop, they heal.

My mother had smoked cigarettes since she was a teenager. After my dad died of cancer, my mother finally decided that she wanted to be healthy, and she was actually able to quit. In a year's time her lungs were almost clear. Her body was healing, Later in life, she took it a step further to eat better and exercise, and her body responded by being in the best shape she had ever been—and she was in her sixties!

So don't think you are too old or too set in your ways to make a change. Small steps can get you there.

BENEFITS OF A HEALTHY LIFESTYLE AFTER 50

- Being active will improve the quality of your sleep.
- Weight-bearing exercise will increase your bone density and reduce your chances of osteoporosis.
- Participating in active programs will keep you alert and sharpen your senses.
- Exercising and eating right will minimize aches and pains.
- Stretching will improve joint movement and improve overall mobility, preventing unnecessary injuries.
- Staying fit will give you more energy and help you be more productive.
- Being in shape will help you feel better about yourself and give you a more positive outlook on life.

Lorraine Bossé-Smith, *Fit Over 50* (Lake Mary, FL: Siloam, 2005), 5–8, 16.

THE BATTLE BETWEEN YOUR EARS

by Ron Kardashian, NSCA-CPT

Y OUR GREATEST BATTLE to gain mastery and manifest a healthy lifestyle occurs in the six-inch area between your ears—your brain. As you continue your journey toward health and fulfilling your vision for fitness, it will be helpful to keep the following *Es* in mind. They will inspire you to maintain your progress in your battle against faulty thinking, which, of course, results in faulty doing and being.

Exercise

Exercise is a gift to you and to the ones you love. Doing ten to fifteen minutes a day of moderate exercise increases your use of oxygen, which enhances your life expectancy. It also improves your quality of life, bathing the skin with natural beauty, reducing anxiety, and diminishing stress.

An ancient proverb says that every time you walk a step, it adds a minute to your life. Consider that the next time you ride an elevator or escalator instead of taking the stairs. A person who exercises regularly knows the true wealth of the health it provides. Do you believe you are worth reducing your risk factor for stroke, heart disease, osteoporosis, bloating, obesity, insecurity, and so on? Then you understand the true wealth of exercise health.

Energy

Energy is a serious asset and a sweet friend. You may relate to the term energy by its scary definition—calorie. But when you are taking in the right kind of calories—energy—you receive the benefit of this sweet friend, which is a satisfying quality of life. You know that it takes energy to enjoy anything in life.

Wrong kinds of calories, like those found in a tall mocha, spike your energy and then cause it to crash a few minutes later. When you choose to consume good forms of calories, you turn the days of your life into memories of a quality lifestyle and a treasury of wealth, manifested in your success in living your dreams and fulfilling your destiny.

Equanimity

Equanimity is a little-used word that refers to being calm and even-tempered.[1] It is a quality that is welcomed on every level of life—spirit, soul, and body. The value of this quiet demeanor cannot be measured in dollars and cents. It guards against panic attacks, depression, and a lack of peace. The apostle Paul instructed believers: "And let the peace (soul harmony which comes) from Christ rule (act as umpire continually) in your hearts [deciding and settling with finality all questions that arise in your minds, in that peaceful state] to which as [members of Christ's] one body you were also called [to live]" (Col. 3:15, AMP).

Americans spend billions of dollars a year on prescription drugs, trying to counteract the effects of life stressors. But peace is absolutely free for those who seek to know the One who is called the Prince of Peace (Isa. 9:6). Choose to become the temple of God and follow His laws of wealth and health. Allow God to empower you to manifest all your healthy lifestyle.

Ron Kardashian, *Getting in Shape God's Way* (Lake Mary, FL: Siloam, 2009), 207–209.

DISEASES and DISORDERS

WHAT IS HEART DISEASE?

by Francisco Contreras, MD

I**F YOU TIE** a ribbon tightly on the base of any of your fingers, your finger will first change color from red to purple. Before long it will become pale, at which point the pain will be very sharp. The same thing happens to your heart during a myocardial ischemic attack—better known as a heart attack.

Let's take a closer look at why heart attacks occur and why they are so dangerous.

Many different types of heart disease exist, some affecting the valves of the heart, some the walls of the heart, and some the chambers—but the most prevalent heart disease involves the coronary arteries—those vessels that feed the heart itself.

To put it simply, heart disease occurs when inflammation and plaque buildup block coronary arteries, causing reduced or stopped blood flow to the heart.

Arteries are supposed to be flexible and smooth, expanding and contracting as the blood flows through. Nearly all coronary artery disease results from *atherosclerosis*, which comes from the Greek words *athero*, meaning "porridge or paste," and *sclerosis*, meaning "hardness."[1] With atherosclerosis, deposits of fats and calcium build up on the inner walls. These fat and calcium deposits are called *plaques*.[2]

When these hard plaques damage the inner layer of the artery wall—causing them to harden, thicken, and lose elasticity—*arteriosclerosis* occurs. These terms can be confusing terms, so just keep this in mind: *arteriosclerosis* and *atherosclerosis*, even though they are not synonyms, for all practical purposes mean hardening of the arteries.

Plaque is like the flaky rust inside of an old water pipe. Building up layer by layer, it can eventually block an artery completely and stop the blood flow, or it can narrow an artery and reduce blood flow enough to form a blood clot, or a thrombus. When a blood clot blocks a coronary artery, a heart attack occurs.[3]

We normally think of atherosclerosis in terms of the heart, but it can seriously impact other parts of the body too. For instance, a diseased carotid artery leading to the brain can cause a stroke. A blocked renal artery leading to the kidney can cause high blood pressure. Atherosclerosis in the arteries leading to the bowel can cause abdominal pain, weight loss, or death of the bowels.

Blockage in the arteries supplying the legs with blood can cause difficulty in walking due to muscle discomfort and can eventually lead to gangrene.[4]

All of these symptoms are caused by ischemia, or lack of blood, and thus lack of oxygen.

Francisco Contreras, *A Healthy Heart* (Lake Mary, FL: Siloam, 2001), 7–8.

SYMPTOMS OF BLOCKED ARTERIES

by Francisco Contreras, MD

A CORONARY ARTERY THAT fails to send enough blood to the heart muscle causes chest pain, which doctors call *angina pectoris*. *Angina* means "pain," and *pectoris* means "chest." This pain, often described as a feeling of pressure or heaviness, is usually located in the center of the chest, but it may occur only in the neck, shoulder, arm, or lower jaw, particularly on the left side.[1] This pain almost always occurs after the heart has been "stressed" in some way, either by physical activity, emotional stress, cold temperatures—or even after a third helping of pork ribs, french fries, coleslaw, and corn on the cob. Anything that increases the heart's workload increases the danger for someone whose coronary arteries are blocked.

If your chest discomfort lasts for less than five seconds or more than twenty minutes, then you are probably not having heart problems (provided it's not a heart attack). If you experience a sharp or "stabbing" pain that is brought on by a sudden movement or deep breath, it's probably not your heart. If your chest pain is confined to a small area, or if it's relieved by rest or by stopping your physical activity, it's probably not your heart (again, provided you are not having a heart attack). In addition, if your chest wall is tender to the touch, it is probably not your heart.[2]

One of the difficulties in diagnosing heart problems is that many of its symptoms are similar to symptoms of less serious afflictions. Signs of a blocked coronary artery can be:

- Indigestion
- Nausea
- Abdominal bloating
- Belching
- Vomiting
- Severe pain in the upper right abdomen
- Discomfort unrelated to eating
- Shortness of breath
- Sweating
- Pain radiating to the jaw, neck, or arm
- Severe pressure, fullness, squeezing, pain and/or discomfort in the center of the chest that lasts for more than a few minutes
- Clammy skin
- Paleness
- Dizziness or fainting
- Unexplained weakness or fatigue
- Rapid or irregular pulse

Few people jump to the conclusion that they are having a heart attack when they have indigestion or nausea. But identifying the cumulative symptoms could save your life and your quality of life.

Francisco Contreras, *A Healthy Heart* (Lake Mary, FL: Siloam, 2001), 9–10.

BEAT THE STATISTICS FOR HEART DISEASE

by Don Colbert, MD

THE PRIMARY FUNCTION of the cardiovascular system is to deliver oxygen and nutrients to all the cells in your body and to remove cellular debris and waste.

Each day your heart beats approximately 85,000 to 115,000 times. About 5,000 gallons of blood travel 60,000 miles through blood vessels, which include arteries, veins, and capillaries. Thus your heart will beat over two billion times if you live an average life span, and it will pump over one hundred billion gallons of blood. This superhighway system is truly wonderful.

Wouldn't it be a good idea to keep this blood superhighway free of traffic jams?

Free radicals are the enemies of the heart and of our bodies' cells in general. Some estimates calculate that the cells in our bodies sustain over 10,000 hits from free radicals each day.

God's plan for winning the battle against heart disease includes a powerful weapon against free radicals—*antioxidants* (such as vitamins C and E). They're amazing substances that prevent oxidation and block or repair free-radical reactions in our bodies.

Here are some other things you can do to help lower your risk for heart disease. Think of them as five steps to a longer life.

1. Limit your fat consumption. Reduce your intake of the saturated fats found in red meat, pork (especially bacon), whole milk, cheese, butter, ice cream, fried foods, and chicken skins. Even more dangerous to the health of your heart than saturated fats are hydrogenated fats, which are found in margarine, peanut butter, processed foods, pastries, cookies, and doughnuts—they can even be found in many so-called "health products." I recommend limiting the amount of fat consumed to less than 30 percent of daily calories.

2. Let go of type A behavior. Type As are often impatient, extremely competitive, and pretty aggressive in almost everything they do. Type As have twice the risk of heart disease as compared with non-Type A individuals. Constant, excessive anger, worry, stress, and anxiety pump up the adrenalin levels, raise the blood pressure, and thereby exert heavier loads on the heart and circulatory system.

3. Don't smoke. Cigarette smoke fills the air with over four thousand chemicals, fifty of which are cancer causing. These chemicals trigger significant free-radical reactions, which damage the linings of the arteries or damage healthy cholesterol and form oxidized cholesterol. Smoking also causes blood platelets to clump together and so raises fibrinogen levels, which increases your risk of both heart attack and stroke.

4. Reduce your stress. When you're overly stressed, destructive changes occur in the chemical makeup of your brain and circulatory system. Reducing stress makes you more physically healthy.

5. Exercise regularly. A well-conditioned heart beats approximately sixty beats per minute. Since the unconditioned heart beats approximately twenty beats more per minute, that's an extra twelve hundred beats per hour, almost twenty-nine thousand extra beats per day, and over ten million extra beats per year! It would be great if your heart could do a little less work during your lifetime. The way to lower your heart rate is to exercise regularly, for at least thirty minutes, four times per week. Exercise and proper diet will also help you lose weight and help to lower your blood pressure.

Don Colbert, *The Bible Cure for Heart Disease* (Lake Mary, FL: Siloam, 1999).

HIGH CHOLESTEROL

by Don Colbert, MD

CHOLESTEROL CAN BE considered the Jekyll-and-Hyde nutrient of your body. There is a good type of cholesterol (HDL)—which prevents heart disease—and there is a bad type of cholesterol (LDL) that is very detrimental to your health and increases your risk of heart disease. HDL (high-density lipoprotein) is responsible for transporting one-third to one-fourth of the cholesterol away from the arteries and back to the liver where it is eliminated from the body. HDL actually removes cholesterol from the arterial lining, which can build up in the arteries, forming plaque, and cause coronary disease and heart attacks.

As I mentioned, HDL acts like a police officer patrolling our arteries, carrying cholesterol out of the arteries and depositing it in the liver so that it can be removed from the body. The higher the level of HDL, the lower the risk of heart disease.

It is well known that regular aerobic exercise, small amounts of red wine (one to two 4-ounce glasses a day) and the B vitamin niacin all raise HDL levels. New research is showing that dark chocolate is able to protect your blood vessels. One ounce of dark chocolate contains ten times more antioxidants than a strawberry, according to Penny Kris-Etherton, ND, PhD, professor of nutrition at Penn State University.[1]

LDL (low-density lipoprotein) is the primary carrier of cholesterol in the blood. If too much LDL is circulating, it can slowly build up as plaque in the arteries and can be especially dangerous in those arteries that supply blood to the heart and the brain. Clogged arteries in these areas can lead to deadly heart attacks and strokes.

Your doctor will determine your cholesterol ratio by dividing your total cholesterol level by your HDL number. This gives him an idea of what your risk for coronary disease due to cholesterol actually is. The ideal ratio to reach is 3.5 to 1 or lower. Decreasing just one unit from this ratio can dramatically reduce your risk for a heart attack.

Simply decrease your intake of saturated fats, avoid all hydrogenated fats, decrease your consumption of high-cholesterol foods, and limit the amount of simple sugars and highly processed carbohydrates in your diet, and your LDL cholesterol levels will begin to decrease naturally.

Eliminate man-made, processed foods from your diet, and choose "God-made" foods such as fruits, vegetables, and whole grains, which are high in soluble fiber. Begin to use extra-virgin olive oil. Choose lean meats, fish, turkey, and chicken without its skin. As you prefer skim milk and skim-milk cheeses and yogurt in place of fatty cheeses, butter, and whole-milk products, your cholesterol levels will come down even further. Increase your intake of soluble fiber, such as beans, peas, lentils, flaxseed, and psyllium seeds.

Start a regular aerobic exercise program by walking briskly three to four times a week for twenty minutes. And take supplements such as soluble-fiber supplements, antioxidants, policosanol, and niacin or no-flush niacin. By following these simple steps, you will begin to notice a dramatic change in your cholesterol levels, and you will be on your way to a happier, healthier life!

Don Colbert, *The Bible Cure for High Cholesterol* (Lake Mary, FL: Siloam, 2004).

LOWER BLOOD PRESSURE

by Reginald Cherry, MD

U SUALLY THERE IS no warning of high blood pressure until something breaks. By then it is a major battle to overcome the problem.

God has a better way! There are three natural supplements that, when used on a daily basis, can lower blood pressure naturally *and with no side effects*!

1. Potassium

Potassium protects the lining of blood vessels from damage. Consuming five or more servings of fruits and vegetables daily is the ideal way to obtain sufficient potassium. We also recommend potassium in the citrate form at a total of 99 mg daily. Taking the supplement will ensure constant blood levels, and your dietary intake of fruits and vegetables can simply build on this consistent level.

2. Polyphenols

Polyphenols found in olive oil lower blood pressure. A study reported in one medical journal noted that patients using 1–2 tablespoons of olive oil daily showed a marked reduction in the required dosage of blood pressure medications.[1] In fact, patients who were on antihypertensive medications were frequently able to cut their medicine dosage in half after only a few months. In these studies, a cold-pressed, extra-virgin olive oil was utilized.

3. Magnesium

Those who consume higher amounts of magnesium in the form of fruits and vegetables have significantly lower blood pressure.[2] Low magnesium levels also correlated with hardening of the arteries and the accumulation of cholesterol plaque in the carotid arteries, which supply blood to the brain. Increased magnesium intake causes blood vessels to dilate, which, in turn, results in reduced blood pressure. Magnesium can also help prevent heart palpitations and improve cholesterol levels. Even greater benefits are noted when the magnesium is taken with a potassium supplement and when salt is restricted in the diet.

TAKE ACTION

Because high blood pressure can creep up slowly on a person, giving no warning signs until it is too late, it is so important to be proactive in preventing potential serious problems before they strike. *Have your blood pressure checked regularly.* If your doctor sees readings in the 130/80 range, it is time to take action. You should lose weight, exercise, increase your consumption of fruit—especially bananas—and consider taking supplements that can lower blood pressure, including garlic capsules (the equivalent of one clove daily).

If your readings are found to be consistently over 140/90, you may need to be on a one-pill-a-day prescription drug such as one of the ACE drugs. Once you start taking a drug, this does not mean that you will be on it for life. When lifestyle changes are made, many patients can decrease and even go off their blood pressure medicine. However, this must be done with close monitoring under the care of a physician.

Reginald Cherry, *Bible Health Secrets* (Lake Mary, FL: Siloam, 2003), 55–58.

PREVENT HARDENING OF THE ARTERIES

by Reginald Cherry, MD

NEXT TO CANCER, hardening of the arteries is one of our most serious concerns. This disease, also known as *atherosclerosis*, is, in fact, the leading cause of heart attacks and strokes, which kill more people in industrialized countries than all forms of cancer combined.[1] Is there anything we can do to stop this process, or is it just "in our genes," an inevitable part of aging? There are multiple things you can do to avoid facing this ravaging problem.

TAKE LOW-DOSE ASPIRIN

Amazingly, half of the people with these plaques, which can clog the arteries, have normal cholesterol levels. It is the initial damage to the artery lining caused by the bad cholesterol that sets the stage for inflammation. This is why one low-dose (81 mg) "enteric-coated" baby aspirin can work wonders in preventing heart disease—it stops the inflammation. (The term "enteric-coated" should appear on the label of the bottle.) Interestingly, regular aspirin (325 mg) may not be as effective as the low-dose aspirin (81 mg).

TAKE ANTIOXIDANTS

Why does the cholesterol damage the arteries? Damage is caused by the oxidation or breakdown of the LDL cholesterol, which enables it to harm the healthy cells lining the arteries. This is why it is so critical to provide antioxidants in the form of vitamin E (800 IU daily), vitamin C (2,000 mg daily), and selenium (200 mcg daily), along with others, such as the carotenes and coenzyme Q_{10}.

LOWER HOMOCYSTEINE LEVELS

Protein is another potential culprit in the development of atherosclerosis. It is not the protein we eat (which is good for us) but the breakdown of certain types of protein (amino acids) into a by-product known as *homocysteine* that can cause problems. High homocysteine levels can damage the arteries, and these levels increase when we lack sufficient amounts of B vitamins in our diet.

To prevent hardening of the arteries, I recommend that you take 600 mcg of folic acid daily, 75 mg of vitamin B_6 daily, and 100 mcg of vitamin B_{12} daily. These amounts of B vitamins keep the homocysteine levels low and thus offer sufficient protection from hardening of the arteries.

Reginald Cherry, *Bible Health Secrets* (Lake Mary, FL: Siloam, 2003), 60–61.

WHY TRADITIONAL CANCER TREATMENTS DON'T ALWAYS WORK

by Francisco Contreras, MD, and Daniel E. Kennedy

THE ENORMOUS FAILURES of conventional therapies do not result from the procedures themselves but from how and why they are used. This is true for two primary reasons.

1. Based on a false premise

First, their application is based on a false premise, that *cancerous tumors are the disease*. In reality, the tumors are but symptoms of the metabolic failures that allowed them to grow.

Thus, removing or destroying tumors is only a half measure. Our failure to restore the organic deficiencies that caused the tumors in the first place is what accounts for most cancer recurrences and deaths.

And yet, success is often still measured by what happens to the tumor, not by what happens to the patient.

2. The criteria with which they are offered

The second reason for failure is the criteria with which chemotherapy, radiation, and surgery are offered. If the cancer is aggressive, the therapy must be aggressive. Maximum tumor mass must be removed or radiated, as much as the patient can tolerate, and chemotherapy will be given.

When it is understood that the disease is much more than the tumor, all of these procedures, in limited cases, can diminish tumor mass. My first criterion for using them is whether I would be willing to be on the receiving end if I was my own patient. My second criterion is whether that procedure is likely to improve the patient's quality of life.

Since the answer to both questions, in most cases, is no, I rarely use them.

Francisco Contreras and Daniel E. Kennedy, *Fighting Cancer 20 Different Ways* (Lake Mary, FL: Siloam, 2005), 45–46.

TWENTY WAYS TO FIGHT CANCER

by Francisco Contreras, MD, and Daniel E. Kennedy

1. Modify your diet to include high-fiber foods such as fruits and vegetables. Consider adopting a Mediterranean diet, or better yet, the Hallelujah Diet![1]
2. Eat plenty of organically grown, pesticide-free tomatoes, garlic, grapes, alfalfa, broccoli, nuts, and artichokes. Aged garlic extract is excellent as well.
3. Drink six to eight 8-ounce servings of freshly extracted vegetable juice every day.
4. Try to keep your intake of dairy products, meats, flour, and refined sugar to a minimum.
5. Cut down on or eliminate cigarettes, excessive alcohol, radiation, and chemically laden, processed junk foods.
6. Exercise as often as possible—walk at least a mile each day, and get plenty of sunshine and fresh air.
7. Consider an eclectic treatment program that includes low-dose chemotherapy, ozone autohemotherapy, ultraviolet blood irradiation, melatonin, and amygdalin.
8. Become familiar with environmental toxins; then do everything possible to avoid them.
9. Inform yourself about cancer, and then take responsibility for your own treatment. Become your own best advocate and your own best hope.
10. Choose to be a victor rather than a victim—find meaning in the crisis. Define your reasons to survive and the purpose of your life.
11. Manage cancer-related stress.
12. Sing, or at least listen to music frequently—don't mind the neighbors!
13. Foster a positive attitude—replace negative thoughts with positive thoughts.
14. Nurture a fighting spirit. Maintain hope and a vision of victory.
15. Talk about cancer issues with loved ones.
16. Stay focused on overcoming cancer, even when you receive a bad report.
17. Laugh frequently.
18. Pray often, and forgive others.
19. Ask God to forgive your sins, even those you are not aware of. Ask Him to heal your spirit and make you whole. Then ask Him to heal your physical infirmities as well.
20. Do all you can that is possible, and let God do the impossible.

Francisco Contreras and Daniel E. Kennedy, *Fighting Cancer 20 Different Ways* (Lake Mary, FL: Siloam, 2005), 4–5.

DIABETES

by Reginald Cherry, MD

D IABETES IS A disease that is reaching epidemic proportions in our society today. According to the Centers for Disease Control, in 2000, approximately 17 million Americans were suffering from the effects of diabetes, but one-third of these—almost 6.5 million people—didn't even know that they had it![1]

The following common symptoms of diabetes should be carefully noted, especially since diabetes consistently goes undiagnosed in people until it has progressed to dangerous phases:

- *Increased thirst.* When the body is facing an unusual amount of glucose in the blood-stream, the kidneys begin to excrete fluid, which increases the need for fluid, hence, increased thirst. Accompanying this symptom is *increased urination*, the kidneys' attempt to flush the bloodstream of the excess glucose.
- *Fatigue.* Because cells are not receiving adequate nutrition due to insulin resistance, most diabetics complain of feeling totally exhausted. Ironically, they have the highest fuel supply in their bloodstream (300–400 glucose levels), but their cells are literally starving to death.
- *Weight loss.* As the body continues to starve, it will begin to feed on its stores of fat and muscle, and the person will begin to lose weight.
- *Blurred vision.* As sugar levels in the blood continue to rise, the blood vessels in the eyes will begin to be adversely affected. If left unchecked, diabetes will lead to partial or complete *blindness*. In fact, diabetes is one of the leading causes of blindness.
- *Neuropathy.* Every nerve in the body is connected to a blood vessel in order to receive life-giving nutrients, which means that every nerve in the body is affected by the high glucose levels of diabetes. As the disease progresses, the person will notice tingling in the extremities as nerves become damaged, a condition known as neuropathy.
- *Kidney failure.* Finally, because the kidneys work so hard to remove excess glucose from the blood, the incidence of renal disease, kidney failure, and dialysis increases dramatically in the diabetic population.

I have listed below the six most important prevention techniques for diabetes.

1. Take daily dosages of chromium, vanadium, and magnesium to make your own body's insulin more effective and decrease your cell's insulin resistance.
2. Take the daily dose of the antioxidants alpha lipoic acid and lycopene—the most powerful antioxidants against the effects of diabetes.
3. Take the essential fatty acids, including fish oil and GLA, to improve glucose tolerance.
4. Cut back on the sugary food that causes glucose levels to spike and then plummet.
5. Exercise. It can dramatically reduce the risk of diabetes.
6. Lose weight. Dropping the pounds will greatly decrease your risk for diabetes.

Reginald Cherry, *Bible Health Secrets* (Lake Mary, FL: Siloam, 2003), 82, 85–86, 91–93.

COLON HEALTH

by Janet Maccaro, PhD, CNC

T HE FIRST STEP in colon health is to cleanse the colon.

There are obvious symptoms of an unhealthy digestive tract: poor digestion, bad breath, lower backache, fatigue, poor skin, body odor, gas, and stomach bloating, to name a few. Internal toxicity has several causes: poor diet with a lack of live foods (fresh fruit and vegetables), lack of proper enzyme activity, constipation, and a lack of water to flush toxins and speed up the digestive and elimination process. Stress also hinders proper digestion, absorption, and elimination.

Overuse of antibiotics has a damaging effect on the intestinal tract as well. Antibiotic therapy removes healthy and unhealthy bacteria in the colon. This causes yeast overgrowth, digestive problems, and elimination problems. Overeating and eating late at night inhibit cleansing and restorative processes and put too much stress on the digestive system.

Dietary considerations

Avoid sugar, animal fats, fried foods, and dairy foods. Drink six to eight glasses of water daily; add fresh lemon to enhance cleansing effect. Add fiber foods to improve transit time, which should be ten to twelve hours. About 40 grams of fiber daily is recommended.

Supplement support for colon health

- Nature's Secret Ultimate Cleanse

After cleansing the colon:

- Magnesium: 400 mg daily
- Bio-K or Kyo-Dophilus to replenish intestinal tract with healthy bowel flora
- Digestive enzyme with each meal
- Milk thistle extract for liver function
- Colon Clenz by Natural Balance, Inc., for occasional bowel sluggishness
- Nature's Secret Ultimate Oil to prevent constipation

Lifestyle choices

Begin a walking program to stimulate circulation. Exercise stimulates the circulatory and lymphatic system. It raises metabolic efficiency and enhances the body's natural cleansing ability. Also, consider colonic irrigations given by a colonic therapist. To relieve stress, you can have a massage.

Janet Maccaro, *Natural Health Remedies* (Lake Mary, FL: Siloam, 2003, 2006), 139–140.

CROHN'S DISEASE

by Janet Maccaro, PhD, CNC

THIS PAINFUL AUTOIMMUNE disease affects over two million Americans today, and the numbers are rising.[1] This is mostly because so many people consistently eat diets that are low in fiber and too high in refined sugar, and they suffer from food allergies, yeast overgrowth, and emotional stress.

Definition

Crohn's disease is a chronic inflammation of the digestive tract, accompanied by painful ulcers that form in one or more sections.

Symptoms

Symptoms include painful ulcers that form in one or more sections of the gastrointestinal tract, diarrhea, abdominal pain, low-grade fever, weight loss, depression, anemia, wheat sensitivity, gas, inflammation, and soreness. Immune system function declines due to malnutrition.

Dietary considerations

Gradually increase your fiber intake until you are eating a substantially high-fiber diet, except during flare-ups of the disease. Drink eight to ten glasses of spring water daily. Consume fresh juices and vegetables daily (grape, carrot, apple, and pineapple are especially therapeutic). Avoid red and fatty meats as well as dairy and fried foods. Eliminate seeds, popcorn, and nuts.

Supplement support for Crohn's disease

- Magnesium: 400–800 mg daily
- Bio-K Liquid Acidophilus during flare-ups, then Kyo-Dophilus capsules
- Glutamine: 500 mg
- Vitamin C
- Royal jelly
- Quercetin
- Kyolic Garlic capsules: six daily
- Green tea
- Flax oil
- Daily green drink
- Peppermint tea sweetened with stevia

Lifestyle choices

- Reduce stress.
- Have regular massages.
- Practice deep breathing.
- Eat early, eat less, but eat often.

Janet Maccaro, *Natural Health Remedies* (Lake Mary, FL: Siloam, 2003, 2006), 142–143.

STEERING CLEAR OF GASTROINTESTINAL DISORDERS

by Reginald Cherry, MD

WHEN YOU INGEST food into your body, digestion begins almost immediately. *Digestion* essentially means the breakdown of food into a form that can be absorbed by the body, and it cannot take place except in the presence of *enzymes*. There are many types of enzymes in the body, but for our purposes, we will examine key enzymes that are crucial to maintain your digestive health. These include the *amylase* enzymes, the *lipase* enzymes, and the *proteases* or *proteolytic* enzymes.

- Amylase enzymes break down carbohydrates.
- Lipase enzymes break down fats.
- Proteolytic enzymes break down proteins.

Through the work of these three types of enzymes, the entire gamut of nutrients available in the four major food groups are available to us. Lactase, an amylase enzyme, is necessary to break down the lactose that is found in milk. Some people do not produce this enzyme and are therefore lactose intolerant, or unable to drink milk without experiencing discomfort such as gas or bloating. Cellulase is another important amylase enzyme; it breaks down various vegetables that we eat.

Although they are produced in smaller amounts in various parts of the digestive tract, these enzymes are primarily secreted by the *pancreas*. The more enzymes the pancreas has to produce, the more it can be subjected to stress and fatigue. Therefore, one of the first steps to take to ensure the health of the digestive system is to supplement these primary enzymes as a part of your daily diet. Two hundred mg each should be taken daily of amylase, cellulose, lactase, lipase, and the protease enzymes.

ENZYME DEFICIENCY

A deficiency in any of these enzymes can result in a host of uncomfortable digestive problems: gas, bloating, diarrhea, or constipation. Without the proper amounts of enzymes necessary for digestion to take place, particles of food will pass through the body, undigested, and create these difficulties. A more serious effect, however, of an enzyme deficiency is fatigue. If problems are occurring at the digestive stage of the process, the food that is eaten is not broken down to a stage where it is absorbable by the body; therefore, the cells will not be receiving the nutrition that they need. Energy sources are quickly depleted, and you feel tired all the time.

One unusual ailment that is in early stages of research is called the *leaky gut syndrome*. This occurs when the proteolytic enzymes (protein digestion) are either not present in sufficient quantities or they are not functioning correctly. Leaky gut syndrome is believed to take place when larger protein molecules that have missed being properly digested migrate to the "gut," or small intestine, and are absorbed there rather than earlier in the digestive tract as God intended. This absorption in an inappropriate area creates an immunological response from the body, and it could be a cause of such immune-related problems as allergies or arthritis.

Reginald Cherry, *Bible Health Secrets* (Lake Mary, FL: Siloam, 2003), 97–99.

TREATING ACID REFLUX

by Reginald Cherry, MD

H ERE ARE FIVE helpful suggestions that have been proven to quench acid reflux or heartburn—without the use of prescription medicine. However, if you are consistently experiencing more than three episodes of acid reflux or heartburn a week, you should see your doctor as soon as possible to help prevent developing scar tissue in your esophagus.

1. Eat large meals early and light meals later.

There is a muscular valve known as a *sphincter* between the esophagus and the stomach. The lining of the stomach is designed to handle a high acid level, but if this acid "refluxes," or backs up, into the esophagus, problems can occur. The cells lining the esophagus are not designed to handle high acid levels. The acid can cause severe damage and even erosions and inflammation in the esophagus that can produce the symptoms of heartburn.

When you eat late in the evening, large amounts of food are in the stomach when you lie down at night, producing pressure on the muscular sphincter. If you are carrying extra pounds, it produces additional pressure on the stomach, which in turn causes more acid to enter the esophagus. The simple habit of eating a light meal early in the evening can dramatically reduce the symptoms of reflux.

2. Raise the head of your bed.

By placing a small block of wood such as a two by four (or even a four-by-four block, in some cases) under the head of the bed, you can elevate the entire bed. This prevents the return of acid into the esophagus and helps contain the acid in the stomach where it belongs. Adding an extra pillow or two under your head can actually make the problem worse because of the angle created between the esophagus and the stomach.

3. Avoid the three "bad guys": peppermint candy, coffee, and chocolate.

There are certain substances that can weaken the tone or strength of the sphincter muscle, allowing acid to reflux. These include coffee, peppermint candy, and chocolate. Isn't it ironic that many times after a meal at a restaurant, we have a cup of coffee, a peppermint candy, or a chocolate mint?

4. Drink more water.

A simple remedy for heartburn that has proven effective is to increase your daily consumption of water. The water tends to wash the acid off the wall of the esophagus.

5. Use antacids with caution.

If you need to use an occasional antacid, remember that the liquid antacids are better than the tablets because they tend to adhere to the esophagus, forming a protective coating. There are over-the-counter medications known as H2 blockers, which include Tagamet and similar medications. These can be used on occasion, but as we get older, the stomach tends to produce less acid, and the chronic use of these medications to neutralize acid can sometimes interfere with digestion.

Reginald Cherry, *Bible Health Secrets* (Lake Mary, FL: Siloam, 2003), 104–106.

two.

IRRITABLE BOWEL SYNDROME

by Reginald Cherry, MD

T HIS UNPLEASANT SYNDROME affects millions of people. It is the number one referral made by family physicians to GI specialists (gastroenterologists).

Irritable bowel syndrome—not to be confused with inflammatory bowel disease, such as ulcerative colitis or Crohn's disease—affects mullions of people. It appears to be a problem with the transmission of nerve impulses affecting the nerve endings to the smooth muscles in the GI tract. We also know that it has been associated with periods of high stress. Symptoms include abdominal bloating and cramping, excessive gas, and either diarrhea or constipation or alternating between the two.

PEPPERMINT OIL

An effective natural treatment for irritable bowel syndrome is enteric-coated peppermint oil. Research has indicated that the oil found in the peppermint plant can relax smooth muscles in the colon. Prescription muscle relaxants (known as *antispasmodics*) can cause numerous side effects, but the peppermint oil found in the plant kingdom has no side effects.[1]

There is one small problem with peppermint oil, however. In the secret #101 I listed peppermint as a major irritant to acid reflux. If you have acid reflux disease as well as irritable bowel syndrome, it is imperative that you take the coated capsule form of the peppermint oil so that the oil will be absorbed in the intestine rather than in the stomach.

Excellent results have been seen with the use of peppermint oil. It tends to stop the excessive spasms in the smooth muscles and helps maintain the muscle tone in the colon. Peppermint oil capsules have been used for several years in Europe for the treatment of irritable bowel syndrome and have been found to be very safe and effective.

Researchers in Britain have recorded a nearly 50 percent reduction in colon spasms after peppermint oil was introduced into the colon. The capsules are available in a standardized, coated form that contains 0.2 ml of peppermint oil. One to two capsules daily between meals were used in the study. Peppermint must be taken properly to avoid the complications associated with acid reflux disease, as I mentioned earlier.[2]

OTHER TREATMENTS FOR IRRITABLE BOWEL SYNDROME

Sometimes a safe prescription medication may be required to relax the smooth muscle. Smooth muscle relaxants that have been proven effective include dicyclomine, cimetropium, mebeverine, and trimebutine. These agents prove to be very effective for relieving the abdominal pain and discomfort of irritable bowel syndrome. At least thirteen out of sixteen studies showed an improvement in symptoms while patients were on these medications.[3]

Other traditional treatments for irritable bowel syndrome include psyllium and wheat bran, although these are not effective and can cause gas in quite a few patients. If peppermint oil capsules do not relieve the symptoms, try adding very small amounts of wheat bran. (An ideal amount would be ¼ cup of Kellogg's All-Bran Bran Buds cereal).

Reginald Cherry, *Bible Health Secrets* (Lake Mary, FL: Siloam, 2003), 108–109.

HEARTBURN AND INDIGESTION

by Don Colbert, MD

A s UNCOMFORTABLE AND embarrassing as they can be, digestive problems are not life-threatening, and the cures are remarkably simple and easy to take. Yes, they can indicate other more serious medical problems. But even the most serious problems usually have treatments that are readily available. Often digestive problems and their accompanying symptoms are related to lifestyle and nutrition. The good news is that you can take positive steps to eliminate this discomfort in your life.

Ideally, if you eat three large meals a day, you should have three bowel movements a day because God designed our bodies to process food at a very consistent pace. Unfortunately, our diets tend to keep our bowel movements from being regular. For instance, high-fat diets will take much longer than necessary to move through our system. Thirty to 35 grams of fiber a day is essential for maintaining a healthy colon. Fiber helps to move food through the colon faster. People with sedentary lifestyles need to increase both their fiber intake and exercise in order to help their digestive processes work more efficiently.

BEGINNING STEPS FOR BEATING DIGESTIVE PROBLEMS

Check which steps you will begin to take right now:

- ❏ Pray, relax, and reduce stress
- ❏ Chew food slowly
- ❏ Focus on God and clear my mind of negative emotions
- ❏ Review how my digestive system works

THE PROBLEM OF DECREASED GASTRIC ACID SECRETION

I believe one of the most common causes of heartburn and indigestion is hypochlorhydria, which is decreased gastric acid secretion or, more simply put, not enough hydrochloric acid. Approximately 50 percent of people over the age of fifty have low stomach acidity.

How often has the pleasure of eating a good meal been ruined for you by painful heartburn? I have wonderful news: you no longer have to endure these problems! It's possible with God's guidance and your own self-control to beat indigestion problems and feel good. Let's explore in greater depth some simple ways you can relieve heartburn through diet, relaxation, exercise, and losing weight.

It all begins with your mental attitude and spiritual outlook. Start by replacing negativity with thanksgiving. Decide to act rather than sit back and suffer. Find a friend who will encourage you in taking the steps mentioned in this chapter. And pray for strength to follow through. Remember, God is not merely a healer. He is your healer. The Bible says, "If you will listen carefully to the voice of the LORD your God and do what is right in his sight, obeying his commands and keeping all his decrees, then I will not make you suffer any of the diseases I sent on the Egyptians; for I am the LORD who heals you" (Exod. 15:26, NLT).

Don Colbert, *The Bible Cure for Heartburn and Indigestion* (Lake Mary, FL: Siloam, 1999).

AUTOIMMUNE DISEASES

by Don Colbert, MD

T HERE ARE MORE than eighty types of autoimmune diseases,[1] with about 50 million Americans are contending with some type of autoimmune disease.[2] You can see that we're in the midst of an epidemic of autoimmune diseases, but why? I believe the reasons usually involve a combination of factors.

First is poor diet. Second is our poor gastrointestinal health. The third factor involves food sensitivities and allergies with which so many Americans suffer. Fourth, and possibly the most significant factor, is the excessive amounts of stress that most Americans are under. Why are women experiencing far more autoimmune diseases than men? In part, it's because of the vital link between these diseases and hormonal imbalances—which is the fifth factor. The sixth reason for this out-of-control epidemic of autoimmune disease is toxic overload. We are laboring under alarming levels of toxicity in this nation. In addition, many individuals' immune systems must also labor against microorganisms, of which they may be completely unaware—the seventh factor. The final is genetics, which you have no control over.

It's easy to see why this is such a mammoth problem in America, and it's growing larger. Nevertheless, autoimmune disease does not have to rob you of the vital health God intended for you to enjoy.

If you are battling an autoimmune disease, the most important thing you can know is that God is on your side, constantly working on your behalf in order to see you well. He desires to see you recover even more than you do. One glimpse of His wonderful love for you would cause you to exclaim as the psalmist did, "This I know, that God is for me" (Ps. 56:9, NAS). God is for you.

The word *auto* is from the Greek word meaning "self." When your immune system is operating normally, it identifies, attacks, and eliminates foreign or invader cells. But when you have an autoimmune disease, the immune system becomes confused, turning the body's attack against itself. Now the immune system targets certain cells, tissues, and organs in your own body.

Sadly, much of today's epidemic of autoimmune disease comes from our poor diets. Instead of eating the vital, living foods that God provided for the healthy maintenance of our bodies, our modern diets are primarily made up of dead foods. Dead foods are grains and vegetables that have been devitalized through processing and storage.

Also, most Americans are overstressed, and many autoimmune diseases follow a very stressful life situation. Many patients with autoimmune disease also have heavy metal toxicity as well as food allergies or sensitivities. My books *The Seven Pillars of Health* and *The Bible Cure for Autoimmune Diseases* shed more light on this subject.

Don Colbert, *The Bible Cure for Autoimmune Diseases* (Lake Mary, FL: Siloam, 2004).

ASTHMA

by Don Colbert, MD

MANY OF THE triggers for asthma are common allergens, pollutants in the home, irritants, recurrent infections, and acid reflux. Common allergens are dust mites, pollen, mold, animal dander, and certain foods. The most common irritants are smoke, fumes, strong scents, and air pollution.

WHAT ACTUALLY TAKES PLACE

When someone is experiencing an asthma attack, this is what occurs:

- The airways become inflamed.
- The airways are constricted.
- The airways have congestion.
- The airways become overly reactive.
- There is dryness in the mouth
- There is tightness in the chest
- The pulse rate increases (unrelated to exercise).
- There is fatigue.
- There are complaints of not feeling well.
- There are feelings of nervousness, anxiety, or irritability.
- There is increased sweating.
- Children become overactive or unusually quiet.

The first line of defense for asthmatics is learning to breathe through their nose. Unfortunately, many asthmatics also have allergies or recurring sinus infections that congest the nasal passages, which is the reason many asthmatics breathe through their mouth.

A SIMPLE BREATHING EXERCISE

Lie flat on your back on the floor with your knees bent. Place a hardcover book on your abdomen so that the binding is touching the bottom of your rib cage. Then breathe in through your nose, and as you are inhaling, try to raise the book as high as you can with your abdominal muscles, at the same time trying to keep your chest flat. Think of your stomach as a balloon that you're filling with air. As you exhale, use the same abdominal muscles to squeeze every bit of air out of your lungs. You should take longer to exhale than to inhale.

As you inhale, try to count to four slowly, and as you exhale, try to count to eight slowly. Practice this exercise slowly so that you take about four to six breaths a minute. It's important that you perform this exercise regularly, preferably on a daily basis for about ten to twenty minutes a day.

Don Colbert, *The Bible Cure for Asthma* (Lake Mary, FL: Siloam, 2004).

SKIN DISORDERS

by Don Colbert, MD

SKIN DISORDERS INCLUDE various forms of acne, psoriasis, and eczema. Approximately six million people in the United States suffer from psoriasis, and about 2 percent of the world's population have psoriasis. Acne affects about 85 percent of all teenagers, and about one-fourth of them will have it so severely that they will be permanently scarred.[1]

Skin disorders attack in a variety of ways, causing painful symptoms for those who suffer them.

Painful psoriasis

Psoriasis is a chronic inflammatory skin disorder that results when skin cells reproduce too rapidly—at a rate approximately one thousand times greater than normal skin. Instead of normal regeneration that takes about a month, psoriasis skin cells regenerate every three or four days. In skin affected with psoriasis, both the epidermis and the dermis are affected by this abnormal cell division.[2]

The epidermis reacts to this abnormal cell reproduction by producing red patches covered with thick, silvery scales. The patches often appear on the backs of the elbows and knees as well as on the scalp, lower back, buttocks, wrists, and ankles.

Addressing issues of acne

Acne is one skin disorder that has made young people miserable for many generations.

Drug treatments that offer relief from symptoms of acne can have harmful side effects that you may choose to avoid. If you suffer from any form of acne, it may relieve you to learn that even the worst cases of acne can be treated by natural methods with very good results.

Enduring eczema

Eczema (also called dermatitis) is an inflammation of the skin that usually results in scaling, flaking, thickening, color changes, and sometimes itching. There are various types of eczema:

- *Atopic dermatitis* is a hereditary form that sometimes becomes apparent in infancy but may occur initially late in life. It usually appears on the face, in the bends of the elbows, and behind the knees; it is marked by itching.
- *Seborrhea* is a form of dermatitis characterized by greasy scales on the scalp as dandruff also affecting the eyebrows, nasolabial folds, and eyelids.
- *Nummular eczema* forms coinlike lesions, most commonly located on the arms, back, buttocks, and legs.
- *Dyshidrotic eczema* is characterized by irritation of the skin of the palms of the hands and soles of the feet. It occurs especially between the fingers and is associated with blisters that burn and itch.
- *Contact dermatitis* is an inflammatory condition of the skin caused from irritants such as detergents, acids, and solvents. Another form of contact dermatitis is allergic contact dermatitis, which is commonly caused by poison ivy, poison oak, poison sumac, and nickel, which is often present in cheap jewelry.

Don Colbert, *The Bible Cure for Skin Disorders* (Lake Mary, FL: Siloam, 2002).

SHINGLES

by Janet Maccaro, PhD, CNC

S HINGLES IS AN acute inflammation of the nerves caused by the *Vericella-Zoster* virus, accompanied by pain and burning over small or large parts of the body.

Symptoms

Fever and chills precede the attack. Then blisters develop around the upper part of the body, after which painful nerves remain irritated for several weeks. Areas affected include hands, neck, face, chest, limbs, and especially the rib area.

Initially, there is an itching or sensitivity in the area of attack, followed by a rash with small raised spots that turn into blisters. These blisters are filled with viral organisms. They are very itchy and extremely painful, often feeling like severe burns. The blisters dry out and leave scabs that eventually fall off, leaving behind scars. Unfortunately, this is not the end of the attack. The pain that lingers can be severe and last for months or even years because it is caused by nerve damage. Shingles that occur on the face or eye area are far more serious because of the possibility of blindness or facial paralysis.

Causes

Shingles is caused by chronic or prolonged periods of stress-compromised immunity, thus allowing the *Vericella-Zoster* virus (which causes chicken pox) to reemerge as shingles. Other triggers include physical stress to the point of exhaustion, lymphoma, Hodgkin's disease, and anticancer drugs.

Dietary considerations

Consider a juicing program for three to five days, followed by eating plenty of fresh vegetables and fruit. Avoid immune-suppressing substances: sugar, caffeine, alcohol, white flour, nicotine, and animal fats. Add fiber to your diet, and drink plenty of water.

Supplement support for shingles

L-lysine: inhibits the spread of the disease	Dr. Janet's Balanced by Nature Glucosamine Cream
Vitamin B_{12}: promotes healing	Reishi, maitake, and shiitake mushrooms: boost immunity
Beta-carotene: enhances immunity	Passionflower: calms the nerves
Vitamin E: promotes healing	Hops: calms the nerves
Echinacea: boosts immunity and has antiviral properties	Valerian root: calms the nerves
Pau d'arco: cleanses the blood and strengthens the liver	Daily green drink

Lifestyle choices

Ice packs can be used to cool and soothe an infected area.	Take long walks in the early morning.
Avoid further stress.	Get plenty of rest.
Listen to peaceful music.	Have weekly or monthly massage therapy.
Practice deep breathing.	Polysporin can help prevent infection.

Janet Maccaro, *Natural Health Remedies* (Lake Mary, FL: Siloam, 2003, 2006), 200–201.

THYROID DISORDER

by Don Colbert, MD

EELING RATHER TIRED lately? Perhaps you've gained weight or just can't seem to lose it no matter how hard you try. Are you cold all the time? Is your skin drier than usual, or have you noticed that you seem extra thirsty or just achy? Maybe you've been kind of down, forgetful, constipated, or unusually irritable. If any of these sound like you, you may be a part of a hidden epidemic: *hypothyroidism or low-thyroid function.*

The main purpose of the thyroid gland is to produce and release two hormones that are vitally important to your body: T3 (or triiodothyronine) and T4 (or thyroxine).

Do You Have Symptoms?

Answer the following questions to determine if you could have symptoms of an underactive thyroid gland:

- Do you have unexplained fatigue?
- Are you weak?
- Are you lethargic?
- Are you experiencing unwanted weight gain?
- Do you have dry skin? Flaky skin?
- Are you experiencing hair loss?
- Are you more irritable lately?
- Are you constipated?
- Are your hands and feet cold?
- Are you depressed?
- Do you have problems concentrating?
- Are you having irregular menstrual cycles?
- Do you forget people's names easily?
- Do you have puffiness and swelling around the eyes, face, feet, or hands?
- Has your voice become hoarse?
- Are you unable to lose weight with proper diet and exercise?
- Do you have a history of miscarriages?
- Have you lost the lateral border of your eyebrows?

In the quiz above, no single question points to a thyroid disorder, but if you answered yes to several of these questions, it is quite possible that you may be suffering from a thyroid imbalance. I strongly recommend that you have your thyroid gland checked by a medical professional who can draw a blood test for TSH and free T4 levels.

The Other Extreme: Hyperthyroidism

What happens if your body gets too much thyroid hormone? You develop the thyroid disease called *hyperthyroidism.* Hyperthyroidism works much the opposite of hypothyroidism. Where hypothyroidism seems to slow down the body's metabolism, hyperthyroidism revs it up. A thyroid on high throttle can cause very distressing symptoms. Take the test below to see if you may be experiencing hyperthyroidism.

- Do you have a rapid or irregular heartbeat?
- Do you feel nervous much of the time?
- Are you more irritable?
- Do your hands shake with tremors?
- Are you always hungry?
- Have you lost weight?
- Do you have a wide-eyed stare?
- Have you experienced more diarrhea?
- Do you have menstrual periods with scant bleeding?
- Are you infertile?
- Do you sweat a lot when others seem to be comfortable?
- Are you intolerant to heat?
- Do you tire quickly?
- Are your muscles weak?
- Are you having trouble sleeping?
- Are you experiencing mood swings?
- Are you experiencing shortness of breath?
- Is your hair fine and straight?
- Is it sometimes difficult to catch your breath?

Because thyroid disorder can hide from even the best medical examiners, no single symptom points to it. But if you answered yes to several of these symptoms, please get examined by your medical doctor or endocrinologist for hyperthyroidism. Remember that your thyroid helps your body to perform many vital functions, so never take a possible problem lightly.

Don Colbert, *The Bible Cure for Thyroid Disorders* (Lake Mary, FL: Siloam, 2004).

CHRONIC FATIGUE

by Don Colbert, MD

THERE IS NO known cure for chronic fatigue syndrome (CFS), also called chronic fatigue, immune dysfunction syndrome (CFIDS). Symptoms include debilitating fatigue that is not improved by bed rest and may be worsened by physical or mental activity, impairment of short-term memory or concentration, sore throat, tender lymph nodes, muscle and joint pain, and headaches. Symptoms must be present for more than six months without any other medical explanation. Individuals with CFS function at a substantially lower level of activity than before onset of the illness, and many continue holding jobs, attending school, or caring for themselves or family members.[1]

COMMON CAUSES OF CHRONIC FATIGUE

- Chronic candida (yeast) infections and other chronic infections often caused by the overuse of antibiotics, food allergies, anemia, low blood sugar, and low thyroid function
- Excessive stress
- Sleep disturbances
- Depression

COMMON SYMPTOMS ASSOCIATED WITH CHRONIC FATIGUE

- Mild fever
- Recurring soar throat
- Painful lymph nodes
- Muscle weakness
- Muscle pain
- Prolonged fatigue after exercise
- Recurrent headaches
- Migratory joint pains
- Neurological or psychological complaints
- Sensitivity to bright light
- Forgetfulness
- Confusion
- Inability to concentrate
- Excessive irritability
- Depression
- Sleep disturbance (either sleeping too much or an inability to sleep)

If you are experiencing symptoms of chronic fatigue, get a complete physical exam by your medical doctor and a thorough evaluation by a nutritional doctor. In addition, chronic fatigue can also be a side effect of certain medications, including antihistamines, blood pressure medications, arthritis medications, antianxiety medications, tranquilizers, and antidepressants.

Don Colbert, *The Bible Cure for Chronic Fatigue and Fibromyalgia* (Lake Mary, FL: Siloam, 2000).

SLEEP DISORDERS

by Don Colbert, MD

IF SLEEP DISORDERS have left you feeling exhausted, depleted, and defeated, rest assured that these things are not God's will for you. You can discover real rest and wonderful refreshing in God. The Bible declared, "Jesus said, 'Come to me, all of you who are weary and carry heavy burdens, and I will give you rest. Take my yoke upon you. Let me teach you, because I am humble and gentle at heart, and you will find rest for your souls. For my yoke is easy to bear, and the burden I give you is light'" (Matt. 11:28–30, NLT).

God never intended for you to push through your days and months feeling increasingly weary. If you are struggling with sleep disorders, there's hope! Sleep disorders fall into two main categories.

- *Dyssomnias* are characterized by problems with either falling asleep or staying asleep, followed by excessive drowsiness during the day. Examples of dyssomnias include insomnia, sleep apnea, narcolepsy, restless legs syndrome, periodic limb movements, hypersomnia, and advanced and delayed sleep phase syndromes.
- *Parasomnias*, on the other hand, are simply abnormalities in behavior that occur during sleep, such as grinding your teeth, night terrors (a frightening activity during sleep), sleepwalking, and sleep talking.

Here are ten tremendous tips you can take to help you sleep.[1] Check the ones you plan to use.

- ❏ Stay away from the big four: caffeine, stress, alcohol, and smoking.
- ❏ Leave time in your schedule for sleep.
- ❏ Set a regular sleep schedule, seven days a week. Get up at the same time every day and go to sleep at the same time each night.
- ❏ Relax before going to bed. Release your stress, and read the Bible or a good book.
- ❏ Use your bedroom for sleep only—no work, study, or eating. If the TV causes insomnia, get it out of the bedroom.
- ❏ Prepare a comfortable sleep environment with a comfortable pillow, mattress, and room temperature. Remove all noise and light from the bedroom.
- ❏ Start a regular exercise program, but don't exercise for three to four hours before bedtime.
- ❏ Observe good eating habits. Don't go to bed hungry, and don't drink excessive fluids before bed.
- ❏ Get up if you can't sleep after twenty to thirty minutes, and go to another room to relax. Return to bed when you are tired.
- ❏ Determine to make sleep a priority and regular part of your life.

Don Colbert, *The Bible Cure for Sleep Disorders* (Lake Mary, FL: Siloam, 2001).

HEPATITIS

by Don Colbert, MD

H EPATITIS CAN BE caused by anything that inflames or damages the liver; however, hepatitis C is caused by a virus. There are several strains of hepatitis, including hepatitis A, B, and C.

Hepatitis A is called "infectious hepatitis" because the virus spreads through contaminated food and water. This type of hepatitis is very common in third world countries. Most of those who contract it recover their health. Victims of hepatitis A do not develop chronic infections.

Hepatitis B is is called "serum hepatitis" because it is transmitted to others through blood and other body fluids. Most adults—95 percent—recover from hepatitis B, though a small percentage develops a chronic infection. Of the nearly two hundred thousand people who are infected by hepatitis B each year, only about ten thousand develop a chronic hepatitis B infection.

Hepatitis C is the most common chronic infection transmitted by the blood in the United States. However, unlike hepatitis B, of those who contract hepatitis C, only 15 percent actually recover. Worldwide, nearly 150 million individuals suffer with chronic hepatitis C.

Approximately 10,000 Americans die each year from chronic hepatitis C. Projections show that mortality rates associated with hepatitis C will triple by the year 2015. According to the Centers for Disease Control, between 28,000 and 180,000 people are infected with hepatitis C each year. It is actually responsible for most liver transplants in the United States. Once infected with the hepatitis C virus, about 20 percent of people go on to develop cirrhosis of the liver in about twenty years.

Hepatitis C is called the silent epidemic because so many people have the disease but are completely unaware of it. In fact, many times severe symptoms do not occur until the last stages of the disease—stages that may take decades to develop. What that means is a person can be walking around with advancing liver disease and never feel it or know it.

SYMPTOMS OF HEPATITIS C

- Flu-like symptoms with fever, chills, sweats, severe fatigue, and nausea
- Pain in the joints
- Tenderness over the liver
- Diarrhea, a spastic colon, indigestion, and abdominal bloating
- Mood swings, confusion, short-term memory loss, depression, restless sleep, and irritability
- Difficulty digesting fatty foods or drinking alcohol
- Fluid retention in the legs and feet
- Headaches and dizziness

The progression of hepatitis C will continue for many years in the body, with or without major recognizable symptoms. Eventually, the effects of the virus will usually lead to more advanced stages of liver disease, such as chronic hepatitis C, cirrhosis of the liver, liver cancer, and fibrosis.

CONTRACTING HEPATITIS C

Blood tainted with the hepatitis C virus must gain entry into the bloodstream through a cut or prick, or from blood splashing onto mucous membranes such as the eyes, nasal passages, or the mouth. It can also gain entry into the bloodstream through the skin from an open sore. Therefore, exposure to other people's blood can cause a person to contract or spread this disease. Here are ways that one can be exposed to infected blood:

- Blood transfusions
- IV drug use, especially from injecting drugs with dirty needles
- Getting a tattoo if the needles, razor, ink, or any other tattooing equipment used during the procedure is not sterile
- Having multiple sexual partners
- Working in the health-care industry—doctors, nurses, firefighters, EMTs, police officers, lab technicians
- Receiving invasive procedures or surgery in third world countries
- Being born to a woman who is positive for hepatitis C

HELP FOR HEPATITIS C CARRIERS

- Avoid alcohol.
- Don't take drugs.
- Shun environmental chemicals.
- Lighten your liver's load by eating organic fruits and vegetables, eating free-range meats, and avoiding fatty foods, all refined vegetable oils, peanuts, dairy products, foods high in sugar, processed foods, and sugar substitutes.
- Eat protein.
- Decrease coffee and tea.
- Get a really good multivitamin, take antioxidants such as vitamin C and alpha-lipoic acid, and supplement amino acids such as N-acetyl cysteine and SAM-e. Take extra selenium.
- Add these healing herbs to your regimen: milk thistle, schizandra chinenis, reishi mushrooms, Chinese bupleurum, burdock root, picrorhiza, dandelion root, and aloe vera.

The most important supplements I have found for hepatitis C are alpha-lipoic acid, milk thistle, selenium, and SAM-e.

Don Colbert, *The Bible Cure for Hepatitis and Hepatitis C* (Lake Mary, FL: Siloam, 2002).

ANDROPAUSE (MALE MENOPAUSE)
by Janet Maccaro, PhD, CNC

FORMALLY KNOWN AS the "male midlife crisis," *andropause* clearly is a time where many men feel that they have lost their vitality, strength, and youth as their muscle mass, energy, and sexual performance decline. If you are in andropause, natural remedies can be an effective way to reenergize every area of your life. Get a complete medical checkup with all of the appropriate health screenings, and use the following recommendations to keep you healthy as you embark on the second half of your journey of life.

Definition
Andropause occurs around that age of forty when testosterone levels begin to decline. These levels continue to fall about 10 percent each decade thereafter.[1]

Symptoms
Symptoms of andropause include fatigue, slow head hair growth, increase in ear hair, loss of muscle mass, frequent urination, postural changes, weight gain around the middle, low sex drive, and depression.

Dietary considerations
Limit red meats, fried foods, full-fat dairy foods, caffeine, and sugar. Brewer's yeast, seeds, nuts, and oysters are good food sources for sexual health.

Supplement support for andropause

- Tribulus terrestris
- For impotence: ginkgo biloba liquid extract three times daily
- For prostate health: saw palmetto and pygeum zinc. Limit or eliminate alcohol (beer especially elevates DHT levels).
- To increase muscle mass: whey protein shake in the morning; L-glutamine stimulates your own growth hormones.
- A daily "green drink," like Kyo-Green

Lifestyle choices
Exercise is a vital part of male sexuality, improving frequency, satisfaction, and performance.

Stress management is vital for sexual health. Stress zaps your adrenal glands. Healthy adrenals are needed at andropause to prevent fatigue and burnout. Adrenal exhaustion in men is linked to depression and anxiety attacks. Limit coffee, and make an effort to get enough hours of sleep each night. Watch your sugar intake. Adrenal support recommendations include B complex, adrenal glandular formula, royal jelly, and pantothenic acid.

Janet Maccaro, *Natural Health Remedies* (Lake Mary, FL: Siloam, 2003, 2006), 102–104.

PROSTATE DISEASE

by Reginald Cherry, MD

MOST MEN SUFFER the *plague* of prostate enlargement as they grow older. I call it a plague because the symptoms it causes bring such aggravation and misery, and the treatments offered by traditional medicine are just as unpleasant—at best. While it is a "natural" phenomenon for the prostate to enlarge with age, because the urethra runs directly through the middle of the prostate, any enlargement causes problems with urination—therein lies the misery. Doctors call this simple enlargement *benign prostatic hyperplasia*, or BPH, which indicates that the cells within the prostate have swollen. Four primary symptoms begin to occur in men who are developing an enlarged prostate gland—all of them unwelcome! Unfortunately, enlargement of the prostate is extremely common in men. Six out of ten men over the age of sixty develop prostate problems. By age seventy, 80 percent of men are displaying symptoms.[1]

SYMPTOMS OF PROSTATE ENLARGEMENT

The first thing that a man might notice is that it begins to take him longer to empty his bladder; his urination is slowing down. This indicates that the swelling prostate is pressing against the urethra and impeding the flow of urine. Second, it becomes harder to cut off the urinary stream, and this causes a dribbling problem that many men start to notice. Third, it becomes harder to start urinating in the first place, and finally, a man finds himself getting up in the night more and more frequently to use the bathroom. I have had patients who literally get up every thirty to forty-five minutes all through the night, every night, to go to the bathroom.

These symptoms can be very frustrating! Not only is it an embarrassing situation for a man, but add to that the fact that he begins to lose sleep, and you also have a cause for other health problems due to the stress and sleep deprivation he experiences regularly.

SEEK EARLY TREATMENT

God's natural provision is available, but it's up to us to begin to walk in the pathway to healing that He has for us. Pray about the problem, ask God what He would have you do, and then obey His instruction. There is no reason to continue suffering in misery. Begin today to find your pathway to healing of prostate problems.

Reginald Cherry, *Bible Health Secrets* (Lake Mary, FL: Siloam, 2003), 150–151, 154.

BLADDER INFECTION

by Janet Maccaro, PhD, CNC

M ANY WOMEN SUFFER at least once a year from the infection. There are several causes, including staph, strep, *E. coli* bacterium, overuse of antibiotics, menopausal tissue changes, lack of fluids, poor elimination, and stress. But most often, the *E. coli* bacterium that travels up the urethra is the culprit. If the infection is not addressed, the kidneys can be infected as well, making it a much more serious condition that can even lead to kidney failure. It is essential to begin attacking the infection at the first sign of infection.

Definition

Bladder infection is an inflammation of the bladder usually associated with *E. coli* bacterium.

Symptoms

Symptoms include painful, frequent, and urgent urination with pain in the lower back and abdominal area, chills, and fever as the body tries to fight the infection. The urine is usually cloudy with a strong smell and, occasionally, with traces of blood. Symptoms are uncomfortable and life disrupting.

Dietary considerations

During the acute stage, take 2 tablespoons of apple cider vinegar and honey in water in the morning.

To alkalize your system, changing your body's pH, eat watermelon and drink Kyo-Green (a green drink), celery juice, and cucumber juice. Avoid chocolate, spinach, sugar, dairy, and red meat, which acidify the system. Drink eight to ten glasses of purified water and diluted fruit juice (especially unsweetened cranberry) daily to flush your system. Eat a yeast-free diet.

Supplement support for bladder infection

- Uva ursi capsules
- Vitamin C
- Acidophilus liquid
- Goldenseal-echinacea extract
- Cranberry capsules
- Grapefruit extract capsules

Lifestyle choices

- Limit the use of a diaphragm.
- Urinate as soon as possible after intercourse.
- Drink a glass of water with 1 teaspoon of baking soda added.
- Place a warm castor oil pack on the abdomen.
- Place a ginger pack on the kidneys.

Janet Maccaro, *Natural Health Remedies* (Lake Mary, FL: Siloam, 2003, 2006), 114–115.

GALLBLADDER DISEASE/GALLSTONES

by Janet Maccaro, PhD, CNC

THE GALLBLADDER HELPS digest fats by producing bile. If the gallbladder bile fluids become saturated with cholesterol, solid crystals form and eventually become gallstones. The key plan of attack is to increase bile solubility to reduce cholesterol levels. In addition, bile flow needs to be increase to aid the gallbladder in expelling small stones.

Definition

Gallbladder disease is an inflammation of the gallbladder caused by saturated bile known as gallstones.

Symptoms

Symptoms include pain in the upper right abdomen during an attack, nausea, cold sweats, possible fever, belching, anxiety, bloating, headache, and anger. The pain becomes more intense as the stones enlarge.

Causes

Causes include chronic indigestion of excessive refined sugar and dairy products, too many fried and fatty foods, food allergies, birth control pills and estrogen replacement therapy (ERT), which cause an increase in cholesterol production, and a sedentary lifestyle.

Dietary considerations

Eat smaller meals that are primarily vegetarian. Avoid red meat, dairy, and eggs because they are high in saturated fats. Each morning take 1 tablespoon of honey and 2 tablespoons of apple cider vinegar in a glass of water. Drink six to eight glasses of water daily, and add lemon to each glass of water that you drink.

Supplement support for gallbladder disease

- Milk thistle extract: for liver function
- Turmeric (curcumin): for inflammation
- B complex
- Chromium picolinate: 200 mcg daily (for weight over 150 pounds, 400 mcg daily)
- Choline and inositol: to regulate cholesterol levels
- Phosphatidylcholine: to regulate cholesterol levels
- Ester C: 3,000 mg daily
- Fiber supplement
- Taurine: keeps bile thinned
- Chamomile tea
- Acidophilus capsules (Kyo-Dophilus)

Lifestyle choices

- Place a warm castor oil pack on the abdomen before bed.
- Start to exercise. Walking every night after dinner is wonderful for digestion and helps to reduce body fat.

Janet Maccaro, *Natural Health Remedies* (Lake Mary, FL: Siloam, 2003, 2006), 165–166.

KIDNEY PROBLEMS

by Janet Maccaro, PhD, CNC

KIDNEY PROBLEMS, WHICH can be prevented through improved diet along with herb and supplement therapy, include inflammation and/or infection of the kidney(s), sometimes accompanied by kidney stones. Symptoms include painful frequent urination, chronic lower back pain, fever, fatigue, chills, and fluid retention. Kidney problems are usually caused by excess sugar, red meat, carbonated drinks, and caffeine in the diet; diabetes; allergies; heavy metal poisoning; excess aluminum; EFA deficiency; overuse of prescription drugs; B-vitamin and magnesium deficiency; and overuse of aspirin, salt, and diuretics.

Supplement support for kidney problems

To reduce kidney inflammation:

- Quercetin: 1,000 mg daily
- Bromelain: 1,500 mg daily
- B complex with vitamin B_6
- Magnesium: 800 mg daily
- Flax oil
- Choline/inositol capsules daily

To help reverse kidney damage:

- Gingko biloba
- Enzymedica Purify capsules
- Spirulina capsule: one daily

For infection:

- Cranberry capsules as directed on the bottle
- Biotic Silver
- Echinacea extract as directed on the bottle

Lifestyle choices

- Avoid NSAIDs (Advil, Motrin, Aleve, etc.), which have been associated with impaired kidney function.
- Avoid smoking and secondhand smoke.
- Take a brisk walk every day.
- Apply castor oil packs to kidney area, alternating with ginger packs to stimulate circulation and flow.
- Do not use antacids (Tums, etc.) for indigestion because they may increase the risk of kidney stones.

Janet Maccaro, *Natural Health Remedies* (Lake Mary, FL: Siloam, 2003, 2006), 188–189.

HEMORRHOIDS

by Janet Maccaro, PhD, CNC

T HIS CONDITION MAY not find its way into your daily conversation, but it certainly gets a lot of attention these days because of the increase in people who suffer from it. Again, it is caused by poor diets filled with low fiber and refined foods. In addition, sitting all day in front of computer screens, not drinking enough water, pregnancy, system toxicity, painkillers, obesity, and allergies contribute to this painful condition.

Definition

Hemorrhoids are clusters of swollen veins in the lining of the anus, usually accompanied by constipation.

Symptoms

Symptoms include itching and rectal bleeding associated with bowel movements, inflammation, and constipation.

Dietary considerations

Eat fiber foods daily, such as bran, vegetables, dried fruit, and cherries. Eat small meals to take stress off of the bowel. Take 1 tablespoon of olive or flaxseed oil before each meal. And drink eight to ten glasses of water daily. Avoid caffeine, sugar, and low-fiber, refined foods.

Supplement support for hemorrhoids

- Enzymatic therapy: Hemotome
- Vitamin E: 400 IU
- Ester C: 3,000 mg daily
- Bioforce Hemorrhoid Relief
- Milk thistle extract
- Colon Clenz to alleviate constipation as needed
- Bromelain
- Vitamin K if bleeding is present
- Magnesium gel caps: 400 mg at bedtime as a stool softener and muscle relaxant
- Carlson's ACES
- A daily green drink

Lifestyle choices

- Take a brisk thirty-minute walk daily to promote healthy circulation.
- If you are overweight, try to lose weight.
- Take a warm sitz bath.
- Use ice packs and witch hazel to help cool the pain and inflammation until improvement comes from natural remedies.

Janet Maccaro, *Natural Health Remedies* (Lake Mary, FL: Siloam, 2003, 2006), 175–176.

LIVER PROBLEMS

by Janet Maccaro, PhD, CNC

A HEALTHY LIVER IS truly vital to a healthy, robust life. This is because the health and vitality of every body system depends on the vitality of your liver. Common causes of liver dysfunction include consuming too much alcohol or drugs, sugar, refined foods, preservatives, and animal protein. It is triggered as well by low-fiber diets, exposure to toxic chemicals and pollutants, stress, candida, and chronic sinus infection.

Fortunately, the liver has amazing regenerative powers. It will take six months to a year to regenerate the liver and improve its function.

Definition

Liver problems consist of inflammation and/or infection of the liver.

Symptoms

Symptoms include poor digestion, tiredness, weight gain, sluggish system, depression, food and chemical sensitivities, constipation, nausea, dizziness, jaundiced skin, skin itching, and congestion.

Supplement support for liver problems

- Milk thistle seed liquid extract
- Dandelion root extract
- Artichoke capsules
- Reishi or maitake mushroom extract
- Royal jelly
- Germanium: 150 mg
- Bio-K or other acidophilus liquid cultures
- Antioxidants are key, especially coenzyme Q_{10}: 100 mg daily; beta-carotene: 10,000 IU daily; and vitamin C (Ester C): 3,000 mg daily.
- Keep bowel function optimal: two to three bowel movements daily.

NATURAL PROTOCOL FOR LIVER SUPPORT

- Exercise daily. Your liver is dependent on high-quality oxygen coming into the lungs.
- Drink eight to ten glasses of pure water with lemon each day.
- Keep fats low in your diet.
- Detoxify your body.
- Avoid acid-forming foods (red meat, caffeine, alcohol, dairy products, and fried foods).
- Increase potassium-rich foods like seafood and dried fruits.
- Increase chlorophyll-rich foods like leafy greens, and have a green drink daily (Kyo-Green from Wakunaga).
- Increase sulfur-rich foods like eggs, garlic, and onions.

Janet Maccaro, *Natural Health Remedies* (Lake Mary, FL: Siloam, 2003, 2006), 189–190.

DENTAL PROBLEMS

by Janet Maccaro, PhD, CNC

TEN MILLION PEOPLE suffer from TMJ (temporomandibular joint syndrome).[1] About 90 percent of all Americans have some form of gum disease or tooth decay, including half of the population over the age of thirty-five.[2] A toothache can cause the worst kind of pain. The best offense is defense when it comes to your dental hygiene.

Proper oral hygiene is essential, which includes proper brushing and flossing. I recommend using HydroFloss and the Dental Herb Company's natural herbal mouth rinse.

Lowered immunity seems to play a part in the development of periodontal disease. Unfortunately, many children are showing signs of gum disease. Stress management and immune enhancement are imperative in the fight against this progressive disorder. Periodontal disease often coexists with cardiovascular problems.

Questions have been raised about the safety of mercury amalgam fillings. Many people are, in fact, sensitive to mercury fillings. However, removal can stir up vapor, making your sensitivity worse. After removal, a detoxification program is essential to cleanse the mercury from your bloodstream. Work with your dentist gradually as you replace your mercury fillings with composite (white) or porcelain inlays.

Definition

Dental problems include toothaches, teeth grinding, decay, TMJ, and periodontal disease.

Symptoms

In all dental difficulties, the two main symptoms are pain and sensitivity.

Dietary considerations

Eat fresh fruits and vegetables to clean teeth. Fill your diet with foods such as apples, broccoli, cauliflower, celery, carrots, peppers, nuts, and seeds. Eat plenty of healthy salads. Drink green tea to help prevent plaque formation. Use stevia to sweeten, as it is also antibacterial. Enjoy strawberry smoothies; strawberries also help prevent the formation of plaque.

Avoid or reduce sugars, fats, dairy products, and candy to minimize the film on teeth that contributes to tooth decay.

Lifestyle choices

- Have regular dental checkups!
- Brush your teeth twice daily (two minutes each time).
- Use natural toothpaste, such as Tom's of Maine or from Dental Herb Company.
- Use Natural Tooth and Gum Tonic from Dental Herb Company.

NOTE: If you suspect mercury toxicity, have a hair analysis performed since mercury does not show up in urine or blood samples.

Janet Maccaro, *Natural Health Remedies* (Lake Mary, FL: Siloam, 2003, 2006), 146–148.

HEARING LOSS

by Janet Maccaro, PhD, CNC

HEARING LOSS IS defined as the loss of ability to perceive sounds as compared with what would be considered normal due to tinnitus, ear malfunction, and excess earwax. Causes of hearing loss include allergies, sinus inflammation, chronic bronchial mastoid inflammation, arteriosclerosis, excess earwax, poor circulation, high blood pressure, metabolic imbalance, low immunity, autoimmune disease, hypoglycemia, and a diet that consists of too many mucus-forming foods.

Dietary considerations

Eat whole grains, fresh fruit, vegetables, and vegetable proteins. Drink six to eight glasses of water daily with fresh lemon for added benefit. Eliminate or limit intake of chocolate, caffeine, and alcohol. And reduce or avoid sugars, salt, and dairy foods.

Supplement support for hearing loss

- Beta-carotene: 150,000 IU daily
- Ester C: 3,000 mg daily
- PCOs from grapeseed or pinebark: 100 mg three times daily
- Coenzyme Q_{10}: 30 mg daily
- Ginkgo biloba: 60 mg daily
- Nature's Secret Ultimate Oil
- Echinacea extract drops to fight infection
- Goldenseal: use only one week at a time to fight infection
- Vitamin B_{12}: 2,500 mcg with folic acid
- Cayenne-ginger capsules for improved circulation
- Magnesium: 800 mg
- Glutamine: 1,000 mg
- Multivitamin/mineral formula
- A daily green drink

Especially for ringing in the ears, take mullein, hyssop, eucalyptus, ephedra, black cohosh, and licorice extract. Also limit aspirin use.

Lifestyle choices

For earwax buildup, make a solution of vinegar, warm water, and three drops of hydrogen peroxide. Drop into ear with a dropper. Wait one minute, then drain. Do this daily until you get relief.

For ear infection, place two to four drops of warm liquid Kyolic Garlic into the ear canal. Eliminate wheat and dairy because they are common food allergy triggers. You should notice a difference in two weeks.

If hearing loss becomes worse or does not improve, a professional evaluation is recommended.

Janet Maccaro, *Natural Health Remedies* (Lake Mary, FL: Siloam, 2003, 2006), 169–171.

VISION PROBLEMS

by Reginald Cherry, MD

D O YOU WEAR glasses or have eye problems? Are you concerned your vision isn't as sharp as it used to be? Your eyes are a delicate and sensitive part of your body, and aging, pollution, and sun exposure can weaken or damage them.

The primary vision problems that people have as they age include cataracts, macular degeneration, glaucoma, and retinopathy (damage caused to the blood vessels of the eyes that is often related to diabetes).

ESSENTIAL NUTRIENTS TO PROTECT YOUR EYESIGHT

NUTRIENT	EFFECT	DAILY DOSAGE
Alpha lipoic acid	Antioxidant that regenerates vitamin C, vitamin E, and glutathione—three powerful antioxidants that help defend the lens, macula, and other eye tissues from free radicals	100 mg
Bilberry	A natural source of anthocyanidins and flavonoids, both of which are powerful antioxidants that help reduce oxidative stress on that eyes	40 mg
Eyebright	Herb used to promote proper eye function and to ease oversensitivity to light	10 mg
L-glutathione	Antioxidant that helps defend the lens, macula, and other eye tissues from free radicals	50 mg
Lutein/zeaxanthin	The most biologically active carotenoids, especially important for promoting macular health	6 mg
Quercetin	Natural antioxidant flavonoid that helps protect the eyes from sun damage	50 mg
Taurine	Amono acid that has been shown to reduce oxidative damage to your eyes caused by sunlight, while simulating your body's ability to remove waste by-products that accumulate in the retina	100 mg
Vitamin C	Essential vitamin and antioxidant that neutralizes free radicals in the lens, macula, and other eye tissues	300–500 mg

The biblical record of the death of Moses tells us something unusual about his health. It records for us the fact that Moses was 120 years old when he died and that his "eye was not dim, nor his natural force abated" (Deut. 34:7, KJV). The Living Bible paraphrase of this verse says, "His eyesight was perfect and he was as strong as a young man." Even in old age, Moses did not experience cataracts, macular degeneration, or other vision problems that most of us experience as we get older. Thank God that we don't have to be like everybody else! He has a better way for His children.

Reginald Cherry, *Bible Health Secrets* (Lake Mary, FL: Siloam, 2003), 142, 144–147.

PAIN RELIEF

PAIN

by Janet Maccaro, PhD, CNC

P AIN SERVES TO signal us to attend to its underlying cause. While painkillers allow you to ignore the pain temporarily so you can work, live, and function better, they do nothing to address the cause of the pain. In addition, pain relievers can be addictive or damaging to the stomach lining as well as the liver and kidneys. There are natural methods to overcome pain in the body. They work at a very deep level in the body, relaxing, soothing, and calming the area in pain. The following recommendations have been proven to aid in the relief of many different pain syndromes.

Dietary considerations

Eat a vegetarian diet, low in fats and high in minerals. Avoid caffeine, sugar, and salty foods that create an acidic system. Also, have a green drink each day, such as Kyo-Green by Wakunaga.

Supplements to support pain relief

Herbal pain relievers:

- White willow bark: anti-inflammatory and analgesic
- Kava: relieves stress from chronic pain or injury
- Valerian: a sedative that will help you relax and sleep

Other natural painkillers:

- DLPA: 1,000 mg daily
- Turmeric
- GABA: 750 mg daily
- Glucosamine capsules and Dr. Janet's Balanced by Nature Glucosamine Cream

Enzymes to reduce inflammation:

- Enzymedica's Purify
- Bromelain
- Quercetin
- MSM
- Boswellia

Lifestyle choices

- Chiropractic adjustments
- Massage therapy
- Therapeutic baths
- Magnet therapy

Janet Maccaro, *Natural Health Remedies* (Lake Mary, FL: Siloam, 2003, 2006), 194–195.

BACK PAIN

by Don Colbert, MD

BACK PAIN IS classified by the length of time it has been present. *Acute* back pain lasts up to six weeks. *Subacute* back pain usually lasts from six weeks to three months. And back pain classified as *chronic* lasts more than three months. Here are some common causes for back pain.

- Herniated disk
- Trauma to the spine
- Strains and sprains
- Osteoarthritis
- Slipping vertebrae
- Compression fractures
- Spinal stenosis
- Piriformis syndrome
- Scoliosis
- Rheumatoid/psoriatic arthritis
- Bone tumors or cancer
- Metastatic cancer
- Infection.

PREVENTING BACK PAIN

- Exercise to lose excess weight.
- Exercise to increase flexibility in your back.
- Exercise to reduce stress and release tightness in back muscles.
- Supplement a healthy diet with glucosamine sulfate, bromelain, MSM, and a good multivitamin/mineral.
- Drink plenty of pure, clean, filtered water.
- Practice relaxation techniques.
- Consider seeing a chiropractor or massage therapist.
- Let go of anger, unforgiveness, bitterness, and other toxic emotions.
- Go to God for total healing—mind, body, and spirit.

Don Colbert, *The Bible Cure for Back Pain* (Lake Mary, FL: Siloam, 2002).

WHICH KIND OF ARTHRITIS ARE YOU OVERCOMING?

by Don Colbert, MD

While there are many different forms of arthritis, I will discuss two of the main forms—osteoarthritis and rheumatoid arthritis.

RHEUMATOID ARTHRITIS	OSTEOARTHRITIS
Is an autoimmune disease that often afflicts those from ages twenty-five to fifty	Caused by the wear and tear of cartilage
Usually occurs in younger adults, but it can attack children, even infants	Usually affects people after age forty
Usually affects joints on both sides of the body (e.g., both knees)	Affects isolated joints, or joints on only one side of the body at first
Causes redness, warmth, and swelling of many joints; attacks many joints, often the small joints of the hands, feet, ankles, knees, and elbows	Causes discomfort in the joints but does not usually cause swelling; particularly affects the weight-bearing joints like the hips and knees
Causes major fatigue of your whole body	Does not usually cause fatigue
Causes prolonged morning stiffness	Causes brief morning stiffness

DO YOU HAVE OSTEOARTHRITIS?

Osteoarthritis is by far the most common form of arthritis and is characterized by joint pain. The joint pain is due to a gradual loss of cartilage and degeneration of the joint. Over forty million Americans suffer from osteoarthritis. Osteoarthritis primarily affects the larger weight-bearing joints. Approximately 80 percent of Americans over the age of fifty suffer from arthritis. There are two main forms of osteoarthritis, primary and secondary.

Primary osteoarthritis usually begins after the age of forty-five, affecting the fingers, neck, lower back, knees, and hips. While the cause is unknown, we do know that obese individuals tend to develop it more commonly. As you gain weight, the pressure on the weight-bearing joints such as the hips and knees increases dramatically. When an obese patient runs or jumps, the pressure on the joints can be as much as ten times a person's body weight. In other words, if a 250-pound man jumped down off of a ladder, the pressure on his hips and knees could be as much as a ton. Is there any wonder why patients who are obese are becoming crippled with osteoarthritis?

Secondary osteoarthritis is simply due to trauma. I commonly see ex-football players in my practice who are crippled with osteoarthritis, especially in the fingers and the knees due to repeated trauma to these joints. Weightlifters commonly get arthritis in their shoulders and knees due to repetitive trauma to these joints. Tennis players commonly get arthritis in their dominant shoulder, whereas golfers commonly get arthritis in their lower back. Continually moving these joints in the same way causes this arthritis, which can eventually lead to chronic trauma and then to degeneration of the joint.

DO YOU HAVE RHEUMATOID ARTHRITIS?

Rheumatoid arthritis is different from osteoarthritis. It affects approximately ten million Americans, striking women three times more often than men. Rheumatoid arthritis is an autoimmune disease; the body is actually attacking itself. It affects not only the joints but also the entire body due to chronic inflammation. The joints affected are usually swollen, tender, warm to touch, and quite stiff.

Don Colbert, *The Bible Cure for Arthritis* (Lake Mary, FL: Siloam, 1999).

NUTRITIONAL ANSWERS FOR ARTHRITIS AND JOINT PROBLEMS

by Reginald Cherry, MD

SOME OF THESE nutritional answers provide more than just relief from the symptoms of arthritis; they can actually *reverse* cartilage damage, restoring health to damaged cartilage caused by the disease. I encourage you to become acquainted with the following natural resources.

Curcuma

Curcuma is a substance that comes from turmeric, a plant root commonly found in curry powder. It controls joint pain and swelling. Curcuma does not create the same kidney problems that common medications such as Celebrex and Vioxx do. I recommend 100 mg daily.

Tart cherries

The kind of cherries that creates benefits for the joints and cartilage are the tart cherries—the kind in cherry pies. Cherries have been used for centuries to alleviate arthritic pain and joint swelling. I recommend 100 mg a day of tart cherry fruit powder.

Holy basil

Holy basil is another ingredient that contains much the same properties as curcuma and tart cherries. It relieves painful, swollen joints. To relieve pain and reduce inflammation, take 150 mg a day.

Boswellia (frankincense)

Boswellia comes from a plant that contains the active chemical boswellic acid, now proven to be a potent anti-inflammatory substance. If you are suffering from arthritis, you understand that mornings are often the worst time of day for joint stiffness; as the day begins and you start to move around, the joint stiffness decreases. Boswellia has been shown to cause that morning stiffness to virtually disappear! Two hundred mg a day is recommended.

Sea cucumber

A sea cucumber is not a member of the plant kingdom but a marine animal, an underwater creature that feeds on plankton in every sea on Earth. They collect certain compounds from plankton that have anti-inflammatory properties. Sea cucumber may be taken at a dose of 100 mg per day.

Glucosamine and chondroitin

When glucosamine and chondroitin are combined (along with the other natural substances that we discussed), relief can begin to occur within a matter of days. Glucosamine works to rebuild the cartilage itself, and chondroitin serves to attract the necessary water to return to the cartilage, inflating like a sponge and building the cushion back up within the joint. Glucosamine should be taken at a dose of 1,500 mg a day, and chondroitin at a dose of 100 mg a day.

Bromelain

Within the stocky portion of the pineapple, the part that most of us choose not to eat, lies a compound called *bromelain*. It too acts as an anti-inflammatory, decreasing the production of the chemicals in the body that cause swelling. Fifty mg a day is a sufficient dosage.

Reginald Cherry, *Bible Health Secrets* (Lake Mary, FL: Siloam, 2003), 114–117.

FIBROMYALGIA

by Don Colbert, MD

Fibromyalgia shares some of the same symptoms and remedies as chronic fatigue syndrome, but it has some additional factors as well. Fibromyalgia is actually a rheumatic type of disorder characterized by diffuse musculo-skeletal pain with trigger points, or tender points throughout the body, sleep disturbances, and fatigue. Common associated symptoms include depression, irritable bowel, irritability, headaches, dizziness, decreased memory, temporal mandibular joint symptoms, and anxiety.

If you are experiencing this condition, your fatigue is accompanied by extremely tender muscles, which usually occur in specific areas of the body. Nine different trigger points are commonly associated with fibromyalgia. These include the muscles in the neck, in the upper back, in the mid-back, at the base of the skull, in the buttocks, in the upper portion of the thigh, just above the lateral elbow, and in the rib cage, especially around the second rib.

The major symptoms include:

- Six or more trigger points of the body that are reproducible
- Muscle aches, pains, and stiffness of a minimum of three different areas for at least three months

Disorders that produce similar symptoms must be excluded. The minor symptoms include:

- Sleep disturbances
- Irritable bowel syndrome
- Generalized fatigue
- Chronic headache
- Tingling or numbing sensations
- Swelling of the joints
- Psychological and neurological complaints
- Symptoms varying in intensity with activity, stress, or changes in weather

Fibromyalgia is much more common in women than in men. Some reports have said that it occurs as much as ten times more often in women than in men. Medical tests such as X-rays and blood tests usually do not reveal any abnormalities.

Chronic fatigue and fibromyalgia are caused by yeast, allergies, antibiotics, and any of the other culprits that may be taxing your immune system and stealing your energy.

Don Colbert, *The Bible Cure for Chronic Fatigue and Fibromyalgia* (Lake Mary, FL: Siloam, 2000).

HEADACHES AND DIZZINESS

by Reginald Cherry, MD

CATEGORIES OF HEADACHES range from simple stress or tension headaches to more severe problems such as brain tumors or temporal arteritis, which can be serious. The simple headache consists of a buzzing or pulsing discomfort in the head, and it can be related to high blood pressure, fever, stress, weather, and other causes. The following list may help you identify the type of headache(s) you experience:

- Ice pick headaches—brief, stabbing headaches, which, although potentially frightening to many patients, are benign.

- Tension headaches—usually begin in the back of the head or neck area, or in the forehead or temple region, and spreads throughout the head. Frequently, tension headaches occur on both sides of the head.

- Cluster headaches—characterized by a piercing or burning pain, often occurring on one side of the head, usually in exactly the same place from one episode to another. These headaches occur on a regular basis for days or weeks at a time and then may disappear.

- Migraine headaches—vomiting, nausea, and vision problems often accompany them. These headaches are due to constrictions and dilations in blood vessels in the brain. Migraines are sometimes very difficult to diagnose as they may present only with blurred vision or partial loss of a vision field on one side.

- Ocular migraine headache—can cause a loss of peripheral vision. It is often hereditary.

- Combination headache—presents as a migraine headache followed by a dull, continuing pain afterward.

NATURAL PAIN RELIEF

Add just a few drops (four to five) of fresh lemon to a cup of black coffee and then sip it slowly. Caffeine is a well-known, plant-derived substance that can help alleviate headaches by dilating the blood vessels in the brain. Another herbal treatment is to add two to three drops of peppermint oil to a cold compress. Place it on the painful area for fifteen minutes to relieve tension headaches.

DIZZINESS

Dizziness is one of the most common neurological symptoms encountered in the medical practice. It is, in fact, second only to fatigue among "nonpain" symptoms. On one end of the scale, dizziness is often a vague complaint that can be very brief and benign. By the same token, it can extend to more serious diseases such as tumors or decreased blood flow to the brain.

Reginald Cherry, *Bible Health Secrets* (Lake Mary, FL: Siloam, 2003), 135–137.

SECRETS to LONGEVITY

HEALTHY BONES

by Reginald Cherry, MD

I N RECENT YEARS in the United States, doctors have begun to connect with the "nutritional world" in recognizing the healing properties of glucosamine and chondroitin, especially in the treatment of arthritis. Now the scientific community has been able to witness cases of arthritis where the disease is *actually reversed*.

One study recorded in the medical journal *Lancet* looked at 212 people who suffered from arthritis. Half of them were given glucosamine, and half were given a placebo. The study followed the patients for three years, and the results were amazing. Glucosamine patients showed at least a 25 percent rate of improvement in their symptoms, while the patients on the placebo got worse! Patients receiving glucosamine ultimately lost 80 percent less cartilage than their counterparts![1] What that means is that the disease was stopped, and even partially reversed, in patients who took 1,500 mg of glucosamine a day.

For years, doctors considered arthritis a progressive disease, meaning that once a person had it, they knew that their joints and cartilage were on a decline that would continue until their lives ended. With the use of glucosamine, however, it is possible to provide patients with a real solution. Glucosamine can stop the debilitating progression of the disease!

It works especially well when combined with chondroitin, a compound found in animal cartilage. When people take glucosamine without combining it with chondrotin, it can take the glucosamine up to three months longer to "kick in." But when the glucosamine and chondroitin are combined (along with other natural substances), relief can begin to occur within a matter of days. The symptoms will be quickly reduced, and over the long run, the disease can be stopped and eventually reversed.

Glucosamine should be taken at a dose of 1,500 mg a day, and chondroitin at a dose of 100 mg a day.

Our God is an amazing God, full of grace and compassion for all of our needs. He has provided a way, within His natural plant and animal kingdoms, for us not only to deal with the symptoms of joint disease but also to know how to repair the damage that was done and restore the joints to the way He intended for them to work. God is in the restoration business!

Reginald Cherry, *Bible Health Secrets* (Lake Mary, FL: Siloam, 2003), 116–117.

ANTIAGING PROTOCOL

by Janet Maccaro, PhD, CNC

YOUTHFULNESS IS NOT a chronological age, and age is not the enemy—disease is! The good news is that God made our bodies able to be rejuvenated at any age, thereby giving us more healthy vibrant years. We can slow the aging process by making sure that we maintain the very best internal environment possible to prevent disease.

While it is true that cell age is genetically controlled, disease or illness is most often the result of poor diet, lifestyle, and environment, not to mention stress! Research in longevity has shown that there are three main causes of premature aging:

1. Enzyme depletion from poor diet and inadequate enzyme supplementation
2. Lowered immune response, which sets the stage for disease
3. Cell and tissue damage from free radicals

Aging is the process by which the body matures and grows old or shows signs of growing old that continue throughout the span of life. It is caused by a breakdown in the replacement process of cells that are continually dying.

Dietary considerations

Good nutrition is the key to adding years to your life and life to your years. First priority is to drink plenty of pure water every day. This will keep you hydrated and help all of your body's systems to work more efficiently. In addition, water will help proper elimination, remove toxins, and lessen arthritic pain. It also helps transport proteins, vitamins, minerals, and sugars for assimilation. Water helps the body work at its peak.

Eat fresh seafood at least twice weekly for thyroid health and balance. Nuts, seeds, beans, fiber, and essential fatty acids are living nutrients. Enjoy fresh fruits and vegetables—enzyme rich and full of vitamins, minerals, and fiber.

Practice caloric reduction. As you age, your body requires fewer calories; it also burns calories at a lower rate. In addition, a low-calorie diet has been shown to protect your DNA from damage. This will thereby prevent organ and tissue degeneration. Try to get more "bang for your caloric buck" by eating only high-quality, densely nutritious foods at each meal.

Avoid fried foods, red meat, too much caffeine, and highly spiced and processed foods.

Supplement support for aging

- Coenzyme Q_{10} for cardiovascular health, periodontal disease, or gum problems
- Multivitamin/mineral supplement
- L-glutathione: antioxidant, amino acid that neutralizes radiation and inhibits free radicals
- Gota kola: brain and nervous system health
- Royal jelly: antiaging superfood, great for chronic fatigue and immune health, great source of pantothenic acid
- Lycopene: anticancer antioxidant that reduces the risk of prostate and cervical cancer
- Vitamins C, A, and E: antioxidants
- Bilberry: protects against macular degeneration
- Germanium: increases tissue oxygenation, thereby preventing disease

- Ginkgo biloba: helps restore circulation, improves hearing and vision, improves memory and brain activity
- Green superfoods: spirulina, chlorella, barley green, kelp, and wheatgrass
- Daily green drink: I recommend Kyo-Green by Wakunaga
- Astragalus: for adrenal health, helps to lower blood pressure, improves circulation
- Reishi, shiitake, and maitake mushrooms: power mushrooms that boost immunity, may help prevent cancer, and are antiviral and antibacterial
- Hawthorn berry: protects the heart from free-radical damage, helps the heart pump blood efficiently
- Plant enzymes: improve digestion, thereby enhancing all other body functions—elimination, assimilation, alertness, and energy levels
- Red ginseng (for men): an adaptogenic herb that provides energy to all body systems, promotes strength, fortifies the body against the effects of stress and fatigue, and promotes testosterone production
- White or American ginseng: helps to stimulate memory centers in the brain
- Siberian ginseng: supports the glandular system, especially the adrenals, circulation, and memory
- Yogurt or acidophilus: daily for nutrient assimilation, helps to boost friendly bacteria

Emotional health

It is a common fact that people who fill their lives with laughter and share an attitude of optimism live longer and healthier lives. To live a long life, it is important to take time to play and pray!

Janet Maccaro, *Natural Health Remedies* (Lake Mary, FL: Siloam, 2003), 96–98.

Q&A ON AGING

by Janet Maccaro, PhD, CNC

Q: CAN EXERCISE really keep me young?

A: Exercise is considered the best "nutrient" of all time. It can prolong fitness at any age. It also helps increase your stamina and circulation, lifts depression, and increases joint mobility.

Q: I have arthritis and am afraid to begin an exercise program. I hurt so badly that I don't want to even try it for fear that I will make things worse.

A: I understand. When you are in pain, you don't want to "rock the boat" and make things worse. I recommend that you begin with deep-breathing exercises daily (outdoors in the morning is especially good). Deep breathing will help. In addition, stretching exercises will help to limber up the body in the morning, and stretching before going to bed at night will help to relax you and promote more restful sleep. You can also begin a walking program. You will be surprised at how great it makes you feel. Begin slowly at first. As you continue, you will see that you can walk faster and for longer periods of time with positive results.

Q. How does my being overweight factor into the aging process? My grandmother lived to be eighty and was overweight. Does it really matter?

A: Let me make this comment. It is widely believed that 10 to 30 pounds of extra weight may take two years off your life. Thirty to 50 pounds of extra weight may result in losing four years, and over 50 pounds may take eight years off your life. This is not to mention all of the diseases associated with obesity, like diabetes, cancer, and arthritis.

Q: I smoke. It is hard for me to quit. Smoking helps to relieve my stress. I want to look younger and feel better. What can I do?

A: Nothing ages you more prematurely than smoking, with the exception of too much sun exposure. Smoking uses up tissue oxygen, which feeds the brain and helps prevent disease. Each cigarette takes eight minutes off your life, one pack a day takes one month off of your life each year, and two packs take ten to fifteen years off of your life. In addition, cigarettes contain over four thousand known poisons.[1]

Q: Can you give me some dietary suggestions that promote longevity?

A: Eat fresh. *If it does not rot or sprout, do without.* Eat as close to the "original garden" as possible. Shop the perimeter of the grocery store where the *live foods* are found.

Janet Maccaro, *Natural Health Remedies* (Lake Mary, FL: Siloam, 2003, 2006), 95–100.

ALZHEIMER'S—THE LONG GOOD-BYE

by Janet Maccaro, PhD, CNC

OLDER AMERICANS HAVE come to fear that Alzheimer's will cause them to be a caregiver to a loved one or that it will attack them personally. Alzheimer's now has been diagnosed in over four million Americans. This means that 25 to 50 percent of all people over the age of eighty-five are likely to have Alzheimer's disease.[1]

Definition

Alzheimer's is a degenerative disease in which the nerve cells of the brain deteriorate, resulting in impaired memory, thinking, and behavior.

Symptoms

The most common symptoms of Alzheimer's disease include disorientation, confusion, memory loss, language impairment, insomnia, irritability, depression, and reversion to childhood. The disease is progressive. Death occurs about ten years after diagnosis. Currently there is no known cure, though natural therapies have been successful in slowing brain deterioration.

Causes

Many cases are the result of too many prescription drugs along with nutritional deficiencies. Proper diagnosis is essential. Other factors that contribute to the disease are poor circulation, arteriosclerosis, thyroid malfunction, aluminum toxicity, mercury toxicity, heredity, and possible viral connections. Genetic predisposition is present in more than half of the cases.

Dietary considerations

Choosing to eat nutritiously can help to overcome the effects of Alzheimer's disease, especially if you make those choices early in life. The following dietary regimen can be helpful.

Avoid red meats and sugar; eat nuts, eggs, and soy. Eat a largely vegetarian diet, choosing organic foods to avoid xenoestrogens from pesticides. Eat foods that block aluminum toxicity such as liver, fish, brown rice, wheat germ, and molasses. Drink spring water only as fluoridated water increases aluminum absorption. Eat avocados, poultry, and low-fat dairy to boost tryptophan levels. Take vitamins, minerals, and nutritional supplements that enhance memory, nourish the brain, protect brain cells, and reduce amyloid protein strings to overcome brain damage.

Supplement support for Alzheimer's

- Vitamin E: 800 IU daily
- Evening primrose: 500 mg three times daily; feed the brain
- Ginkgo biloba: 60 mg three times daily; symptom stabilizer
- Neuro-Logic by Wakunaga: improves memory and mental acuity
- Huperzine A: enhances memory retention
- Daily green drink
- Phosphatidyl choline: 5,000 to 10,000 mg; helps overcome brain damage
- Royal jelly: to improve memory
- Omega-3 flax oil: nourishes the brain
- Lysine: 1,000 mg to preserve brain cells
- DHA: natural calcium channel blocker

- Carnitine: 500 mg two times daily; a brain nutrient, reduces mental decline
- Coenzyme Q_{10}: 100 mg daily; cellular energy
- Thiamine (vitamin B_1): 100 mg daily; increases mental power
- Vitamin B_{12}: 2,500 mcg daily; increases mental power
- Purify by Enzymedica: take as directed to help overcome brain damage by reducing amyloid strings

Lifestyle choices

Since higher than normal mercury levels have been found in the brains of people with Alzheimer's disease, mercury exposure, which occurs mainly through dental amalgams, should not be overlooked as a potential contributor to Alzheimer's disease. Mercury toxicity releases into the brain and affects brain health. Consider removing silver amalgam dental fillings.

Most biological dentists have amalgam removal protocols that are followed before, during, and after the removal process that involve chelators and cleansers. These protocols are necessary to keep your system from reacting adversely to the removal of this heavy metal.

Janet Maccaro, *Natural Health Remedies* (Lake Mary, FL: Siloam, 2003, 2006), 100–102.

ZAPPING THE BIG EIGHT AGE-MAKERS—PART 1

by Janet Maccaro, PhD, CNC

WHEN I USE the term *new midlife crisis*, I am referring to the alarming rate of degenerative diseases that occur to people in their middle years of life. The good news is that it is now believed that consuming the right supplements in the optimal dosages may greatly reduce a fifty-year-old's risk of developing cancer, Alzheimer's disease, arthritis, cataracts, and cardiovascular disease, and it may redefine the aging process.

The following eight age accelerators should be addressed by all persons fifty and older. Once they are addressed, your chances of becoming fabulous at fifty are excellent! I'll be explaining the first four in this secret and giving recommendations for preventing them, followed by the last four in secret #133.

1. Inflammation
2. Hormonal imbalance
3. Digestive enzyme deficiency
4. Oxidative stress
5. Fatty acid imbalance
6. Immune dysfunction
7. Excess calcification
8. Excitotoxicity[1]

Inflammation

By age fifty, several lifestyle areas contribute to chronic inflammation, including diet, obesity, smoking, and a sedentary lifestyle. Chronic inflammation is related to most chronic disease processes, such as inflammatory disease of the skin, bowels, central nervous system, rheumatoid arthritis, allergies, asthma, atherosclerosis, cancer, and diabetes.

Curcumin is one of the most potent known anti-inflammatory agents.[2] Take 500 mg twice a day.

Hormonal imbalance

Aging itself causes a hormonal imbalance that may be a contributing cause of many diseases associated with aging, such as osteoporosis, loss of libido, depression, and coronary artery disease (CAD). The key to restoring hormonal balance is using bioidentical natural hormone supplementation.

Bioidenticals are hormone supplements that work with your body to enhance and reestablish your natural internal balance. Since they complement your natural hormones, your body accepts and uses them to reestablish your natural balance without the dangerous and uncomfortable side effects of synthetic hormones. Examples of bioidenticals would be natural estrogen or progesterone derived from plant sources such as soy or Mexican wild yam. Or you may use herbs like black cohosh and vitex that are standards in natural medicine.

To determine whether you need to take these supplements to restore your hormonal balance, you should have your doctor perform a formal assay (blood work) on you every year. The results of your assay will help your health-care provider determine a hormone-balancing protocol tailored to your specific needs. This yearly assay will serve as a guide to insure that balance is achieved and maintained. This assay should determine your levels of DHEA sulfate; progesterone; E1, E2, E3 (estradiol, estrone, and estriol); T3; T4 (thyroid panel); TSH; testosterone, FSH, and LH. Men should also have a PSA (prostate specific antigen) test done yearly. Women should receive Pap and pelvic exams yearly and, after age fifty, annual mammograms.

Digestive enzyme deficiency

The aging pancreas often fails to secrete enough digestive enzymes. The aging liver sometimes does not secrete enough bile acids. This can result in chronic indigestion that can lead to various digestive diseases such as gastroesophageal reflux disease (GERD), nausea, bloating, gas, and poor food assimilation.

Supplementing with digestive enzymes will help eliminate digestive problems and boost nutrient assimilation, which will in turn boost your immune system. Take enzymes from a plant source at the beginning of each meal.

A digestive enzyme supplement should be broad spectrum so that it can facilitate the digestion of protein, fat, carbohydrates, fiber, and milk lactose. Two capsules of enzymes taken with meals help to replace naturally occurring enzymes that are destroyed in highly processed and cooked foods.[3]

Oxidative stress

Aging causes a loss of endogenous antioxidants. This allows free-radical damage to escalate. Free radicals are chemically reactive atoms with unpaired electrons. They attack cells and cause cellular damage caused by exposure to radiation, overexposure to sun, and exposure to cigarette smoke and toxic chemicals. Free-radical damage has been implicated with the aging process and the development of degenerative disease. It is therefore prudent to supplement with antioxidants such as alpha-lipoic acid (ALA), especially at midlife. The recommended dosage of ALA is 250 mg, once or twice daily. People with a deficiency of vitamin B_{12} should not take alpha-lipoic acid.[4]

Janet Maccaro, *Fabulous at 50* (Lake Mary, FL: Siloam, 2003), 19–23.

ZAPPING THE BIG EIGHT AGE-MAKERS—PART 2

by Janet Maccaro, PhD, CNC

CONTINUING OUR DISCUSSION of the eight big age-makers, I am listing the last four conditions with their suggested remedies.

Fatty acid imbalance

Fatty acids maintain cell energy output. The effects of a fatty acid imbalance may be felt as low energy, irregular heartbeat, painful joint degeneration, and other age-related conditions. Supplementation with fatty acids can suppress chronic inflammation.

Fatty acids are part of our makeup. They live in our healthy cells, muscles, nerves, and organs. They are essential for life—which is why they are called *essential* fatty acids. Sources of these essentials include oils from nuts, vegetables, and some fish. These are unsaturated healthy fats. Without proper levels of good fats, dangerous saturated fats from animal fats and dairy products will replace the good fats in our cells. The healthy fats include GLA (gamma-linolenic acid), DHA (docosahexaenoic acid), and EPA (eicosapentaenoic acid).[1] Take 450 mg of GLA, 500 mg of DHA, and 750 mg of EPA twice daily with meals.

Note: Do not take essential fatty acids if you are on anticoagulant medications. Also, note that for optimal absorption, do not take these with fiber supplements.

Immune dysfunction

As we age, the immune system loses its ability to attack viruses, bacteria, and cancer cells as it could in years past. It is at midlife that the immune system often turns on its host (you) and creates autoimmune diseases, such as rheumatoid arthritis. Immune boosting is mandatory at midlife.

Modern research has validated what has been known for centuries: garlic can support the immune system by increasing natural killer cells. I recommend 1,000 mg of Kyolic garlic and 500 mg of olive leaf extract twice daily to support immunity and promote a healthy intestinal environment with plenty of beneficial bacteria. Several studies have demonstrated that components of garlic are immune boosters. Pharmaceutical-grade olive leaf extract contains the highest concentration of oleuropein. Oleuropein is a bitter compound isolated from the olive leaf. It is a powerful phytochemical that strongly supports the immune system. Olive leaf extract also provides natural protection and a healthy environment for cells without suppressing immune system function or harming beneficial intestinal microflora.[2]

Excess calcification

Aging disrupts calcium transport, resulting in calcium being deposited into the heart valves, brain cells, and the middle arterial wall—which can cause arteriosclerosis. Calcium is an essential nutrient in the maintenance of human bone integrity, but it is important to keep it out of the arterial walls. Calcium buildup on arterial walls can begin as early as the second decade of life and can continue throughout adulthood.

It has been revealed that vitamin K may help keep calcium in the bone, where it does a great job of building strong bones.[3]

Note: Do not take vitamin K if you are on anticoagulant medication. The recommended dosage is 9 mg of K_1 (known as phylloquinone) and 1 mg of K_2 (called menaquinone). Taking 3 mg of boron will also aid in retaining calcium in bones. Take these once a day.

Excitotoxicity

Excitotoxicity occurs when the brain ages and loses control of its release of neurotransmitters, such as dopamine and glutamate. This can result in brain cell damage and destruction. This also causes brain aging and degenerative neurological disease. This can produce symptoms such as a loss of ability in thinking, remembering, and reasoning.

Vitamin B_{12} (methylcobalmin) is a brain cell protector. It has been shown to protect the brain against excitotoxic neuronal damage. Vitamin B_{12} comes in pill or liquid form. For best effectiveness, it should be dissolved under the tongue (sublingually) in order to bypass the liver during its first pass through the bloodstream. The daily dose for healthy midlifers is 1 mg, while the dose for those with neurological impairments is from 20–80 mg daily, depending upon severity of symptoms.[4]

I have outlined supplements that every fifty-year-old should consider. Please consult your physician before beginning this regimen. Your doctor needs to know what you are taking and how often, especially if you currently take prescription medications or have ongoing medical conditions for which you have been in a physician's care.

Janet Maccaro, *Fabulous at 50* (Lake Mary, FL: Siloam, 2007), 19–28.

ANTIAGING SELF-EXAM

by Janet Maccaro, PhD, CNC

Take this quiz to help determine if you are aging faster than necessary.

- Have you noticed brown spots on the back of your hands or around your eyes and nose?
- Is it more difficult for you to lose weight?
- Do you have frequent indigestion, heartburn, or gas after eating a meal?
- Do you have insomnia?
- Do you have heart palpitations or chest pain?
- Do you have poor eyesight?
- Have you experienced hearing loss or ringing in the ears?
- Are you frequently constipated?
- Is your hair turning gray?
- Have you lost height?
- Is your skin becoming dryer or thinner? Are you noticing more moles, bruises, or cherry angiomas (red blood blisters)?
- Is your recovery time slow from a cold or flu?
- Do you have poor circulation?

Janet Maccaro, *Fabulous at 50* (Lake Mary, FL: Siloam, 2007), 31–32.

DIETARY KEYS TO LONGER LIFE

by Janet Maccaro, PhD, CNC

H ERE ARE SOME of the latest findings from Dr. Michael Roizen, who introduced the Real Age concept—a scientific way of calculating a number that reflects your overall state of health rather than calendar age:[1]

- Use 9-inch plates—smaller plates mean smaller portions. Age reduction equals 3.1 years.
- Eat fiber early in the day—fiber at breakfast slows the rate at which the stomach empties. This will help you not to snack and get excessive calories late in the day. Age reduction equals 0.6 years.
- Eat flavonoid-rich foods—green tea, broccoli, and strawberries can equal lower risk of breast and prostate cancer. Green tea has also been linked to a reduced heart disease risk. Age reduction equals 3.2 years.
- Combine vitamins C and E—they are more powerful when taken in combination. Age reduction equals up to 1 year.
- Get enough folate (a B vitamin)—it lowers homocysteine, an amino acid linked to heart disease. Age reduction equals 1.2 years.
- Laugh more—it reduces stress, lowers cancer risk, and lowers levels of heart disease, stress, and hypertension. Age reduction equals 1.7 to 8 years.

Janet Maccaro, *Fabulous at 50* (Lake Mary, FL: Siloam, 2007), 40–41.

NATURAL REMEDIES FOR YOUNGER-LOOKING SKIN

by Janet Maccaro, PhD, CNC

IT IS AN undeniable fact that beautiful skin is the result of a healthy, toxin-free, balanced body. The skin is the largest organ of the body. It receives great benefit from an enzyme-rich circulatory system. Skin that is well enriched by oxygen and high-quality nutrients will always look smooth, firm, and velvety.

Enzymes are the digestive catalysts that make nutrients available to the blood for their journey to every cell in the body. To feed your cells, detoxify your system, slow the aging process, oxygenate, and boost your circulatory system, you must make midlife enzyme supplementation a priority.

MIDLIFE SKIN-BEAUTIFYING ENZYMES

- Protease—breaks down protein foods that feed the cells of the dermis; also improves distribution of all nutrients to the skin
- Amylase—reduces skin inflammation
- Lipase—keeps skin cells plump to reduce wrinkling
- Cellulase—breaks down fiber and allows nutrients access to the skin

Stress, excessive sun exposure, liver malfunction, hormone depletion, smoking, alcohol, sugar, fried foods, caffeine, and poor circulation all contribute to the condition of our skin. Age spots, wrinkles, dry sky, uneven skin tone, sallow complexion, and acne are the result of how well our systems handle wastes. Free-radical damage is another major contributor to poor skin.

DIETARY THERAPY

- Drink plenty of water (six to eight glasses each day).
- Add fresh lemon to your water for added benefit.
- Make a fresh "liver cocktail" each day: 2 ounces beet juice, 3 ounces carrot juice, and 3 ounces cucumber juice (use a juicer).
- Avoid sugars, caffeine, and red meat to prevent dehydration.
- Eat fresh fruits and vegetables each day; fruits are wonderful cleaners.
- Use alpha-hydroxy acids (fruit acid) to exfoliate the skin.

BODY THERAPY

- Reduce or prevent wrinkles by rubbing papaya skins on the face. (Papain is an enzyme that exfoliates the skin.)
- Manage stress.
- Practice deep breathing.
- Have a massage with almond oil, sesame oil, or wheat germ oil to soften the skin.
- Moisturize immediately after bathing.
- Rub lemon juice on age spots, or use 2 percent hydroquinone topical cream to reduce and fade age spots.
- Limit sun exposure; always use a sunblock of SFF-15 or higher to prevent further damage and to prevent age spots from darkening.

Janet Maccaro, *Fabulous at 50* (Lake Mary, FL: Siloam, 2007), 114–118.

WAYS TO EXTEND YOUR DAYS—PART 1

by Janet Maccaro, PhD, CNC

1. Cancer prevention: indole-3-carbinol

Indole-3-carbinol is a powerful phytochemical found in cruciferous vegetables, providing breast, cervical, and prostate cell support by activating detoxification enzymes, promoting healthy estrogen balance and cellular metabolism, and scavenging free radicals.[1]

2. Mood elevator: 5-HTP

5-hydroxytryptophan is derived from the *griffonia simplicifolia* plant. Supplementation with 5-HTP encourages brain serotonin levels that can lead to positive effects on emotional well-being, appetite control, and sleep/wake cycles. Clinical studies have shown that 5-HTP increases serotonin levels.[2]

3. Antianxiety: L-theanine

L-theanine is an amino acid derived from green tea that has been recognized for centuries as having relaxant properties. In addition to promoting relaxation, L-theanine helps to moderate occasional stress and the effects of caffeine on the central nervous system. L-theanine is a unique amino acid that eases irritability and nervous tension without causing drowsiness.[3]

4. Natural hormone replacement: black cohosh

Black cohosh (*cimicifuga racemosa*) offers support during menopause and reduces hot flashes. It helps maintain healthy levels of LH (luteinizing hormone), which contributes to physical well-being. Black cohosh has mild estrogenic properties by binding to estrogen receptors, thereby supporting healthy estrogen levels during menopause.[4]

5. Joint health midlife marvel: glucosamine, chondroitin, MSM

This trio of substances—glucosamine, chondroitin, and MSM—helps to strengthen cartilage and promote comfortable joint movement. These naturally occurring substances build and maintain the matrix of collagen and connective tissue that forms the ground substance of cartilage.[5]

6. Prostate support: lycopene

Lycopene is a natural tomato extract. Studies show that lycopene from consumption of tomato or tomato-based products may help digestive, lung, stomach, cervical, prostate, and breast health. In a study involving thirty male subjects, supplementation with lycopene promoted healthy prostate function. It is interesting to note that the study also found that lycopene supplementation, rather than dietary tomato consumption, supported prostate health. In addition, lycopene is an antioxidant that supports cellular health.[6]

7. Stress, cardiovascular, immune, cognitive, and joint health: ashwaganda

Ashwaganda is a four-thousand-year-old adaptogenic herb that belongs to the pepper family. In animal studies, ashwaganda has been shown to support the activity of lymphocytes and macrophages, moderate occasional stress, enhance memory and cognitive function, provide neuroprotection by scavenging free radicals, and support thyroid function. Ashwaganda's adaptogenic properties provide multifunctional support for promoting mental and physical wellness, occasional stress, and healthy lipid and glucose metabolism.[7]

8. Nerve health and glucose metabolism: alpha-lipoic acid

Alpha-lipoic acid is a potent antioxidant that neutralizes harmful free radicals and enhances the activity of vitamins C and E. It is a key player in the metabolic process that produces energy in muscles and directs calories into energy production. In addition, alpha-lipoic acid supports the nervous system and provides support for healthy liver function. It also helps to sustain normal blood sugar levels and promotes healthy glucose metabolism in both lean and overweight persons.[8]

9. Healthy lipid metabolism: policosanol

Policosanol is derived from sugar cane. It supports cardiovascular health, provides antioxidant protection, promotes healthy platelet function, and supports healthy lipid metabolism. Policosanol is a well-tolerated supplement that has been the subject of both short- and long-term research over the past decade.[9]

10. Cardiovascular protection: CoQ_{10}

CoQ_{10} provides benefits for cardiovascular health (recommended by many cardiologists), gum disease, prostate, and breast cancer protection. Additionally, CoQ_{10} offers the following health benefits: immune health, skin health, cognitive and nerve health, cellular health, and cranial vascular health.

11. Antiaging superfood: royal jelly

Royal jelly is a superfood for antiaging that stimulates immunity and deep cellular health, boosts circulation to the skin, and supplies key nutrients like pantothenic acid for energy and mental alertness.

12. Immune support: zinc

Zinc helps to limit free radicals your body naturally produces and plays an important role in supporting the body's defense system. Zinc plays a fundamental role in collagen formation and healthy tissue development. This mineral also contributes to healthy prostatic function.

Janet Maccaro, *Fabulous at 50* (Lake Mary, FL: Siloam, 2007), 183–186.

WAYS TO EXTEND YOUR DAYS—PART 2

by Janet Maccaro, PhD, CNC

13. Powerful antioxidant: oligomeric proanthocyanidins (OPC)

OPCs are powerful antioxidants that strengthen capillaries and connective tissue. They reduce LDL cholesterol that can accumulate in arteries, which can contribute to atherosclerosis.

14. Antioxidant for immune system support: selenium

Selenium is both an antioxidant and a trace mineral that protects the body from heavy metal toxicity, increases glutathione, and reduces the risk of cancers, such as lung, esophagus, prostate, and colorectal cancers.

15. Primary antioxidant: vitamin C

Vitamin C boosts immunity. It is a primary antioxidant that offers protection against heart disease, allergies, cancer, high blood pressure, arthritis, and infection. In addition, it safeguards against toxic heavy metals, radiation, and pollutants.

16. Arterial protection: bioflavonoids

Bioflavonoids are a natural anti-inflammatory component of vitamin C that prevents hardening of the arteries; strengthens connective tissue, veins, and capillaries; and helps control bruising. In addition, bioflavonoids help stimulate bile for better digestion and help lower cholesterol.

17. Antiaging antioxidant: vitamin E

Vitamin E is an antiaging antioxidant that reduces the risk of heart attack by acting as an anticoagulant and vasodilator against blood clots. It retards cellular and mental aging.

18. Potent antioxidant: tocotrienols

Tocotrienols are compounds related to vitamin E's tocopherols that have powerful antioxidant effects, lower cholesterol, and have anticancer properties. In addition, tocotrienols protect against damage to the arterial walls and have a strong lipid-lowering ability.

19. Prime immune booster: L-glutathione

L-glutathione is an antioxidant amino acid that works to neutralize radiation and/or drug toxicity and inhibits free radical formation. A potent detoxifier, it cleanses the blood from the effects of liver toxins, chemotherapy, and X-rays. In addition, it is protective against age-related eye disease, such as macular degeneration and cataracts.

20. Antiaging brain and energy stimulant: ginkgo biloba

The ginkgo leaf is shaped like the human brain. Interestingly enough, ginkgo biloba has been confirmed to boost circulation to the brain, improving memory and cognitive function. It is widely used in Europe and Asia as a longevity tonic.

21. Anti-inflammatory: turmeric

Turmeric has a bold yellow-orange color that is familiar to anyone who has eaten curry. As in traditional Indian medicine, turmeric is used to treat arthritis, bursitis, and tendonitis. It also improves circulation!

22. Heart health: hawthorn

European studies have confirmed hawthorn's cardiovascular benefits, which include lowering blood pressure during exertion, strengthening the heart muscle, and improving blood flow to the heart and throughout the entire body. It has also been shown to aid in lowering cholesterol.

23. Antiaging brain nutrient: acetyl-L-carnitine

Acetyl-L-carnitine is an amino acid that reduces age-related mental decline and increases alertness, attention span, and memory-learning ability.

24. Broad spectrum adaptogenic herb: Panax ginseng

Panax ginseng is an antiaging wonder that increases energy and stamina. It has been used medically in Asia for over five thousand years. It is considered an "adaptogen," meaning it enhances body functions and the immune system to help people adapt to the negative effects of stress, both mental and physical.

Janet Maccaro, *Fabulous at 50* (Lake Mary, FL: Siloam, 2007), 186–188.

MEMORY LOSS

by Reginald Cherry, MD

UNTIL JUST RECENTLY, the medical community has believed that once a neuron, a nerve cell, died—including the cells of the brain—it could never be regenerated or brought back to life. They believed the body could heal itself in every other tissue or organ, but once damage was done in the brain, it was irreversible.

Within the last two to three years, scientists have begun to learn that brain cells can and do regenerate under the proper conditions. The following natural substances are proven remedies for improving memory function as well as stopping the progress of the devastating Alzheimer's disease.

Huperzine-A (club moss)

The chemical that communicates memories between neurons in the brain is called acetylcholine. As you age, the level of acetylcholine in your brain begins to decrease, and as a result, your memory function begins to deteriorate.

A natural source of the chemical huperzine-A, which amazingly has been found to increase acetylcholine levels just as effectively as prescription drugs, is synthesized from the club moss plant. It does this by inhibiting the enzyme that breaks down acetylcholine in the brain, thus allowing the levels to increase. The club moss plant has increased memory, thinking ability, focus, and concentration in many Alzheimer's patients. The recommended dosage is 0.1 mg daily.

Periwinkle (vinpocetine)

For years, periwinkle, because of a chemical found in it called vincristine, has been used in traditional treatments for cancer. But about twenty years ago, scientists began to learn that another potent chemical in periwinkle, vinpocetine, has helpful properties in dealing with memory loss. Its primary function in the body is as a vasodilator, meaning that it causes the blood vessels to dilate, or open up, to a greater extent. The reason this improves memory function is that it enlarges the blood vessels to the brain, allowing more oxygen and nutrient supply to the brain.

Vitamins B and E

Vitamin B_{12} has such a potent effect on preventing the effects of aging nerve cells that it has actually been called the "senility vitamin"! Vitamin B_6 is commonly known as a nerve supplement and has been used successfully in the treatment of nerve damage in the wrist. This same nerve repair can be done in the brain through a dose of vitamin B_6 taken at 6 mg per day, while vitamin B_{12} should be taken at 12 mcg per day.

Among people who were taking vitamin E for rheumatoid arthritis, scientists began to find less and less incidence of Alzheimer's disease or other mental difficulties. Eventually it was determined that its anti-inflammatory properties, which were so helpful in dealing with the arthritis, were also helpful in decreasing any slight inflammation within the brain that could impair its functioning.

Reginald Cherry, *Bible Health Secrets* (Lake Mary, FL: Siloam, 2003), 121, 123–128.

WOMEN'S HEALTH

THE BODY GOD DESIGNED

by Gregory L. Jantz, PhD, with Ann McMurray

Y OUR PHYSICAL BODY houses an amazing spiritual treasure, but you've really been focusing in on your flesh-and-blood body—what you eat, what you drink, what you do. After all, that's where you're living right now, and that's what you have to contend with. Achieving the body God designed for you is a major step in discovering your true shape in God, but there's more to it than just your physicality.

The best part of this adventure is the true destination of all of this work, sacrifice, learning, and understanding. The whole reason to achieve the body God designed is so that you can declare victory over your preoccupation with the physical and really rev your spiritual engine. Listen to Paul's reminder in 1 Timothy 4:8: "For physical training is of some value, but godliness has value for all things, holding promise for both the present life and the life to come" (NIV).

Do you realize that all this time you've been engaged in training for your physical body you've been learning about godliness too? You've been multitasking in the best sense of the word.

God didn't just create "people," the vast billions and billions who have ever lived; He created you individually. Through His will, He designed a body just for you and nobody else. God knows you intimately, in ways you don't even know yourself. Because of this intimacy, you are learning to trust Him with your struggles about weight and health, as well as about the other challenges you have in life.

God is a God of diversity and expansive creativity through all of the different shapes, sizes, and styles of bodies He created. Through this, you learned the *acceptance* of God for who you are right now. God is not some captain of a divine softball team, choosing which "players" He wants and doesn't want from a global lineup. God doesn't play favorites. He doesn't choose only the "attractive" people to use in His kingdom. If you doubt that's true (especially after watching some of the well-coiffed, practically perfect-in-every-way televangelists), consider the description of Jesus written down by the Old Testament prophet Isaiah: "He had no beauty or majesty to attract us to him, nothing in his appearance that we should desire him" (Isa. 53:2). By worldly standards, Jesus would have been chosen last. But as God often does, He throws our expectations a curveball and makes Jesus first.

God throws us a curveball so we'll understand the world's ways are not His ways. The world may not accept who you are (*you* may not accept who you are), but God does. He's not interested in your six-pack abs or your firm behind unless your preoccupation with them compromises your spiritual growth. His acceptance of you is about who you ultimately are on the *inside*. And as your inside becomes transformed slowly by godliness, your outside will reflect that change.

God instead wants you to be transformed through a process of obedience. Slow and steady wins this race as you consistently turn over to God your challenges and struggles with your weight and body.

It's important to see yourself and your body as a creation of God with the same majestic attributes as the mightiest mountain or stunning vista. You reflect God's majesty; wear it proudly.

Gregory L. Jantz with Ann McMurray, *The Body God Designed* (Lake Mary, FL: Siloam, 2007), 218–219.

EATING DISORDERS

by Linda Mintle, PhD

WE ALL DIET now and then. But dieting can become a way of life or, worse yet, an obsession that prevents you from enjoying life. Dieting is often an entrée to an eating disorder. Eating disorders are serious and usually require treatment by a mental health multidisciplinary team. Early intervention is best because of the potential for serious medical problems, the extreme being death. Eating disorders affect men and women of all ages but are especially present in young women.

Abnormal eating patterns may include self-starvation, compulsive eating, and self-induced purging. Simple starvation leads to anorexia nervosa; binge eating and purging to bulimia nervosa. In some cases, people have a combination of anorexic and bulimic symptoms.

Anorexia involves severe weight loss, excessive exercise, body image disturbance, fear of getting fat, and food avoidance.

A fear of food accompanies a fear of weight gain. Thus, there is usually a tendency to exercise excessively or to take laxatives, water pills, diet pills, or to vomit as a way to keep from gaining weight.

Anorexia involves self-starvation, and it can cause a number of physical and medical problems, such as loss of menses (amenorrhea), an increase in infections, irregular heartbeat and heart failure, mild anemia, and swollen joints.

Bulimia is an eating disorder characterized by binge-purge cycles. During a binge, large amounts of food are consumed while feeling out of control. Purging usually follows. Many methods of purging (getting rid of the food) are used. These methods include vomiting, taking laxatives, diuretics (water pills), diet pills, exercising excessively, using enemas, fasting, or drinking Ipecac syrup to induce vomiting.

Unlike anorexics, you can't easily spot a bulimic because she is usually at normal weight.

Bulimia can bring on medical problems such as stomach or esophagus rupture (rare, but it happens), heart irregularities due to loss of vital minerals such as potassium, wearing away of the enamel on teeth from acid when vomiting, scarring on the backs of hands from using fingers to induce vomiting, inflamed esophagus, and more.

Many things can influence the development of eating disorders—the tremendous cultural pressure to be thin and beautiful, gender role expectations and changes, family patterns, personality factors, physiological predispositions and experience around loss, abuse, and other trauma.

Here is a brief overview of how to break free from these eating disorders:

1. Admit you have a problem. Confront your denial.
2. Ask for help. By faith, believe that you can be healed and your life different.
3. If necessary, be willing to work with a team of people who will address all aspects of the eating disorder.
4. Get a complete physical examination by a physician.
5. Track your symptoms in order to identify triggers and work on thoughts and emotional responses.
6. Be willing to look below the surface of eating problems for root causes.
7. Base your image and esteem in Christ.
8. Practice healthy eating patterns.

9. Set realistic goals and expectations.
10. Stop trying to be perfect.
11. Daily renew your mind.
12. Find your voice.
13. Directly express and confront negative feelings.
14. Practice assertiveness and problem solving.
15. Lose your "all-or-nothing" thinking.
16. Learn to regulate your emotions.
17. Stop living in fear.
18. Identify the lies that keep you trapped.
19. Face the normal developmental tasks of growing up—independence, budding sexuality, forming an identity and leaving home.
20. Resolve relationship issues. Begin with your family.
21. Work through trauma and loss and any other "tagalong" conditions.

Linda Mintle, *Breaking Free From Anorexia and Bulimia* (Lake Mary, FL: Siloam, 2002).

WHAT TO EXPECT ON YOUR FIRST OB/GYN VISIT

by Scott Farhart, MD, and Elizabeth King, MD

VISITING THE GYNECOLOGIST for the first time can be a scary experience. Most women fear the pelvic exam, and many are embarrassed to be examined. But the gynecologist will be one of the most important physicians in a woman's life. He or she can be a confidant, a counselor, a trusted friend, an ally, and an instrument in healing. The gynecologist is there to offer advice in selecting birth control, planning for a baby, care during pregnancy, help through the changes of life, and treatment for any gynecological diseases that may come your way. But it all starts with the first visit.

Many mothers ask us when their daughters should see the gynecologist for the first time. This is an individual decision and is based on the need of that young woman. Anyone who is sexually active or planning to become sexually active needs a visit. Those who are already sexually active need screening for sexually transmitted diseases and cancerous changes of the cervix. If they do not desire pregnancy, counseling for birth control is given.

Many girls will transition from the pediatrician or family physician to the gynecologist in their teen years. We are seeing more teenagers since the HPV (human papillomavirus) vaccine was introduced because many mothers desire vaccination for their daughters before they become exposed to that STD. Mothers also bring in their daughters to discuss birth control. Our city has some of the highest rates of teenage pregnancy in the country. If a girl is planning on becoming sexually active, we certainly want the opportunity to discuss the options of birth control before she becomes pregnant.

Young women who are still virgins can also benefit from a visit to the gynecologist. They generally will not need a pelvic exam, and it can be a time to get to know one another. When she feels comfortable, a young woman is free to ask questions and receive valuable information.

Remember to ask your physician lots of questions. If your physician is going to treat you, then good communication is the key to discovering how to properly maintain your health. Here is a sample checklist of questions to ask:

- How do I do a proper breast exam?
- What is a Pap smear?
- How do I prevent STDs?
- Can you tell if I have an STD?
- What is a normal menstrual cycle?
- What are my options for birth control?

Scott Farhart and Elizabeth King, *The Christian Woman's Complete Guide to Health* (Lake Mary, FL: Siloam, 2008), 27–28.

YOUR ANNUAL EXAM

by Scott Farhart, MD, and Elizabeth King, MD

THE ANNUAL EXAMINATION includes several things. The first is a review of lifestyle issues that may need to be addressed. Personal habits such as smoking, alcohol and drug use, and sexual practices are addressed. Counseling in these areas is designed to prevent disease.

A physical exam includes height, weight, blood pressure measurement, and on some occasions a urine specimen.

We generally palpate the neck to feel the thyroid gland and determine if it is enlarged. Women are five to nine times more likely to have thyroid disease than men, with most being undiagnosed.[1] A swollen thyroid gland can be a sign of disease.

Often the physician will listen to the heart to check for murmurs or abnormal rhythms.

A breast exam is then done to evaluate for lumps or other abnormalities. This is also a great opportunity to educate a woman on the technique of breast self-examination. This can be accomplished both standing and lying down. It has been suggested that it be done in the shower as a way of developing a routine. How, when, or where it is done is not nearly as important as simply doing a self-exam.

Breast self-examination is an important tool in the detection of breast cancer. Many of our patients rely on their annual gynecologic exam to screen for breast disease. This leaves them vulnerable the rest of the year.

Abnormalities detected during the breast exam may require evaluation with sonography or mammography to exclude breast cancer.

Next, the abdomen is palpated for any tumors or hernias.

An inspection of the vulva is done to evaluate for abnormalities or diseases, including herpes, genital warts, or cancer. An internal examination of the vagina and cervix is accomplished with a device called a *speculum*. The speculum is inserted into the vagina and opened to reveal the vaginal walls and the cervix. An inspection is done for the presence of vaginal discharge, which could indicate infection ranging from yeast or bacterial overgrowth to sexually transmitted diseases. If discharge is present, a sample may be taken for evaluation under a microscope or for laboratory analysis. Often a diagnosis is available by the end of the visit, but some laboratory assays and cultures make take two or three days.

Inspection of the cervix is followed by a Pap smear. This consists of a brush or swab that is twirled around the opening of the cervix to collect cells for evaluation. The primary goal is to identify cells that are precancerous. With regular Pap smears we hope to avoid the diagnosis of full-blown cancer. Once the smear is taken, the speculum is removed and one or two gloved fingers are inserted into the vagina while the other hand is pressed against the lower abdomen. This is called the *bimanual examination.* The uterus and ovaries are palpated between the two hands for any abnormalities in shape or size.

If necessary in younger women, and many times in those over fifty, the last component of the pelvic exam is the insertion of a gloved finger into the rectum. This is done to evaluate behind the uterus for nodules that could indicate endometriosis. In older women, a stool specimen is taken for evaluation for blood in the screening of colorectal cancer.

Menstrual Cycles

A common component of the gynecologic history is the evaluation of the menstrual cycle. Every visit will record the last menstrual period and whether it was normal. One reason for an office visit, or for a referral from a family physician, is the evaluation and treatment of abnormal menstrual cycles. Every day in our offices we see women who are unhappy with their menstrual cycles, and we can often bring them great relief.

In taking the menstrual history, it is important to determine if the patient could be pregnant, as we never want to treat someone with medications who might be pregnant. Your doctor may ask to do a urine pregnancy test as part of his or her evaluation. There may be blood work to check for hormone imbalance of the ovary, pituitary, or thyroid gland.

A bimanual pelvic examination will be done to feel for abnormalities in the size or shape of the uterus. A pelvic ultrasound may be offered either in the office or at a radiology facility to check for the presence of uterine fibroid tumors or polyps that could be causing abnormal bleeding patterns.

Scott Farhart and Elizabeth King, *The Christian Woman's Complete Guide to Health* (Lake Mary, FL: Siloam, 2008), 28–31.

HEALTHY EXPECTATIONS

by Pamela M. Smith, RD

THINK OF PREGNANCY as a twelve-month experience—a minimum of three months to prepare a healthy body for a healthy baby, and nine months to build a strong baby with food and love. It is also just a beginning; not only is a baby being brought into the world, but so is a mother. Be encouraged that the same way of eating that provides optimal health for you is the same kind of eating that keeps your baby healthy, happy, and well nourished. Your baby can start life with an advantage that carries on throughout a bright future. Every aspect of your baby's life will be affected by nutrition that starts long before birth.

Much of the same nutrition you learned in fifth grade still applies today, but in your pregnancy, it will be more focused. There are still six essential nutrients—the body's fuel and recipe mix for a healthy life. Every human needs protein, carbohydrates, vitamins, minerals, water, and even fat (in limited amounts); pregnancy only intensifies the need. In order to support the tremendous amount of growth and development that takes place during these special nine months, you will need a diet sufficient in calories and rich in nutrients.

There is much that you can do to take charge of the experience—and make it simply the most positive time possible. The factors that contribute to a positive experience include:

1. *Your general health.* Being in good overall physical condition gives you the best shot at having a comfortable, vitality-filled pregnancy. Ideally, get chronic conditions like allergies, asthma, diabetes, or back conditions at their stable best before conception. Clear up lingering infections such as urinary tract or yeast infections. Once you become pregnant, continue to take *great* care of you!

2. *Your eating plan.* Following a well-balanced eating plan gives you the best chance for a terrific pregnancy. Not only can it better your chances of avoiding or decreasing the miseries of morning sickness and heartburn, but it also can help fight excessive fatigue, combat constipation and hemorrhoids, prevent constant bladder infections and anemia, and get you over the hurdle of leg cramps. Not only are you impacting your well-being and enjoyment of this amazing time, but you are also giving your baby the best gift of all—contributing to that sweet one's developing well and being born healthy.

3. *Proper weight gain.* Gaining weight at a steady rate and keeping the gain within the recommended levels (25 to 35 pounds) can greatly improve your odds of escaping or minimizing such misery factors as hemorrhoids, varicose veins, stretch marks, backaches, fatigue, heartburn, and shortness of breath.

4. *Fitness.* Getting enough of the right kind of exercise can help improve your overall well-being. Exercise is important at any time, but especially in repeat pregnancies; abdominal muscles tend to be laxer, making you more susceptible to lots of aches and pains.

5. *The pace of your life.* Living life in the frenzied lane can greatly aggravate—or even cause—many of the most horrific pregnancy symptoms such as morning sickness, heartburn, fatigue, and backaches. These symptoms are magnified when there are other children to care for in addition to the general cares of life.

Pamela M. Smith, *Healthy Expectations* (Lake Mary, FL: Siloam, 1998), 4–7.

PREGNANCY: THE FIRST TRIMESTER

by Scott Farhart, MD, and Elizabeth King, MD

FOR MANY WOMEN, one of the first signs that they are pregnant is feeling nauseated. Morning sickness is, like its name, more pronounced in the morning, though it can occur at any time during the day. People who experience it often get some relief once they eat, and they do not have problems unless they have an empty stomach. Eating several small meals throughout the day to keep your stomach from being empty can help. Most people who suffer from morning sickness will vomit on occasion. There are several medications that can help relieve these symptoms, including some over-the counter preparations that your doctor can recommend. Usually nausea and vomiting do not cause any serious problems and will subside as the first trimester ends.

Occasionally, what initially began as morning sickness can progress into a more serious condition known as hyperemesis gravidarum. This is severe nausea and vomiting where patients are unable to tolerate any food or liquids. This can lead to extreme dehydration and weight loss and requires hospitalization with intravenous (IV) fluid administration.

BODY CHANGES

One other prominent symptom early in pregnancy is breast tenderness, which is caused by hormonal stimulation of breast tissue. The ducts in the breast are stimulated to grow in both quantity and size in preparation for milk production. By six weeks of pregnancy, your breasts may grow one whole cup size and may keep growing in size and weight during the first three months.[1] If you plan on nursing, it is a good idea to buy nursing bras when you are pregnant.

Another common symptom in the beginning of pregnancy is feeling bloated. As the uterus grows, there is less room in the abdominal cavity for the bowel, and pressure is exerted on the bladder. This leads to the need to urinate frequently. Some of the hormones produced during pregnancy slow the bowels down, leading to constipation and problems with gas. Drinking plenty of water, eating high-fiber foods, or taking a stool softener can all help relieve this discomfort.

EMOTIONAL CHANGES

In addition to undergoing physical changes, your emotions will fluctuate too. You may be happy that you are pregnant, yet still experience sadness or moodiness. Getting plenty of rest will help, as will reaching out to family and friends for support. It is very common, especially for first-time parents, to worry about their baby and whether or not they will be good parents.

Many women faced with childbirth fear the birthing process itself. Attending classes that prepare you for childbirth and discussing the birthing process with your doctor may help allay those fears.

It is a life-changing event to bring a child into the world. It is normal to feel that your life will never be the same, and that doesn't have to be a bad thing. You will experience a whole new world and a new perspective on life. It truly is a gift from God, and you will experience countless blessings.

Scott Farhart and Elizabeth King, *The Christian Woman's Complete Guide to Health* (Lake Mary, FL: Siloam, 2008), 163–166.

ABNORMALITIES DURING PREGNANCY

by Scott Farhart, MD, and Elizabeth King, MD

S OMETIMES YOUR FEARS may be justified, and there is a problem with your pregnancy. We sometimes have patients tell us they "don't feel pregnant" or they are having pain and bleeding. We take these concerns very seriously as they may be a sign of an abnormal pregnancy.

MISCARRIAGE

It is estimated that between 12 and 15 percent of all pregnancies end in miscarriage;[1] however, it is difficult to estimate because some will occur before a woman even knows she is pregnant. Most miscarriages occur during the first trimester and are caused by chromosome abnormalities. These are usually due to chance and not because of an underlying genetic disorder of the parents. Because the rate of chromosome abnormalities increases with a woman's age, the chance of having a miscarriage increases as you get older.

The most common sign of a miscarriage is vaginal bleeding. Most women who experience vaginal bleeding or spotting during the first trimester of pregnancy go on to deliver healthy infants. However, anytime a woman experiences bleeding early in pregnancy, it is referred to as a threatened miscarriage. Other signs that you may be having a miscarriage are low backache and cramping along with bleeding. Occasionally, a woman will not have any symptoms of miscarriage, and it will be discovered at a routine doctor's visit that there is no heartbeat in the fetus.

If you think you may be having a miscarriage, it is important to contact your doctor. He or she will perform a pelvic exam and usually an ultrasound. If there is any tissue left in the uterus, or if you are experiencing heavy bleeding, your doctor may recommend a procedure called a *D&C*, which stands for "dilation and curettage." This is when your cervix is gently opened and the contents of the uterus removed. Sometimes medications are prescribed to aid in the process as well.

You should not worry that you did something to cause a miscarriage. There is no proof that engaging in everyday activities such as exercise, working, or sex causes miscarriage. Birth control pills do not cause a woman to miscarry. You should be able to get pregnant again and carry the baby without any problems following a miscarriage. In fact, you can ovulate as soon as two weeks following a miscarriage, so if you do not want to become pregnant, you should ask your doctor about birth control options.

ECTOPIC PREGNANCY

Sometimes, the embryo can be trapped in the fallopian tube or float out into the abdominal cavity. When the developing pregnancy grows outside the uterus, it is known as an ectopic pregnancy. This occurs in about one of every fifty pregnancies and is almost always in the fallopian tube.[2]

As the fetus begins to grow, it can cause the fallopian tube to expand and can lead to rupture of the tube. This is a surgical emergency and can lead to hemorrhage and death if not treated. If the fetus is still small and the tube is not ruptured when an ectopic pregnancy is found, medication can be used to treat you by dissolving the pregnancy. There is no way to transplant the developing embryo from the tube into the uterus.

A prior ectopic pregnancy, previous tubal surgery such as tubal ligation, other abdominal or pelvic surgery (which can lead to scar tissue formation), pelvic inflammatory disease, STDs, infertility, and endometriosis can all increase the chance of a woman developing an ectopic pregnancy.

Symptoms of an ectopic pregnancy include vaginal bleeding, lower abdominal discomfort (often more pronounced on one side), weakness or dizziness (due to blood loss), and shoulder pain (due to the buildup of blood underneath the diaphragm).

If you think that you may have an ectopic pregnancy, you should contact your doctor immediately. Testing may take time and may need to be repeated to establish a definitive diagnosis.

GENETIC TESTING

Many couples worry that their child may be born with a problem, or birth defect. Birth defects are rare, occurring in only three to four per one hundred births.[3] Some birth defects are caused by environmental factors (exposure to a harmful agent), others are passed from the parents to the affected child, and some are a combination of the environment and inheritance.

Chromosome disorders can be caused by a damaged, missing, or extra chromosome and occur when the egg and sperm are joining together. One of the most common chromosome disorders is Down syndrome, which is caused by an extra copy of chromosome 21. These disorders occur more commonly as a woman ages. You may be at increased risk for having a child with a birth defect if you are thirty-five or older when your baby is due.

Other factors that increase your chance of having a baby with a birth defect are having a family or personal history of birth defects, having a previous child with a birth defect, taking certain medications during your pregnancy, and having diabetes that is not well controlled.

There are tests that can be performed to assess your risk for certain birth defects. Carrier testing is offered if either parent carries a genetic defect or if you are at an increased risk of carrying the genetic defect based on your history. Cystic fibrosis is a common genetic disorder that all women should be offered testing for. If a woman is found to be a carrier for a recessive disorder, her partner can be tested to see if the baby is at risk of being affected.

As a Christian, you may struggle with the thoughts of pursuing these tests. A child is truly a gift from God, and you may feel that you should accept whatever gift is given to you. While that may be true, some people find that it is easier to prepare for how their life will be changed if they are caring for a child with special needs. Rest assured that God will give you the strength you need to make it through this time, and He has prepared a special life for you to care for.

Scott Farhart and Elizabeth King, *The Christian Woman's Complete Guide to Health* (Lake Mary, FL: Siloam, 2008), 163–171.

PREGNANCY: THE SECOND TRIMESTER

by Scott Farhart, MD, and Elizabeth King, MD

T HE SECOND TRIMESTER is usually the most enjoyable time during a pregnancy. By the start of the second trimester, most of the time morning sickness resolves. This is also when you will begin to look pregnant, or to "show." And best of all, you now can feel your baby move. If this is your first pregnancy, you may make it almost halfway through your pregnancy before you feel your baby move. Usually you will feel the first little flutters around eighteen weeks. At first, the movements you feel may seem like trapped gas or butterflies in your stomach. If you have been pregnant before, you may feel movement a little earlier, around sixteen weeks. However, do not worry if you do not feel movement until twenty weeks.

As your baby grows, the movements will become more distinct. By the time you reach your third trimester, you may be able to identify specific body parts protruding under your skin.

GENETIC TESTING

A maternal serum screening is offered in the second trimester. This is a blood test that is done between fifteen and twenty weeks to screen for neural tube defects, abdominal wall defects, trisomy 18, and Down syndrome (trisomy 21). It is commonly referred to as the quad screen because it looks at the following four substances in a woman's blood to help estimate her risk of carrying a fetus with one of the above disorders:

1. Estriol—a hormone similar to estrogen, found in the mom, baby, and placenta
2. Human chorionic gonadotropin (hCG)—a hormone made by the placenta responsible for maintaining the pregnancy
3. Alpha-fetoprotein (AFP)—made by the fetus but passed into the maternal bloodstream in small amounts
4. Inhibin A—a hormone produced by the placenta

If the screening test is positive, indicating an increased risk of having a baby affected with one of the above disorders, a diagnostic test can be performed.[1]

ULTRASOUND

Most doctors will perform a basic ultrasound between eighteen and twenty weeks to evaluate the fetal position, size and number, placental location, amniotic fluid volume, heart rate, and anatomy. This is when you can learn the sex of your baby, if you desire. Most of the time a transabdominal ultrasound is performed, with the probe of the ultrasound placed on the abdomen. However, in special situations, such as evaluating the cervix or placenta and during the first trimester, a transvaginal ultrasound may be performed. There are now centers offering keepsake ultrasound videos and pictures using the new 3-D and 4-D technology. This offers a "lifelike" look at your baby inside the womb.

Scott Farhart and Elizabeth King, *The Christian Woman's Complete Guide to Health* (Lake Mary, FL: Siloam, 2008), 172–177.

PREGNANCY: THE THIRD TRIMESTER

by Scott Farhart, MD, and Elizabeth King, MD

T HE THIRD TRIMESTER is an exciting time as the fetal movement is a lot stronger and you can see the movements through your skin. Your husband can also begin to feel the baby, which makes him more a part of this process. Up until now, he has had to take your word for things and watch your body change from a distance. But now he can experience some of the things you do when he feels the baby kick through your skin.

This trimester is also the time of rapid fetal growth. From about the seventh to ninth months, the baby doubles in size. Just when you think you can't possibly hold any more or stretch any further, he or she sprints up the growth chart to prove you wrong.

The rapid growth may bring some unpleasant side effects to your skin, such as stretch marks. These are actually tears in your skin that resemble scars and are bright pink. Over time, these fade to a more natural skin tone and shrink in length and width.

Most women will also notice a brown line begin to form in the middle of their abdomen that starts at the bottom and progressively rises higher as the pregnancy goes along. This is called the *linea nigra* and is a normal sign of pregnancy.

Hands and feet may begin to swell in the late third trimester. Some of this is from the weight of the baby pressing on your lower pelvic blood vessels. The blood pumps down the legs, but it gets harder to get it back up. This causes the blood vessel to "leak" fluid into the surrounding tissues. Salt can also leak out, causing water to follow it. This is one reason women swell. If you work outside the home or are on your feet a lot, swelling will almost surely happen. We only get concerned about it if it is accompanied by high blood pressure. If you have sudden swelling, you may be asked to come to the office to check your blood pressure.

As the third trimester comes to an end, you will notice more contractions occurring, especially in the evening. Some may be mild, tightening only, and some may be stronger, the so-called Braxton-Hicks contractions, which are relatively painless and are usually felt as a tightening or hardness in the abdomen. However, sometimes they are painful, making it difficult to tell them apart from true labor contractions.

Braxton-Hicks contractions are also known as false labor pains, because they do not usually cause the cervix to dilate much. They do get your body ready for labor and can soften and open your cervix a little. They usually become more frequent the closer you get to your due date and are more common following sexual intercourse, physical activity, and in the evening. They can also occur when a woman is dehydrated, so it is important to drink plenty of fluids. If you are having Braxton-Hicks contractions prior to thirty-seven weeks, it is important to monitor them. If you have more than four or five in an hour, you should call your doctor.

Scott Farhart and Elizabeth King, *The Christian Woman's Complete Guide to Health* (Lake Mary, FL: Siloam, 2008), 179–186.

CHILDBIRTH

by Scott Farhart, MD, and Elizabeth King, MD

L ABOR AND DELIVERY is a process that makes it hard to maintain your dignity. You will feel exposed and vulnerable. Your husband and any other family or friends you choose to involve in the process will see you in a light you may feel is less than desirable. Many people get nauseous during labor, and you may throw up. During the process of pushing the baby out, you use some of the same muscles used to have a bowel movement, and you may in fact do so while pushing. In the past, enemas were used in the early stages of labor to help evacuate any stool prior to the birth of the baby. Now, most obstetricians have abandoned that process, as it served no benefit to either mom or baby.

As for episiotomy, it is sometimes necessary to assist in delivery of the baby. This is where your doctor may need to cut to widen the vagina so the baby will fit. Sometimes this is done in an attempt to keep the vagina from tearing badly. We used to think it was preferable to perform this procedure rather than letting the woman tear; however, current studies have shown women are more likely to suffer complications of incontinence following episiotomy because it can create a weak point, making further tearing more likely.[1] Most obstetricians now try to avoid episiotomy for these reasons. If you do tear or need an episiotomy, stitches will be placed to repair the area. These sutures will dissolve on their own but will require some care and avoiding intercourse for a time while they heal.

After delivery, your body will be overcome with a rush of adrenaline, causing extreme shaking. This normal and natural response worries some moms. After the baby is born, the delivery is not yet complete. The placenta, or afterbirth, needs to be delivered. This often does not require any work or pushing from the mom, but it can be felt and, when completed, provides a sense of relief.

INDUCED LABOR

Sometimes your doctor may allow induction of labor for elective purposes. Induction of labor is not without risks, however. Being induced can put you at an increased risk of needing a cesarean section. This is especially the case if your cervix is not "ripe." Your cervix will be examined by your doctor to evaluate both dilation and effacement (thinning). If your cervix has not dilated or effaced much, he or she may use a cervical ripening agent the evening before to begin the induction process. This is usually placed into the vagina and helps to soften the cervix.

If your cervix has already started to dilate, your doctor may strip your membranes to get you to go into labor. This is done by sweeping the examining finger over the membranes that connect the bag of water to the lower part of the uterus. This causes your body to release chemicals that ripen the cervix and may cause contractions. Other ways to induce labor include breaking your water and giving a medication called pitocin through the IV. To break your water, your doctor will perform a vaginal exam and then make a hole in the amniotic sac. Pitocin is a hormone that is found naturally in the body (oxytocin) and is responsible for causing contractions.

ASSISTED DELIVERIES: VACUUM AND FORCEPS

Most of the time, deliveries occur without any problems. However, there are some cases where your doctor may need to intervene for your health or the health of your baby. There are certain medical conditions affecting the mother that can make pushing hard on her body. Sometimes the mom just becomes exhausted after hours of pushing and is too tired. The baby's position may make it difficult for the mom to push, and sometimes the heart rate will drop down, necessitating a quick delivery.

One way your doctor can assist in the delivery of your baby is by placing forceps around its head. These look like big spoons and work by guiding the head under the pubic bone through the birth canal. Another device that is sometimes used is a vacuum extractor. This is a suction cup that attaches to the baby's head with an attached handle that allows your doctor to pull as you push. Most of the time when these devices are used, there are no problems.

CESAREAN SECTION

About one out of every four babies is born by cesarean section in this country, making it a very common procedure these days. Sometimes it is planned, while in other cases it is performed because of a problem or emergency that arises during labor. Some reasons for performing a cesarean delivery include the following circumstances: previous cesarean delivery, breech presentation, placenta previa, infections, multiple pregnancy, failure to progress, and fetal distress.

If you undergo a planned cesarean delivery, a spinal block is usually used for anesthesia. This is similar to an epidural in that medication is put next to the spinal cord; however, a catheter is not placed, so it is a single dose. In the case where a cesarean is performed for a problem arising during labor, an epidural can usually be used if already in place. The anesthesiologist simply injects additional medication into the catheter to numb the lower abdomen and pelvis. If an emergency cesarean needs to be performed, you may have to undergo general anesthesia (get put to sleep).

Most of the time, a cesarean section is performed through a small horizontal incision on the lower abdomen just above the pubic bone. This is commonly referred to as a "bikini cut." A similar, small horizontal incision is usually then made on the uterus, through which the baby is delivered. The placenta is then removed, and the uterus is then sewn back up. The procedure takes about thirty minutes to do. If you are awake, you may feel some pressure or tugging as your baby is pushed out of you by the assistant or doctor performing the surgery, which is normal. Most of the time, you are able to see your baby immediately and may even be able to hold him or her in the delivery room.

Scott Farhart and Elizabeth King, *The Christian Woman's Complete Guide to Health* (Lake Mary, FL: Siloam, 2008), 187–197.

INFERTILITY: CAUSES AND TREATMENTS

by Scott Farhart, MD, and Elizabeth King, MD

WHILE AGING IS a primary factor of infertility, especially after age thirty-five, medical diseases can play a role as well. Polycystic ovarian syndrome (PCOS) is a common reason women do not ovulate. There is speculation that local insulin levels may be too high and suppress ovulation. Body fat stores estrogen and sends false messages to the brain that estrogen levels are sufficient, altering the signals sent by the brain to the ovaries to spur ovulation. Thyroid disease can send similar false signals from the brain, which disrupts ovulation. Certain medications for psychiatric or neurological conditions impact ovulation at the level of the brain. Even strenuous exercise and anorexia play a role in these brain chemistries.

Besides ovulation, other factors causing female infertility involve reproductive organs such as the cervix, the uterus, and the tubes. Uterine abnormalities come into play when it is time for the embryo to implant. A final factor in female infertility is endometriosis.

FERTILITY EVALUATION FOR WOMEN

The first thing that is evaluated is ovulation. If an egg is not released, there can be no pregnancy. There have been charts made of basal body temperature measurements to predict when ovulation will occur and to document that it did indeed occur.

Secondly, we evaluate the female organs themselves. Transvaginal ultrasonography may be used to assess if the egg was ovulated, to look for ovarian cysts or tumors, and to evaluate uterine abnormalities such as fibroids. Another test is a hysterosalpingogram, or HSG. This is an X-ray of the uterus and tubes done by injecting radioactive material through the opening of the cervix into the uterus. The dye is then spilled out of the tubes if they are open. Abnormalities of the lining of the uterus, such as polyps, fibroids, or embryonic defects, can also be identified. If tubes are scarred closed or if the dye collects at the end of the tube, this signifies reduced fertility.

The third area is surgical tests. An abnormal HSG of the uterus requires hysteroscopy. This involves placing a scope attached to a camera through the cervix to visualize the uterine cavity. The patient is generally asleep. Any abnormalities are directly seen and often treated in the same operative setting to enhance the ability of the embryo to implant. Laparoscopy is a surgical procedure where the same camera is placed through a scope in the navel to evaluate the internal pelvic organs. This is useful in verifying any tubal disease, adhesions, fibroids, or endometriosis. Often treatment can also be done in the same operative encounter.

Treatment for female infertility

The most common treatment for female infertility is clomiphene citrate (or Clomid). This medicine causes ovulation by acting on the pituitary gland. It temporarily decreases the level of estrogen in the body and causes the pituitary to "yell louder" at the ovaries, enhancing ovulation. It is often used in women who have PCOS or other problems with ovulation.

Human menopausal gonadotropin (Repronex, Pergonal) is often used for women who do not ovulate on oral medication. Human menopausal gonadotropin (hMG) acts directly on the ovaries to stimulate ovulation and is an injected medicine. A similar injectable medication is follicle-stimulating hormone, or FSH (Gonal-f, Follistim). It works much like hMG by directly causing the ovaries to ovulate. These medicines are usually injected by the patient's husband.

Negatives for these drugs include pain from daily injections, significantly higher cost, and a sharp increase in the possibility of multiple fetuses: twins, triplets, or greater. Women who are pregnant with multiple fetuses have more problems during pregnancy, and their fetuses have a high risk of being born prematurely with all of the health and developmental problems that go with it.

MALE INFERTILITY

Male infertility comprises one-third of cases and focuses on sperm. Certain conditions may be associated with male infertility. These conditions include infection of the prostate or testicles from STDs or other bacterial causes. The prostate gland is the main organ responsible for making semen, the vehicle that carries sperm out of the man with ejaculation. Infection alters the semen quality. It also brings white blood cells that mistakenly attack swimming sperm in their attempt to destroy harmful bacteria.

Other conditions include varicocele. These are varicose veins of the scrotum. It is thought that the pooling of blood from these veins causes an increase in the local temperature of the testes, impacting sperm survival.

Abnormal male chromosomes impact sperm formation. One such condition is known as Klinefelter's syndrome. Instead of the usual XY chromosomes that most men have, these men have an extra X chromosome, making them XXY. This may be from a faulty egg or fertilization by two sperm instead of one. While not every man with extra chromosomes has infertility issues, some do.[1]

There are other sources of male infertility. Some men have undergone radiation treatment for cancer therapy and have sustained damage to the testes as a result. Others have had diseases such as mumps that can cause shrinking of the testicles, or they have experienced traumatic injury to the testicles. Even previous surgical procedures from childhood such as hernia repair can impair blood flow to the testes.

Fertility evaluation for men

An analysis of the man's semen is a key part of the basic workup. He is asked to abstain from intercourse for at least three days. The sample is obtained by masturbation into a sterile cup that is then analyzed in a lab about one hour later. The sperm is evaluated for mobility. It is of no use to have sperm that cannot swim and make the journey needed to fertilize the egg. Other values measured include the pH and any signs of infection.

If a low sperm count or a high percentage of sperm abnormalities are found, blood tests may be done to measure testosterone or a biopsy of the testes may be ordered.

Fertility treatment for men

One of first things that a urologist will recommend to men who are trying to conceive a child is to minimize those factors that impair sperm production.

Some urologists and fertility specialists advocate intrauterine insemination (IUI) as another type of treatment for male infertility. IUI is known by most people as artificial insemination. In this procedure, the woman is injected through the cervix with specially prepared sperm from her husband to concentrate and place those sperm as close to the opening of the fallopian tube as possible. This reduces the tremendous loss in numbers that occurs in the normal journey from the vagina to the tubes and shortens the "swim" necessary to the waiting egg. Because the timing of this procedure is critical to its success, the woman must also be ovulating on the same day.

Finally, for those with very low counts, poor motility, or high numbers of abnormal shapes, a technique called intracytoplasmic sperm injection (ICSI) can be offered. In this technique, a single sperm is extracted and inserted into an egg to achieve fertilization. This embryo is then placed into the uterus. This technique is sometimes used in those couples where the man has had a previous vasectomy and there is no other way to extract sperm from him.

Scott Farhart and Elizabeth King, *The Christian Woman's Complete Guide to Health* (Lake Mary, FL: Siloam, 2008), 151–162.

BIRTH CONTROL

by Scott Farhart, MD, and Elizabeth King, MD

CONTRACEPTION IS AN extremely sensitive issue among believers of differing doctrines. While we realize that some reading this may be offended, our objective is only to help readers. Just as marriage takes two people, the choice for contraception and having children should also be a mutual decision.

NATURAL FAMILY PLANNING

A popular form of birth control is natural family planning (NFP). Also called "the rhythm method," it is the exact opposite of the method used to enhance fertility. To use NFP, a woman attempts to discover the most fertile times of her cycle and avoids having intercourse on those days of the month. This method requires no drugs or devices and is absolutely free. It does not interfere with the body's own reproductive cycle.

BARRIER METHODS

The next class of birth control is called the "barrier method." It involves blocking the entrance of sperm into the cervical canal to prevent fertilization of the egg. There are four types of products used in this method: spermicides, diaphragm, cervical cap, and condoms.

BIRTH CONTROL PILLS

Most birth control pills come in four-week packets that contain three consecutive weeks of hormones, followed by one week of placebo or "sugar" pills that signal the uterus to menstruate. When that menstrual week is over, a new round of pills begins again.

There is a form of birth control called the "morning-after pill" (or emergency contraception in the medical community) specifically designed for cases where the condom breaks or a woman has not used contraception prior to intercourse and desires pregnancy prevention after the fact. It must be taken within three days of intercourse. If taken as prescribed, it is 89 percent effective in preventing pregnancy. If the woman is already pregnant, it will not cause abortion. Even if taken correctly, 11 percent of women will still conceive. The earlier the pill is taken following intercourse, the better it will work.

OTHER BIRTH CONTROL PRODUCTS

Another from of contraception is Ortho Evra, a patch that is worn once a week for three weeks followed by one week off to allow menstruation. Women who are healthy and do not smoke can use the patch with very little real-life risk.

Another form of contraception is the NuvaRing, a flexible plastic ring the size of a fifty-cent piece. It is inserted by the woman into the vagina and left there for three weeks. It is removed in the fourth week to allow menstruation. Neither the woman nor her partner can feel the ring when it is properly placed.

A new contraceptive rod called Implanon has recently been introduced. It is a single flexible rod inserted under the skin of the arm to release progesterone for up to three years. It is a very effective method of birth control that is easily reversible.

Another product, Depo-Provera, is an injection of progesterone given every three months in the doctor's office. The injection usually results in a cessation of menses after a few months and can be of great benefit to those women who suffer from heavy monthly bleeding, severe menstrual cramping, or PMS.

The side effects are irregular bleeding and weight gain that averages 10 to 15 pounds over a year. In general, it provides some of the most effective contraception available that is still reversible.[1] Because the injections last for up to six months but must be overlapped every three months, there are at least six to nine months from the last injection before a woman can conceive. This must be accounted for in any contraceptive strategy a woman makes with her physician.

Continuous Birth Control

A product called *Seasonique* is a thirteen-week pill pack that contains twelve weeks of birth control pills followed by one week of placebo pills. This pattern will give a period every three months, or four times a year. A similar product called *Lybrel* is a monthly pack with no placebo week that is taken daily throughout the year to completely avoid periods.

The IUD

There are two types of IUDs in the United States: the ParaGard and the Mirena. The Mirena is a progesterone-containing device that releases the hormone locally. It does not cross into the blood-stream. The device causes the uterine lining to become thin and does impede implantation. Because the lining is thin, most women will cease menstruating. The Mirena can last up to five years.

ParaGard is a T-shaped device that contains copper, a naturally occurring spermicide designed to kill any sperm that enter the uterus. It is effective for up to ten years. It does not change the uterine lining, but should the sperm live in spite of the spermicidal effect of the copper, implantation may be prevented by the T-shaped design blocking entrance of the embryo into the uterus.

If pregnancy does occur, it is more likely to be ectopic. This is a serious situation that demands immediate attention. Fortunately it is very uncommon. Should pregnancy occur in the womb, the IUD must be removed if one hopes to prevent damage to the developing fetus. Removal of the IUD can carry a 25 percent miscarriage rate, depending on the proximity of the fetus to the IUD.[2] The IUD is used in our practice primarily for married couples who think they may be finished with childbearing but do not want to make a permanent commitment to sterilization.

Permanent Sterilization

The options are tubal ligation for the woman or vasectomy for the man. Vasectomy is simpler and safer, but a vasectomy does not become effective for several weeks. Tubal ligation involves interrupting each fallopian tube and preventing the union of egg and sperm. This can be done laparoscopically through a small incision in the navel by clamping or burning the tubes. A variation called Essure involves blocking the tubes from inside the uterus and can be done in an office setting with some sedation, eliminating the need for an incision or general anesthesia.

Scott Farhart and Elizabeth King, *The Christian Woman's Complete Guide to Health* (Lake Mary, FL: Siloam, 2008), 106–117.

STDS

by Scott Farhart, MD, and Elizabeth King, MD

S EXUALLY TRANSMITTED DISEASES can be divided into categories: bacterial or viral, or acquired by skin contact or through bodily fluids. Here are some common STDs.

CHLAMYDIA

Chlamydia is transmitted through oral, vaginal, or anal intercourse. Symptoms include pus or discharge from the penis or vagina and, in men, may result in painful urination. These symptoms present within one to three weeks after exposure to the bacteria.

If left untreated, chlamydia may develop into pelvic inflammatory disease (PID), a serious infection of the reproductive organs. The infection spreads from the cervix to the uterus, through the fallopian tubes, and into the pelvic cavity where it circulates throughout the abdomen. PID causes tremendous pain, fever, chills, nausea, and vomiting, requiring hospitalization for many to receive intravenous antibiotics and pain medication.

PID can cause scarring of the fallopian tubes, which can block the tubes and prevent fertilization from taking place. PID is the chief cause of ectopic pregnancy, where the embryo gets "stuck" in the fallopian tube. The placenta then penetrates the wall of the tube, causing it to rupture. The hemorrhage caused by this rupture can be substantial, making ectopic pregnancy the leading cause of death in women due to pregnancy.[1]

GONORRHEA

Gonorrhea causes infections in the genital tract, mouth, and rectum—anywhere that bodily fluids are exchanged. It is often diagnosed in the same individual who has chlamydia, prompting laboratories to include gonorrhea testing whenever chlamydia is also sought.

Symptoms of the disease usually manifest within seven to ten days after exposure. For women, symptoms include bleeding after intercourse, painful urination, vaginal discharge, and PID. The most common and serious complication of gonorrhea in women is PID. Cervical mucus prevents the spread of sexually transmitted diseases (STDs) inward except during ovulation, when the organism may be carried on the backs of sperm, and menses, when the cervix opens to let menstrual blood escape. STDs in the vagina can also be pushed upward during the douching process. For that reason, among others, douching is not recommended by most gynecologists.

Men infected with gonorrhea experience pus draining from the urethra and painful urination. Infants exposed to gonorrhea at birth can develop eye infections, which are now routinely prevented by giving antibiotic ointments at birth in most states in this country. Prolonged exposure to gonorrhea can lead to arthritis, damage to heart valves, and inflammation of the brain.

SYPHILIS

Syphilis is caused by a form of bacterium that infects through skin-to-skin contact and is poorly prevented by condom use.[2] It initially leaves an ulcer on the skin and then moves inside the body, eventually damaging internal organs if left untreated. While it is fairly easy to treat with antibiotics if caught early, it is often not diagnosed because it resembles so many other diseases.

Scott Farhart and Elizabeth King, *The Christian Woman's Complete Guide to Health* (Lake Mary, FL: Siloam, 2008), 60–73.

HPV—HUMAN PAPILLOMAVIRUS

by Scott Farhart, MD, and Elizabeth King, MD

O NE OF THE most common STDs in the world today is the human papillomavirus, or HPV. An estimated 20 million Americans are currently infected, with 6.2 million new cases diagnosed each year. At least 50 percent of sexually active men and women acquire genital HPV infection at some point in their lives. According to the CDC, by age fifty, at least 80 percent of women will have acquired genital HPV infection.[1]

How is genital HPV contracted?

Genital HPV is spread primarily through sexual contact, either skin to skin or through bodily fluid exchange. Risk factors include the number of sexual partners, age at first intercourse of sixteen or younger, number of sexual partners her male partner has had, and smoking.[2]

What are the symptoms of HPV?

While visible genital warts are the most easily recognizable form of the disease, half of all women and the majority of men have no symptoms. Most women are diagnosed at their annual gynecologic examination when their Pap smear returns abnormal. HPV is highly contagious by oral, genital, or anal sex, and two-thirds of people exposed to it will develop the disease within three months of contact. Most teens and adults will clear their infections spontaneously, but the virus may remain dormant for years. This has made determining when and with whom the virus was contracted a nearly impossible task. For women, the common sites of HPV infection are the cervix, the vaginal opening, and the anus. Men can experience lesions at the penis, scrotum, and anus.[3]

What are the possible complications?

Two main complications of HPV can occur. The first is cancer of the genital organs in both males and females. Precancerous lesions, formerly called dysplasia, can be detected in women by a Pap smear of the cells lining the cervix. Other lesions may be diagnosed on the genitals of both men and women through biopsy of abnormal skin lesions. For women, a yearly Pap smear beginning with the onset of sexual activity, along with a visual inspection of the genital region by a health-care provider, is the best defense against genital cancers.

What treatment options are available?

Genital warts may clear spontaneously, remain the same, or grow in size. These lesions can be treated with topical agents, freezing, electrocautery, or laser. Most of these treatments require medical application in either an office setting or an outpatient surgical suite, depending on the extent of the lesions. Smaller warts can be treated at home if the patient desires and can safely self-administer the topical solution available by prescription under the name Condylox or the gel under the prescribed name of Aldara.

Treatments can be painful and expensive. They are designed to rid the body of the visible warts but not the invisible virus. HPV can persist in the body for a lifetime with periodic recurrences.

Scott Farhart and Elizabeth King, *The Christian Woman's Complete Guide to Health* (Lake Mary, FL: Siloam, 2008), 60–73.

HIV AND AIDS

by Scott Farhart, MD, and Elizabeth King, MD

HUMAN IMMUNODEFICIENCY VIRUS, or HIV, is the agent responsible for AIDS. HIV damages the immune system, rendering its victims unable to defend themselves against infectious diseases or cancer.

While the largest population of individuals infected with HIV continues to be gay men, women now account for nearly 30 percent of all new cases. Of the HIV/AIDS diagnoses for women during 2001–2004, an estimated 15 percent were for women aged thirteen to twenty-four years.[1]

The HIV virus is actually difficult to contract. It dies when exposed to the air, cannot be left behind on toilet seats or telephone receivers, and cannot be passed by shaking hands with someone. It must travel inside bodily fluids such as semen, blood, vaginal secretions, and in some cases saliva. It is often not contracted by those exposed to it.

HIV acts slowly and silently. Many of its victims are without symptoms for months or even years, outwardly appearing completely normal to everyone else. With the hosts unaware of their infectious state and free to mingle with the uninfected, the virus is silently passed from one person to another.

Many people contract the disease from a single individual. In every country where its origins have been traced, the virus is concentrated first in homosexual men and intravenous drug users. These people frequently share blood-tinged needles or have sex with multiple partners over a short period of time. Soon, the girlfriend of the IV drug user contracts it from heterosexual sex or the bisexual male brings it home to his suburban wife, and the virus has entered a new arena.

AIDS

AIDS, or *acquired immunodeficiency syndrome*, is a condition caused by HIV. The virus becomes incorporated into the genetic makeup of the human cell, preferring the white blood cells called lymphocytes. These cells are a major part of our immune system, protecting us against infection and cancer. The virus progressively destroys the immune system, leaving its victim vulnerable to unusual infections and rare cancers that a healthy person would not encounter. The infected person develops AIDS. The diagnosis is based on the development of certain infections in the presence of HIV that signals a critical loss of the immune system. A person does not die directly from HIV itself but from the infections and tumors he cannot defend himself against.[2]

There are antiviral medications that can reduce the number of viral particles in the blood because the higher the viral count, the more infectious the person. Also, the higher count usually reflects a poorer immune system. Drugs to decrease the viral load are not curative, but they have been crucial to the fight to make HIV/AIDS a chronic disease one lives with for decades. It will eventually kill the individual, but not as rapidly as when first diagnosed in the 1980s.

Antiviral medications are critical to preventing the spread of HIV from a mother to her infant at birth, called perinatal transmission. Nearly all HIV transmission to newborns and children in the United States could be prevented if the mother were diagnosed and treated early with these medications. Often cesarean section is recommended to avoid contact by the baby with his mother's blood. Breast-feeding is also discouraged as the virus can be transmitted through breast milk.[3]

Scott Farhart and Elizabeth King, *The Christian Woman's Complete Guide to Health* (Lake Mary, FL: Siloam, 2008), 60–73.

YEAST INFECTIONS

by Don Colbert, MD

Y**EAST IS ACTUALLY** a single-celled organism that under normal conditions lives in our bodies without causing us any problems. Nearly three pounds of friendly bacteria in our intestines help to keep it in check. These friendly bacteria help our bodies maintain a balance of power between the good bacteria and the yeast.

That's until we upset this delicate balance with antibiotics, prednisone, hormones such as estrogen and progesterone, too much stress, diabetes, or by eating too much sugar and highly processed foods. These things can swing the balance of power, causing an overgrowth of yeast to occur.

SYMPTOMS OF YEAST OVERGROWTH

Here are the symptoms according to the system that is affect by yeast.

- Nervous system: fatigue, memory loss, insomnia, depression, mood swings, sleepiness, attention-deficit disorder, hyperactivity, autistic tendencies
- Endocrine system: extreme fatigue as a result of adrenal exhaustion, which can lead to chronic fatigue; overactive or underactive thyroid; skin problems such as eczema, hives, psoriasis, and acne
- Immune system: food allergies and food sensitivities
- Digestive system: difficulty breaking down proteins into amino acids, intestinal permeability or leaky gut syndrome, inability to absorb vital nutrients through the small intestines
- Reproductive system: tinia cruris (jock itch), yeast infections, vaginitis, prosatitis

TREATMENT FOR YEAST OVERGROWTH

There are several ways to bring bacterial balance back to your body, including diet, supplements, medications, detoxification, and lifestyle changes.

Dietary recommendations

- Limit sugar intake.
- Avoid dairy products that contain lactose.
- Avoid refined carbohydrates.
- Avoid foods that contain yeast, mold, or vinegar such as certain breads and cheeses, condiments, preserved and processed meats, nuts when stored improperly, mushrooms, leftovers more than a day or two old, and alcoholic beverages.
- Avoid allergy-causing foods such as chocolate, wheat, corn, and citrus fruits.
- Eat raw, steamed, or stir-fried veggies that have a low glycemic index.
- Consume high-quality protein such as free-range beef or chicken and fatty fish with omega-3 fatty acids such as salmon, mackerel, herring, or sardines.
- Add the right kinds of fat to your diet: extra-virgin olive oil, flaxseed oil, organic butter, and cold-pressed vegetable oil.
- Add fiber to your diet with psyllium seed, fruit pectin, oat bran (if tolerated), and rice bran.

- Try plain, organic goat's milk kefir or organic coconut-milk kefir. (Kefir is similar to yogurt but contains more strains of good bacteria.)

Supplements

- Garlic
- Goldenseal
- Grapefruit seed extract
- Caprylic acid
- Oil of oregano
- Tanalbit
- Chlorophyll (green food)

Medications

- Nystatin

Detoxification

- Take a comprehensive multivitamin.
- Eat at least one serving a week of cruciferous vegetables such as broccoli, cauliflower, brussels sprouts, and cabbage.
- Restore your liver with milk thistle, glutathione, and lipoic acid supplements.
- Restore friendly bacteria with supplements of Lactobacillus acidophilus and Bifido bacteria. Other good probiotics include Theralac, Sustenex, and QuantaBiotica.

Lifestyle changes

- Get at least eight hours of sleep.
- Minimize stress.

Don Colbert, *The Bible Cure for Candida and Yeast Infections* (Lake Mary, FL: Siloam, 2001).

KNOW YOUR BODY

by Janet Maccaro, PhD, CNC

A s A WOMAN with so many things to keep in balance, it is imperative that you take inventory of your body and see just where your weaknesses are. You may find that some of your complaints seem to run in your family or are hereditary. Don't let this alarm you. This simply means that those weak areas need more attention or strengthening. For each biological system listed, check the appropriate boxes that correspond to your body.

KNOW YOUR BODY SELF-ASSESSMENT SCREENING

Your gastrointestinal system	Your respiratory system
❑ Stomach pain	❑ Chronic cough
❑ Fatigue after eating	❑ Asthma
❑ Frequent heartburn	❑ Emphysema
❑ Frequent constipation	❑ Recurrent head colds
❑ Irritable bowel syndrome	❑ Recurrent sinus problems
❑ Hemorrhoids	❑ Recurrent bronchitis
❑ Vomiting	❑ Smoking (cigar or cigarettes)
❑ Colitis	**Your genitourinary tract**
❑ Gallbladder trouble	❑ Too frequent urination
❑ Frequent burping	❑ Blood in your urine
❑ Nausea	❑ Recurrent kidney or bladder problems
❑ Ulcers	❑ Kidney stones
Your structural/neurological system	❑ Inability to control bladder
❑ Headaches	**Eyes and ears**
❑ Muscle cramps	❑ Recurrent ear infections
❑ Neck pain	❑ Eye infections
❑ Jaw pain	❑ Floaters in your eyes
❑ Dizziness	❑ Glaucoma
❑ Back pain	❑ Macular degeneration
❑ Shoulder, elbow, wrist pain	❑ Cataracts
❑ Knee, hip pain	**Your endocrine/glandular system**
❑ Joint pain or loss of function	❑ Cold hands and feet
❑ Osteoporosis or osteomalacia	❑ Low blood pressure
❑ Tendonitis, bursitis	❑ Weight problems, over or under
Your cardiovascular system	❑ Thyroid problems
❑ Irregular heartbeat	❑ Diabetes
❑ Heart murmur or palpitations	❑ Irritability if meals are missed

❏ High or low blood pressure	❏ Dizzy upon standing too quickly
❏ Chest pain	❏ Depression
❏ Poor circulation	❏ Frequent headaches
❏ Previous heart surgery	❏ Digestive complaints
❏ Varicose or spider veins	❏ Recurrent urinary tract infections
❏ Cold hands and feet	❏ Yeast infections
Your immune system	❏ Menstrual irregularity
❏ Frequently sick	❏ Cramping
❏ Swollen glands	❏ Mood swings, depression
❏ Sore throats	❏ Premenstrual syndrome
❏ Depression and/or anxiety	❏ Infertility
❏ Achy joints, muscle pain	❏ Frequent miscarriages
❏ Headaches, migraines	❏ Hot flashes
❏ Recurrent digestive complaints	❏ Currently taking hormone medications
❏ Chronic fatigue	❏ Currently taking birth control pills
❏ Food allergies	❏ Lumps in your breast
❏ Eczema or hives	❏ Uterine fibroids, ovarian cysts
❏ Allergies	❏ Leaky bladder
	❏ Endometriosis

Janet Maccaro, *A Woman's Body Balanced by Nature* (Lake Mary, FL: Siloam, 2006), 5–11.

A WOMAN'S GASTROINTESTINAL SYSTEM
by Janet Maccaro, PhD, CNC

A WOMAN'S GASTROINTESTINAL SYSTEM is delicately balanced and can be disrupted by stress, both good and bad, which can lead to emotional overeating and poor food choices or combinations, such as fried, fatty, or sugary foods that can slow down transit time and lead to constipation. Bowel flora imbalance and digestive enzyme deficiency can create uncomfortable bloating and gas.

Achieving gastrointestinal balance

If you checked any of the symptoms for your gastrointestinal system in the Know Your Body Self-Assessment Screening, you should consider taking digestive enzymes from a plant source with every meal. Digestive enzymes are *crucial* for proper food assimilation. DicQie Fuller, in her informative book *The Healing Power of Enzymes*, has stated: "Any time we suffer from an acute or chronic illness, it is almost certain an enzyme depletion problem exists."[1]

Did you check the box for *frequent heartburn*? Many cases of heartburn, acid reflux, and acid indigestion are the result of insufficient hydrochloric acid production in the stomach. Anytime you experience insufficient stomach acid for proper digestion, food begins to ferment. Fermentation in the stomach creates gas. When your stomach expands from this gas, the gas travels upward toward the esophagus. As it continues to push into the esophagus, stomach acid enters with it. When stomach acid reaches the esophagus, a burning sensation occurs in the throat and creates heartburn. Over-the-counter antacids actually compound digestive problems by neutralizing stomach acid. This is not conducive to a healthy digestive tract. When your stomach becomes less acidic, your system can become a welcoming home to bad bacteria, candida, parasites, and intestinal toxemia.[2] Use Betaine HCL at mealtimes, which will help to insure that your stomach contains enough acid for proper digestion and relief of troublesome digestive disturbance symptoms.

If constipation and hemorrhoids are a problem, you should know that a poor diet plays a huge part in the development of these two conditions. Too little fiber, too many fried foods, too much sugar, and too much red meat, caffeine, and alcohol are the biggest culprits. Not drinking enough water (especially when traveling), lack of exercise, hypothyroidism, and the use of antidepressant drugs are major factors for women. Proper elimination is crucial.

Another common condition that seems to strike women more often than men is irritable bowel syndrome (IBS). This may be due to the fact that most contributing factors are common to the lifestyle of women today. Most IBS sufferers are women between the ages of twenty and forty years old, with A-type personalities and stressful jobs or lifestyles. Women who are anxious, tense, coffee drinkers, lactose sensitive, or who have taken repeated courses of anti-inflammatory drugs or suffer from yeast overgrowth due to antibiotic use are most commonly afflicted.

Colitis is a very painful condition that develops in stages. It may begin with weakness, fatigue, and lethargy, and then be followed by abdominal cramps, distention, and pain, which are relieved by bowel movements. Soon a woman may experience recurrent constipation, alternating with bloody diarrhea and mucus in the stool. Rectal hemorrhoids, fistulas, and abscesses; dehydration; mineral loss; and unhealthy weight loss with abdominal distention occur as this condition progresses.

STEPS TO GASTROINTESTINAL HEALTH

- Eat smaller meals, and chew food well.
- Take a daily walk to stimulate regularity.
- Avoid antacids; often they neutralize HCL in the stomach.
- Reduce stress in your life.
- Clean up your diet by avoiding coffee, caffeinated foods, sodas, nuts, seeds, dairy, and citrus, especially while trying to heal from colitis.
- Eliminate sugary foods, fried foods, sorbitol, and dairy foods (lactose intolerance often affects IBS sufferers). Eliminate wheat (another irritant), and avoid antibiotics, antacids, and milk of magnesia, which destroy friendly bacteria in the intestinal tract.

I recommend that you enjoy some of the delicious herbal teas available to help with digestive problems. Peppermint tea, spearmint tea, and alfalfa mint tea are especially helpful to aid digestion.

QUICK FIXES FROM NATURE

SYMPTOM	REMEDY
Heartburn	Aloe vera juice
Sour stomach	Lime juice with a pinch of ginger
Bloating	½ teaspoon baking soda in water
Poor absorption	Glass of wine with dinner
Flatulence	Slippery elm tea or as an enema; or cinnamon, nutmeg, ginger, and cloves in water

Janet Maccaro, *A Woman's Body Balanced by Nature* (Lake Mary, FL: Siloam, 2006), 12–21.

A WOMAN'S STRUCTURAL/NEUROLOGICAL SYSTEM
by Janet Maccaro, PhD, CNC

D O YOU SUFFER from frequent headaches? Headaches have many causes and fall into several categories. (See secret #127.)

One type of headache called *hormonal headache* is experienced by many women near their cycle or around menopause due to high or excessive estrogen levels. To relieve hormonal headaches, rub natural progesterone cream on your temples.

Structural/neurological problems may also cause muscle cramps and spasms. *Muscle cramps and spasms* are usually caused by vitamin or mineral deficiencies, as well as metabolic insufficiency of magnesium, potassium, calcium, iodine, trace minerals, and vitamins D, E, and B$_6$. In addition, other factors include a lack of adequate HCL in the stomach, allergies, high blood pressure medication, and poor circulation.

GUIDELINES FOR GETTING RID OF HEADACHES

Follow these dietary guidelines:

- Avoid headache triggers such as alcohol, wine, beer, dairy foods, caffeine, sugar, chocolate, wheat, sulfites, nitrates, MSG, and pizza.
- A cup of black coffee can relieve a headache once it has begun.
- Have a green drink daily (Kyo-Green).
- Have a cup of green tea sweetened with stevia.
- Add nuts (almonds), dark leafy greens (for magnesium), broccoli, pineapple, and cherries (for vitamin C).
- Eat turkey to boost serotonin levels.

Make these lifestyle changes:

- Massage therapy
- Therapeutic baths: sea salt, baking soda, and lavender oil
- Chiropractic
- Deep breathing
- Exercise
- Laughter is the best medicine!
- Ice pack applied to the back of the neck; for nausea, place ice pack on the throat
- For tension headache, take a brisk walk and breathe deeply.
- Take time out to focus on relaxation each and every day.

Janet Maccaro, *A Woman's Body Balanced by Nature* (Lake Mary, FL: Siloam, 2006), 21–23.

A WOMAN'S CARDIOVASCULAR SYSTEM

by Janet Maccaro, PhD, CNC

HIGH BLOOD PRESSURE is a major health problem for American women. Middle-aged women have a 90 percent chance of developing high blood pressure.[1] It is often called *the silent killer* because many cases go undiagnosed.

Symptoms of hypertension

- Dizziness
- Swollen ankles
- Great fatigue
- Ringing in the ears
- Red streaks in your eyes
- Frequent headaches and irritability
- Depression
- Kidney malfunction
- Respiratory problems
- Chronic constipation
- Weight gain and fluid retention

High blood pressure goes hand in hand with *circulatory problems* such as varicose and spider veins and cold hands and feet. Symptoms include high cholesterol and triglyceride levels, swollen ankles, chronic headaches, poor memory, dizziness, and shortness of breath.

If your blood pressure is continually 100/60 or below, you have low blood pressure. With it come fatigue, low energy, light-headedness when standing up, nervousness, allergies, and low immunity. The causes for low blood pressure include endocrine or nerve disorders, reaction to medications, electrolyte loss, weak adrenal function, and emotional stress.

The most commonly recognized symptom for cardiovascular problems is chest pain. *Chest pain should always be evaluated by your health-care provider.* Heart attack symptoms are different in women. If you experience any of the following symptoms, you should visit your doctor.

HEART ATTACK SYMPTOMS IN WOMEN

The following symptoms can occur up to a month before a heart attack happens:

- Unexplained shortness of breath, often without pain
- Unusual attacks of indigestion, accompanied by teeth, jaw, ear, and/or back pain
- Poor sleep patterns with accompanying anxiety
- Unexplained unusual fatigue

The following symptoms may indicate a heart attack is imminent:

- Extreme fatigue, weakness, and dizziness
- Shortness of breath with palpitations and cold sweats

Janet Maccaro, *A Woman's Body Balanced by Nature* (Lake Mary, FL: Siloam, 2006), 23–25.

A WOMAN'S IMMUNE SYSTEM

by Janet Maccaro, PhD, CNC

WOMEN WHO LIVE in today's world are all susceptible to stress. Stress, when not managed and dealt with properly, can lower immunity. One sure sign of lowered immunity is chronic infections like colds or respiratory allergies. If you add antibiotic therapy into the mix, you are depressing immunity even more, opening the door to candida yeast infections.

Your immune system is a miraculous healing machine made up of microscopic cells. It attacks and destroys disease-causing invaders and abnormal or infected cells. Your immune system is key to defending you from parasites, toxins, and bacteria. Furthermore, the immune system plays a significant role in helping prevent or reduce the effects of various diseases and much more. A compromised immune system can hinder your body's ability to guard against disease and toxins. It is vitally important for you to restore, strengthen, and balance your immune system. Your immune system requires the right materials to produce the internal medicines to safeguard you from illness. If you are experiencing any of the symptoms of low immunity, the following guidelines will support and strengthen your immunity.

SUPPORTING YOUR IMMUNE SYSTEM

Follow these guidelines to support your immune system for optimal health:

- Consume a diet as close to the "original garden" as possible with plenty of fresh fruits and vegetables, high-fiber foods, seafood, yogurt, and kefir.
- Add garlic and onions to your favorite dishes for added immune-boosting benefit.
- Avoid sugary foods (pies, cakes, etc.), which depress immunity.
- Eliminate fried foods, refined foods, and red meat.

Be aware that sugar consumption inhibits immune function, starting just thirty minutes after consumption and lasting more than five hours. One hundred grams of sugar in any form—honey, table sugar, fructose, or glucose—can reduce the ability of your immune system to engulf and destroy invaders. Women typically reach for sugar in times of stress or tension. This is especially detrimental to our balance, because it makes our bodies acidic and strips us of stabilizing B vitamins. Diseases that are known to be caused in part by excessive sugar consumption are hypoglycemia and diabetes.

Janet Maccaro, *A Woman's Body Balanced by Nature* (Lake Mary, FL: Siloam, 2006), 25–27.

A WOMAN'S ENDOCRINE SYSTEM

by Janet Maccaro, PhD, CNC

A WOMAN'S ENDOCRINE SYSTEM is by far the most delicate and most crucial when it comes to vibrant health, balance, and well-being. The extensive list of symptoms included in the Know Your Body Self-Assessment Screening should tell you that your endocrine system helps to regulate everything from energy flow (thyroid and adrenal glands) to inflammation to your monthly cycle.

Womanhood is a wonderful experience when a woman's system is in balance. The endocrine system is delicately tuned and can become imbalanced, causing discomfort and poor function. From puberty to premenopause to menopause to postmenopause, many women in today's stress-filled world are affected by significant imbalances and fluctuations in their endocrine system, which make life difficult. Fibroids, headaches, PMS, endometriosis, depression, low sex drive, and infertility are all indicative of the need for endocrine balance. Finding and maintaining your hormonal balance is not easy in today's world. In addition to extreme stress, today's environment contains estrogen mimics known as *xenobiotics* or *xenoestrogens*. Xenobiotics have a profound impact on hormone balance. Most of them are petrochemically based. Perfumes, pesticides, soaps, clothing, medicine, microchips, plastics, and medicines all have a petrochemical connection. In addition, growth-promoting hormones are injected into our food supply, particularly in beef and poultry products. This contributes to estrogen dominance in relationship to progesterone levels.

When you add a high-stress lifestyle, which depletes your adrenal glands, you add in another huge player in the endocrine imbalance picture. A natural protocol for balancing your endocrine system complete with lifestyle therapy can help you rebalance your thyroid, adrenal, and reproductive hormone levels gently, thereby bringing harmony to your body and quality of life. An endocrine hormone-balancing program is especially beneficial after periods of stress, trauma, a hysterectomy, childbirth, serious illness, or surgery.

Janet Maccaro, *A Woman's Body Balanced by Nature* (Lake Mary, FL: Siloam, 2006), 30–31.

TEN THINGS WOMEN NEED TO KNOW ABOUT ESTROGEN
by Scott Hannen, DC

HERE ARE TEN things women need to know about estrogen:

1. Many women are estrogen dominant (have too much estrogen), not estrogen deficient.
2. Estrogen dominance is produced in perimenopausal women because of ovulation or lack of ovulation, followed by insufficient production of progesterone.
3. Estrogen dominance is produced in perimenopausal women (ages thirty to mid-fifties) due to erratic cycles or lack of ovulation, when estrogen levels fluctuate rapidly from high to low in the absence of adequate progesterone.
4. Estrogen dominance is produced in postmenopausal women from an excess of estrogen to progesterone ratio. In waning reproductive years, when ovarian production of estrogen declines by 40 to 60 percent, progesterone levels can drop to nearly zero.
5. Estrogen dominance can lead to lowered thyroid function, causing cold intolerance (hands and feet are always cold, low body temperature), depression, anxiety, decreased libido, hair loss, evening fatigue, and acne.
6. Some women have high levels of xenoestrogen (toxic estrogen that is produced from chemicals in our foods, especially meat and dairy, that have biochemical structures that mimic estrogen).
7. Cholesterol is converted into sex hormones (progesterone, estrogen, and testosterone).
8. Adrenal hormones (cortisol and DHEA) can affect the balance of estrogen.
9. Unlike progesterone, which is a single hormone, estrogen is actually used as a general name to represent up to twenty different female hormones of like structure and function. Estrone, estriol, and estradiol are the most researched and appear to be the most important types.
10. The worst type of estrogen is estradiol (E2), yet most hormone replacement therapies (HRT) consist of high levels of this kind of estrogen, with low levels of the other types that are shown to be beneficial.

Scott Hannen, *Healing by Design* (Lake Mary, FL: Siloam, 2003, 2007), 107–108.

PMS

by Reginald Cherry, MD

ANY WOMEN SUDDENLY find themselves weeping, screaming with anger and frustration, or feeling unusually tense with no real external cause. Although the exact causes for premenstrual syndrome are not fully understood, researchers suspect that they are the result of a hormonal imbalance and an increased sensitivity to those unbalanced hormones.

If you are suffering the terrible symptoms of PMS, if it is making you miserable—along with everyone around you—begin to pray and seek God's wisdom as to what path He would have you take to find relief. You don't have to waste one single day to cramps, irritable moods, or discomfort! Begin to pray specifically for the serotonin levels within your brain, that they would come into balance, along with the levels of estrogen and progesterone in your body. Pray for the successful absorption of the necessary vitamins and minerals to help ease your symptoms.

Don't stop at just bringing the problem before the Father in prayer. Do what things you can do naturally to take care of the situation. I recommend that you try the following:

- Get enough rest.
- Try to reduce your stress levels, especially when you sense the onset of symptoms.
- Take a hot bath to ease the cramps.
- Exercise consistently.
- Cut back on the caffeine.
- Begin taking vitamin and nutrient supplements.

Once you have done all that you know to do in following your pathway to healing, stand in faith for it, and expect God to keep His promise.

Reginald Cherry, *Bible Health Secrets* (Lake Mary, FL: Siloam, 2003), 166–168.

PERIMENOPAUSE

by Janet Maccaro, PhD, CNC

PERIMENOPAUSE OCCURS IN women around the age of forty and continues until the early fifties when the menstrual period becomes a thing of the past, signaling the beginning of menopause. During this stage of life, many women experience a decrease or even cessation in their progesterone production because of irregular ovarian cycling and ovarian aging. At the same time, estrogen levels may be excessively or moderately high, causing a troubling continual state of imbalance. This condition is now recognized as "estrogen dominance." And therein lie most of the midlife woman's complaints.

Women may experience a plethora of symptoms, some for years on end. These may include fatigue, breast tenderness, foggy thinking, irritability, headaches, insomnia, decreased sex drive, anxiety, depression, allergy symptoms (including asthma), fat gain (especially around the middle), hair loss, mood swings, memory loss, water retention, bone loss, endometrial cancer, breast cancer, slow metabolism, and many more. Hormonal imbalance has far-reaching effects on many tissues in the body, including the heart, brain, blood vessels, bones, uterus, and breasts.

The key to smooth perimenopause is bringing the levels of estrogen and progesterone back into balance as well as managing stress. Once this is accomplished, women feel wonderful again, complete with vitality, alertness, and optimism. They become more sociable and more nurturing to themselves and others.

In order to bring your estrogen and progesterone back into balance, I recommend using natural progesterone. It not only helps to restore balance, but it also helps to regulate thyroid activity. Natural progesterone is essential for the production of cortisone in the adrenal cortex, and it helps prevent breast cysts.

Natural progesterone has been found to be effective at combating perimenopause anxiety and mood swings. In addition, it plays a very important part in the prevention and reversal of osteoporosis. Natural progesterone offers a woman all of these benefits without a high risk of side effects commonly found in conventional hormone replacement therapy (HRT). The recommended dosage for women in perimenopause is ¼ to ½ teaspoon applied to any clean area of the skin twice a day (morning and evening).

Janet Maccaro, *A Woman's Body Balanced by Nature* (Lake Mary, FL: Siloam, 2006), 185–187.

NATURAL SUBSTANCES TO RELIEVE HORMONAL CHANGES DURING MENOPAUSE

by Reginald Cherry, MD

THERE ARE BASIC substances found in nature that have been proven to provide relief for women who are experiencing hormonal changes in their bodies. They also serve to protect women from developing deadly diseases as they grow older.

Soy and red clover

Soy, especially as an ingredient in tofu and miso, has two primary isoflavins, genistein being the most prominent, and red clover has four. So when these two are taken in combination with each other, the results are powerful!

In addition, soy blocks the receptor sites that would generally bind with the prescription estrogen and cause either breast or uterine cancer.

The genistein present in both soy and red clover inhibits the breakdown of bone in the body and stimulates the formation of new bone. Amazingly, soy and red clover provide powerful symptom relief from menopause and, unlike traditional medical treatments, do not cause breast or uterine cancer or heart problems. In fact, they actually *protect* women from these diseases!

Fifty mg daily of the soy isoflavones and 500 mg daily of red clover leaf extract will bring the greatest benefit.

Black cohosh

Black cohosh, a phytoestrogen (estrogen derived from a plant), comes from a buttercup plant that was used for centuries by the American Indians to relieve menopausal symptoms. The chemicals within the black cohosh bind to the receptor sites and help to prevent uterine or breast cancer.

Black cohosh seems to alleviate headaches, heart palpitations, depression and anxiety, and vaginal dryness, thus preventing urinary tract infections. It also alleviates dizziness, high blood pressure, and high blood sugar. A dose of 80 mg per day is recommended.

Dong quai (angelica)

Dong quai is an Asian herb that is most helpful when combined with the other treatments we are discussing. Its primary benefits are associated with stopping the hot flashes and vaginal dryness. A dose of 300 mg per day is best.

Ginseng

Siberian ginseng will improve the mood and stress relief of a woman, especially when her hormone levels begin to drop off as she grows older. The recommended dose is 200 mg a day.

Boron

Boron is a mineral that helps the body absorb calcium and therefore proves helpful in strengthening bone structure and protecting women from osteoporosis. Boron should be taken at a dose of 3 mg per day.

Bromelain

Bromelain is primarily an anti-inflammatory. It is especially helpful in curbing the edema, or swelling, caused by fluid retention. The recommended dose is 45 mg per day.

Reginald Cherry, *Bible Health Secrets* (Lake Mary, FL: Siloam, 2003), 160–162.

OSTEOPOROSIS

by Don Colbert, MD

WOMEN ARE PARTICULARLY susceptible to osteoporosis, which means "porous bones." It is progressive loss of bone mass that leads to decreased bone density. How prevalent is it? Approximately one in four postmenopausal women have been afflicted with it—which is over twenty million people in the United States. Osteoporosis often results in painful, unnecessary fractures to the spine, forearms, hips, shoulders, and ribs.

Some major risk factors for osteoporosis in women include:

1. Inactivity
2. Low calcium intake
3. Postmenopause
4. Premature menopause
5. Caucasian (white) or Asian
6. Smoking history
7. Slenderness and leanness
8. Short stature and small bones
9. Never pregnant
10. Family history of osteoporosis
11. Heavy alcohol use
12. Hyperthyroidism
13. Hyperparathyroidism
14. Long-term use of corticosteroids
15. Long-term use of anticonvulsants
16. Gastric or small bowel resection

Here are some suggestions you can implement to prevent osteoporosis:

- Let half of your daily diet consist of fresh fruits and vegetables. This will create an alkaline environment in your body.
- Do not eat a lot of meats, since they tend to form acid in the body.
- Foods that are high in oxalic acid include chocolate, spinach, rhubarb, almonds, cashews, asparagus, beet greens, and chard. Therefore, don't take your calcium supplements while eating these foods at the same time. These foods will inhibit the absorption of calcium.
- Whole grains and fiber can also bind calcium. Therefore, it is best not to take calcium or calcium-containing foods at the same time as eating whole grains or fiber.
- Avoid or decrease your intake of alcohol, coffee, tea, colas, and other caffeinated beverages since they create acidity that can leach calcium out of the bones.
- Avoid aluminum in any form.
- Exercise can help prevent osteoporosis, and it can help treat it by providing strength to your bones and muscles. Exercise will slow mineral loss, help you maintain posture, and improve your overall fitness, which reduces the risk of falls.

Don Colbert, *The Bible Cure for Osteoporosis* (Lake Mary, FL: Siloam, 2000).

VARICOSE VEINS

by Reginald Cherry, MD

MANY PEOPLE NOTICE swelling in their lower extremities after they have been sitting for long periods of time. They have not contracted these muscles in order to help circulation. Even minor contractions of the calf muscles while sitting—raising the foot and rotating the ball of the foot, for example—is sufficient to return blood back up the leg to the heart. However, if blood is allowed to accumulate in the lower extremities (a condition known as *venous stasis*), the risk of blood pooling and, potentially, blood clotting is greatly increased. This can become a serious problem, particularly if it involves the deep veins of the leg.

Decreased physical activity and a sedentary lifestyle puts us more at risk for blood pooling. Blood pooling increases the pressure in the veins, which can break down the one-way valves designed to carry blood back to the heart. When this happens, the vessels below the valves swell, causing what we know as *varicose veins*.

Varicose veins cause fluid to accumulate in the lower extremities (edema), change the skin color, and, in severe cases, cause ulceration. Leg pain, tiredness in the lower extremities, and itching can follow. Doctors refer to this problem as *chronic venous insufficiency* (CVI). It occurs in 10 to 15 percent of males and 20 to 25 percent of females.

The conventional treatment for this condition has been the use of support stockings (which provide compression), accompanied by periodic elevation of the legs to relieve pressure in the veins. Occasionally, doctors will recommend vascular surgery, such as vein stripping or sclerotherapy.

However, there is a natural extract from horse chestnut seed (*aesculus hippocastanum*). The common name of "horse chestnut seed" was given because the seeds resemble a horse's eyes. The primary function of the chemicals in horse chestnut extract is to reduce fluid loss from capillaries, which results from increased pressure in the veins. Research shows that the extract can help stop enzymes that weaken the walls of capillaries and improve circulation by increasing the flexibility of the blood vesses, which in turn improves blood flow.[1]

These chemicals prevent edema and swelling. Studies have shown that they can increase the tone of the veins and help prevent leakage from the capillaries. Study results show a reduction in the swelling in the legs and significant improvements in such problems as itching, pain, and the feeling of fullness in the lower extremities. The horse chestnut extract is safe and well tolerated, as demonstrated by the results of numerous studies, some of which involved over five thousand patients.[2]

The extract is available in tablet or capsule form. In fact, a major pharmaceutical company in the United States introduced a product known as Venastat, made from horse chestnut extract, to promote leg vein health. Take 48 mg twice daily.

If you suffer from varicose veins, it is often helpful to raise your feet at or above the level of your heart for at least forty-five minutes at the end of each day to take pressure off of the veins.

AUTHOR'S NOTE: If you have renal or kidney problems, you should use caution in taking any kind of herbal medicines since all orally ingested chemicals go through the liver and are filtered by the kidneys. In the case of varicose veins, I would urge you, as always, to consult with a physician who is familiar with both natural as well as conventional treatments.

Reginald Cherry, *Bible Health Secrets* (Lake Mary, FL: Siloam, 2003), 170–172.

BREAST CANCER

by Reginald Cherry, MD

HERE ARE THE top ten ways you can keep yourself from becoming a breast cancer statistic.

1. Eat that tofu!

The phyotoestrogens, known as isoflavones, in soy are actually cancer preventives. These isoflavones bind to estrogen receptor sites and actually guard against the development of breast cancer.

2. Take red clover extract.

Red clover contains four major isoflavones that, when taken daily, appear to be a promising and effective method for women to protect their bodies against the potential of breast cancer.

3. Eat lots of fish.

The omega-3 fatty acids found in salmon, cod, mackerel, herring, sardines, and trout are really oils that the human body can convert to a chemical known as *prostaglandins*, which keep breast cells from multiplying and dividing.

4. Avoid cooking with corn oil.

Certain types of oils, such as saturated fats and other vegetable oils containing omega-6 fatty acids, may actually promote breast cancer. Polyunsaturated oils, like corn oil, may contribute to this also.

5. Add kiwifruit to your diet.

Kiwi provides twice as much vitamin C as an orange! Studies show that vitamin C can inhibit breast cell division, thus reducing the risk of breast cancer.

6. Go orange.

Hesperetin and *naringenin*, chemicals contained in citrus fruits, and especially in oranges, prevent cancer cell division and also help neutralize cancer-causing chemicals in the body. Another chemical found in oranges, *limonene*, has potent cancer-fighting properties.

7. Fiber, fiber, fiber.

Fiber tends to bind cancer-causing agents in the gastrointestinal tract and keep them from being absorbed. Sources of fiber include fruits and vegetables, pinto beans, kidney beans, whole-wheat products, and psyllium.

8. Eat cabbage and broccoli.

A unique chemical compound, indole-3-carbinol, stops human breast cancer cells dead in their tracks. It is found in cabbage, broccoli, and brussels sprouts.

9. Stock up on yogurt.

Yogurt contains high amounts of calcium, which can inhibit the division of breast cancer cells. Yogurt also stimulates gamma interferon, which helps fight cancer by enhancing the function of the immune system.

10. Take vitamin A.

Beta-carotene is the best source of vitamin A. Studies consistently show that populations that consume the most vitamin A have the lowest levels of breast cancer.

Reginald Cherry, *Bible Health Secrets* (Lake Mary, FL: Siloam, 2003), 174–177.

MENTAL HEALTH

THE BLESSED MIND-SET

by James P. Gills, MD

A LIGNMENT—THE KEY TO inner healing—really means abandonment to God and the Holy Spirit reigning within your heart and mind. The Lord created you in a wonderful way, yet the many aspects of your consciousness must be kept in check, continually, by your proximity to God and His will. Ungodly, destructive, and negative thoughts proclaim that we are bound rather than freed by the Holy Spirit. Developing God's blessed mind-set is your first step toward true alignment with His design and desire for you. Aligning by adopting God's blessed mind-set allows us to experience the consequent inner healing that every one of us seeks—whether we are aware of our need or not.

The mental attitudes that produce mental health are those in alignment with the Creator—and these are outlined most explicitly in the Beatitudes found in Matthew 5:3–11. They present what is probably the best summary of the mind-set blessed of God, which is the mind-set of inner health. That mind-set produces a life that stands in direct opposition to the life produced under a burden of sin.

In Jerusalem there was a very special pool where there "lay a great multitude of sick people, blind, lame, paralyzed, waiting for the moving of the water" (John 5:3, NKJV). The pool of Bethesda (*Beth* [house] *hesed* [of mercy]) drew those seeking healing. It provided cooling waters to those living in the middle of the city. This pool of Bethesda was a great mercy to the people of Jerusalem for its healing and restorative powers through God's grace.

The anguish and neuroses that we feel so deeply arise out of the time we spend overly focused upon ourselves. We tend to exaggerate our discomforts rather than enjoying peace and anointing. To dip in the pool is to dispense with all of your preoccupation with pain and simply rest in the Lord's arms. This is where you find physical, mental, and spiritual healing. You need to have a deserted place or a pool of healing in which to rest. God's Word is such a place of rest and restoration, for it is there that faith and grace abide. There, under God's sovereign hand, can be found every promise of God, sufficient for all your healings. Or your place of rest may be the place of prayer, meditation, and reflection upon God's gorgeous creation. Perhaps a simple walk on the beach or in the mountains is all that is necessary from time to time for you to slow down, relax, and reorient yourself in the Lord.

The whole purpose of aligning your mind in such a way is to feel that the unction of God lives within you. You can only accomplish this in quiet, personal times spent in God's presence.

James P. Gills, *God's Prescription for Healing* (Lake Mary, FL: Siloam, 2004), 109, 113–115.

THE HEALING POWER OF OPTIMISM

by David B. Biebel, DMin, and Harold Koenig, MD

P ERHAPS YOU'VE HEARD the story about the optimist and pessimist who went duck hunting with the constant companion of the optimist, a Labrador retriever. When the first duck was bagged, the dog's master said to his friend, "Watch this." To the dog he said, "Fetch." The dog jumped overboard, walked across the water, retrieved the duck, stepped into the boat, and laid the bird at the feet of his master. The pessimist made no comment. When the second duck was downed, the dog repeated the amazing feat; still no comment from the pessimist. The third time, however, the pessimist could no longer contain his enthusiasm. "Can't swim, can he?" he said.

According to Webster's dictionary, *optimism* is "an inclination to put the most favorable construction upon actions and events or to anticipate the best possible outcome." An optimist thinks that a half-full glass of water is in the process of being filled, but a pessimist sees it as half-empty on its way to being completely drained. The difference is not in reality—the glass is both half-full and half-empty; the difference is in the interpretation one puts on what one sees.

Although reality is ultimately the same for optimists and pessimists—life will always have its ups and downs—optimists enjoy the journey so much more, and they are likely to be happier, healthier, and live longer, more enjoyable lives as well!

Laura Kubzansky, PhD, a health psychologist at Harvard's School of Public Health, tracked 1,300 men for ten years and found that heart disease among optimistic men was half the rate for men who weren't optimistic. "It was a much bigger effect than we expected," she said. "We also looked at pulmonary function, since poor pulmonary function is predictive of a whole range of bad outcomes, including premature mortality, cardiovascular disease, and chronic obstructive pulmonary disease." Optimists were much healthier. "I'm an optimist," she said, "but I didn't expect results like these."[1]

The bottom line is that optimism contributes to happiness and happiness is health-enhancing, so the next time you see a glass of water, try to view it with realistic optimism. You'll be happier for it.

David B. Biebel and Harold G. Koenig, *Simple Health* (Lake Mary, FL: Siloam, 2005), 119–120.

LAUGHTER

by David B. Biebel, DMin, and Harold Koenig, MD

O NE OF THE simplest ways to improve your quality of life immediately is to laugh. A sense of humor is essential to wellness, and it may even contribute to longevity.

So how can you make laughter a greater part of your life? Here are a few ideas for brightening the world around you through humor and laughter:

- Spend time with people who help you to laugh. In a family setting, try having a "joke night" often.
- Watch or read humor on telvision or in movies, plays, books, or comic strips.
- Don't sweat the small stuff. Try using a humorous calendar, such as a Far Side calendar by Gary Larson, on your desk to help keep things in perspective.
- When work is getting to you, take a laugh break instead of a coffee break. Take some time out to read jokes on the Internet or listen to a comedy CD in your car.
- Keep a file of good jokes handy in case of a "humor emergency"!
- Visit humorous Web sites on the Internet. Keep the best Web sites bookmarked for later.
- Share what you find with others, and very soon you'll be forming a comedy club of your own!

David B. Biebel and Harold G. Koenig, *Simple Health* (Lake Mary, FL: Siloam, 2005), 11, 17.

"HAPPY" OCCASIONS

by Gregory L. Jantz, PhD, with Ann McMurray

I'D LIKE YOU to think back over your life and, on a separate piece of paper, write down significant events that most people would consider ones of celebration and joy. These could be births, weddings, graduations, promotions, birthdays, family reunions, first job, first apartment, first house, etc. Write down what most people would typically consider a happy occasion, even if you don't necessarily feel that way about it yourself.

Now, ask yourself the following questions about each:

1. Did you experience joy at this event?

2. Did you experience other emotions as well? If so, what were they?

3. Looking at the list of any other emotions, what category could you put them into:

   - Perfectionism
   - Fear
   - Anger
   - Shame

4. As you think of each event, which emotion is forefront in your mind?

5. Have you ever been surprised at your reaction to one of these events? Did you expect to be influenced by perfectionism or feel fear, anger, or shame but actually felt more joy than you thought?

6. Can you pinpoint what might have been different about this event that allowed you to feel more joy than you anticipated?

7. How has your ability to experience joy changed over the years? Is it becoming easier or harder? Why do you suppose that is?

I'd like you to do this for all of the events you wrote down. What I'd like you to do is look for an obstacle pattern. What is the shape of your obstacle? What is its name? Once you've determined its shape, it's time to determine where it came from.

Your greatest resource, of course, is a deep and personal relationship with God. He is the reason for lasting optimism, hope, and joy in this world. This attitude isn't something you can manufacture and maintain on your own; it is a gift of God. This gift is one available to you through His Spirit and one He desires for you to have. You don't have to earn it; just accept it and reach for it. Then, having obtained it, use it to your heart's content and God's glory.

Gregory L. Jantz with Ann McMurray, *Happy for the Rest of Your Life* (Lake Mary, FL: Siloam, 2009), 220–231.

JOYFUL HOPE

by Gregory L. Jantz, PhD, with Ann McMurray

WHAT I'VE COME to understand is that for you to rejoice over some of the challenges you face in life, you need to maintain a banked fire of joy. That fire is up to the task of warming your heart at all times and perfectly capable of exploding in fireworks at others. In order to keep the fire going, you need to offer up all of the experiences of your life for joy to consume—the good and the bad, the happy and the sad, the understood and the inexplicable.

Joy is one of the fruit of the Spirit (Gal. 5:22). This is not innate human nature here; rather, it is divine intervention and provision. God Himself is able to empower you with joy as a gift.

Joy, like hope, is most often evident in situations that are far from joyful. When you are joyful over understandable, recognizable, commonplace things and situations, it's still joy, but the challenge is having joy when times are hard. When you learn to rejoice in whatever your circumstances, you strengthen your ability to hope and to persevere.

I have had the privilege to be around joyful, optimistic people who were undergoing hardship of incredible proportions. I have gone to visit them, fully intending to try, in some small way, to offer comfort and instead found myself receiving much more comfort. Here they are, in dire physical or circumstantial straits, and they end up doing more for my attitude and me than I ever did for them. Their complete reliance on God and the Holy Spirit to get them through the situation is crystal clear. I go to give them comfort, and they wind up giving me hope.

Their attitude is summed up for me in a passage from one of the minor prophets, Habakkuk. Habakkuk doesn't understand why God is working the way He is (using the Babylonians to punish Judah and Jerusalem), seeming to allow evil to oppress His people. In the end, Habakkuk comes to understand that God really does have the final say and will make sure justice prevails, even though it will not come about in Habakkuk's lifetime.

> Though the fig tree does not bud and there are no grapes on the vines, though the olive crop fails and the fields produce no food, though there are no sheep in the pen and no cattle in the stalls, yet I will rejoice in the LORD, I will be joyful in God my Savior. The Sovereign LORD is my strength; he makes my feet like the feet of a deer, he enables me to go on the heights.
>
> —HABAKKUK 3:17–19, NIV

I don't know what you personally are going through; please know my heart goes out to you. And if it were only my heart I could give you, frankly, it wouldn't be enough. What I can offer you is to embrace the attitude of Habakkuk. Pray and ask God to empower you through His Spirit to experience joy within your situation. For God, nothing is impossible. The reality of this world is set; hardships and suffering are a given. God will not always remove the impossible situation from you, but He is always able to fill your heart with joy.

Gregory L. Jantz with Ann McMurray, *Happy for the Rest of Your Life* (Lake Mary, FL: Siloam, 2009), 220–231.

BREAKING ADDICTION

by Douglas Weiss, PhD

Step 1: Self-honesty

Self-honesty is your first step out of the cycle of out-of-control behavior. This is where you just choose to be honest about a flaw in your life. You humble yourself and admit to yourself exactly what is true. Self-honesty is by far the easier of the two paths to humility.

Step 2: Cleansing the temple

I have seen many courageous men and women identify and receive healing from the wounds that others have inflicted on them. All forms of abuse, neglect, infidelity, addictions, and shame can be successfully overcome with the desire to do so.

Regardless of the past, healing can take place. It requires work and patience, but the results are nothing short of marvelous. We serve a great God, and as we colabor with Him, all things are possible.

Step 3: Forgiving others and yourself

The next step to healing is forgiveness, and we begin by dealing with unforgiveness toward others. Releasing your offenders will free you if you complete your cleansing the temple work first.

The next step in dealing with this issue of forgiveness is asking forgiveness from yourself. This might sound peculiar, but I have found that if people can own their behavior and forgive themselves for it, they are much more likely to gain control of what has been controlling them.

Step 4: The power of disclosure

One of the most powerful steps in getting a grip on what's controlling you is disclosure. The Scriptures state that if we bring something to the light, it becomes light. (See Ephesians 5:13.)

Step 5: Exercise positive behavior

There are five ways to exercise your "positive behavior muscles": praying, reading, group meetings, daily calling, and prayer. With these, you can see your positive behaviors develop. There is something else that is growing while you exercise these five positive behaviors, and it is your will. As you will gets stronger, it can help control the behavior you are currently trying to get a grip on.

Step 6: The "power-up" principle

I want to take you to a passage in the Bible that gives us the foundation for the power-up principle: "Two are better than one, because they have a good return for their work: If one falls down, his friend can help him up. But pity the man who falls and has no one to help him up!" (Eccles. 4:9–10, NIV).

Douglas Weiss, *Get a Grip* (Lake Mary, FL: Siloam, 2007), 104–191.

THE ROAD LESS TRAVELED

by Gregory L. Jantz, PhD, with Ann McMurray

IN THIS WORLD of difficulty and doubt, of struggles and hardships, of compromises and second choices, of injustice and affliction, each person comes to a crossroads in life. There are two roads with signposts on each that say, "Way to Happiness." On the one hand is the road championed by the world, which promises much and delivers little. Instead of happiness, though, this road can lead to depression, anxiety, and addiction.

There is another choice, another road. However, this road can appear less attractive when compared with the first. Because of this, it is a road less traveled. This is the road of faith, which uses a cross for a talisman. It does not say, "Take this road to avoid your pain." It says, "Take this road because of your pain." The one road promises you'll be in control. The other says you must give it up. The one appears all about pleasure. The other appears all about sacrifice.

In other words, you've come to a fork in the road—two paths promising to lead you to your desired destination. However, the one you choose may not be the most popular, but it may lead you to *true* happiness.

I want to encourage you to take the road less traveled because it will make all the difference. The world's road eventually leads to a literal dead end. God's road leads to eternity. Because it can be so difficult to choose the road less traveled, here are just a few things to remember as you stand at the crossroads each day:

- Happiness is a response to life that comes from the inside of a person, not from outside circumstances.
- Depression isn't something you live with; it's something you get help for.
- Worry and anxiety are a learned response to life that can be acknowledged, understood, and overcome.
- Addictions both mask and amplify pain; they never heal it.
- What you tell yourself becomes who you are, so be careful what you say.
- Relationships are meant to support you, not drag you down.
- An attitude of optimism is a choice.
- Joy is the spark that uses the tinder of optimism to ignite the fuel of hope.

Each of these statements becomes a powerful present you give to yourself. Each takes essential truths and understandings and packages them together into a short sentence or phrase. Just by reading or saying the sentence or phrase, you can unwrap and release the whole meaning in your mind. This is a vital way you provide encouragement, motivation, and comfort to yourself. Memorize them. Put them on sticky notes on your bathroom mirror or refrigerator, on the dashboard of your car. Start each day by reciting them, agreeing all over again that they represent how you choose to live today.

Gregory L. Jantz with Ann McMurray, *Happy for the Rest of Your Life* (Lake Mary, FL: Siloam, 2009), 232–235.

RECOGNIZING THE SIX STAGES OF OUT-OF-CONTROL BEHAVIOR

by Douglas Weiss, PhD

I N LIFE, IT is helpful to have identifiable signs to see if you are headed toward becoming out of control. Let's take a look at the six stages of the cycle of out-of-control behavior.

1. Hopelessness

When you begin to feel hopeless in an area of your life, it might be more than just emotion. For some of us, the area that is out of control in our lives can be feelings inside such as hatred, arrogance, or intolerance of others. For others it is external—food, alcohol, sex, work, or entertainment.

2. Denial

Denial is the second stage of out-of-control behavior. I know it sounds silly, but denial is one of the easiest ways to tell if someone needs to get a grip on their behavior. Nobody wants to admit that they are out of control, and so we just don't believe it.

3. Defensiveness

When someone addresses the area that is out of control in our lives, we become defensive about the behavior. If they continue to press us on the matter, often we use our emotions to defend our behavior.

A defensive response to even the gentlest "reality check" is further proof that you are in a cycle of out-of-control behavior.

4. Rationalization

Rationalization is when you make up reasons for why you do the things you do: "Everyone does it." "It's not a problem." "I can stop anytime." "I only do it when I am tired."

You rationalize the other person's perceptions so you don't have to look at the pride that others see in you.

5. Sadness

Many have had moments of sadness about an out-of-control area. Sometimes this sadness occurs once and is felt very deeply. My experience is that for many people, this sadness occurs again and again. Sometimes this sadness moves a person to the last stage of the cycle, but often times, people just remain "stuck" in deep sadness for years.

6. Motivation

The last stage of the out-of-control behavior is motivation—you know, that feeling you get when you are ready to fight again. When you are in motivation mode, you fully accept that you have an out-of-control area of your life. You are armed with new strategies or information, and you are going to nail this area of your life for good.

Douglas Weiss, *Get a Grip* (Lake Mary, FL: Siloam, 2006), 37–41.

DEPRESSION

by Linda Mintle, PhD

C HRISTIANS SHOULD NEVER get depressed!" Believe it or not, people say this! How wrong it is to make this kind of judgment, especially since it is hurtful and born out of ignorance. There are many causes of depression—sometimes directly related to spiritual issues, other times not.

For example, people can become depressed when they are disobedient and living in rebellion to God's Word.

But rebellion is not always the cause of depression. More often, negative thinking is the culprit. It develops out of life experiences. When depression hits, your relationship with God is usually depressed as well. Part of the work is to restore your belief that God is working for you despite the troubles around you. He still cares and wants you whole. In fact, He is your healer.

Sometimes the causes of depression can be easily seen. At other times, depression seems to spring out of nowhere. Stress, heredity, and genetics all play a role. Here are common causes of depression.

- Loss (relationships, circumstances and situations, expectations and dreams)
- Significant life transitions
- Chronic medical conditions
- Physical changes in the body—stroke, heart attack, cancer, hormonal disorders
- Personality traits such as perfectionism, pessimism, and being overly dependent
- Stressful changes in life patterns
- Unresolved anger
- Unrepentant sin and disobedience
- Occult involvement
- Negative thinking patterns
- Alcohol and drug intoxication and withdrawal
- Diet—specifically, low levels of folic acid and vitamin B_{12}

"How do I know if I'm depressed?" There isn't a biological or physical test you can take to determine if you are depressed. However, there are clear signs and symptoms. Physicians and mental health professionals can evaluate you if you are unsure. It is also important to talk about any suicidal feelings or thoughts you may have.

If you are suffering from depression, usually five or more of these signs are present for a period of two weeks or more:

- Feeling sad and anxious, in a depressed mood
- Loss of interest or pleasure in activities
- Weight changes with changes in appetite
- Sleep changes
- Agitation
- Fatigue and loss of energy
- Feeling worthless, with inappropriate guilt

- Problems concentrating, indecisiveness
- Suicidal thoughts and/or plans[1]

BREAKING FREE

When you face depression, here are some things to keep in mind:

1. Acknowledge the depression (Prov. 12:25).
2. Trust God to help you (Ps. 46:1).
3. Praise Him despite the circumstances (Ps. 34:1).
4. Speak hope into the situation (Ps. 39:7).
5. Renew your negative thoughts by asking God to speak truth to you. Think on good things (Phil. 4:8). Stand on His Word.
6. Take steps to correct your behavior.
7. Address the causes of the depression.
8. Spend time with your Father. Get to know Him intimately.
9. Praise Him because He's already done everything you need.
10. Be transformed by the ongoing renewing of your mind.

Linda Mintle, *Breaking Free From Depression* (Lake Mary, FL: Siloam, 2002).

OVERCOMING A NEGATIVE SELF-IMAGE

by Linda Mintle, PhD

HAVE YOU EMBRACED a distorted view of yourself? Have you used the cultural standards of beauty and success to judge your worth? For the Christian, there is no such thing as a self-image. We are made in God's image to reflect His glory.

Christian self-evaluation is done as an act of responsibility. The Bible tells us how to think of ourselves and how to act. Jesus challenges us to be more like Him and less like our human nature. We understand that we are all sinners in need of redemption.

When you contrast this to the secular, stark differences are apparent. Modern views of the self are based on the idea that each person decides what is right and should know himself or herself well enough to determine the course of action for his or her life. This is called self-reliance. But we are not self-reliant; we need divine guidance to accomplish the purposes for our existence. The more we try to live apart from God, the more we fail.

BREAK FREE TO HIS IMAGE

God invites us to a personal relationship in which we can find ultimate acceptance. With His help, we can break free from a negative self-image. Read these points in order to correct your image.

1. Have a proper understanding of what a self-image is.
2. God esteems you when people do not.
3. At the root of a negative self-image is a lack of true identity.
4. Daily renew your mind with the Word of God.
5. Change your behavior.

Don't get caught up in the lie of building self-esteem. You are already esteemed because you are a child of God. Sit at His feet. Obey His Word, and be transformed by His love. Your worth comes from God, no other source.

Linda Mintle, *Breaking Free From a Negative Self-Image* (Lake Mary, FL: Siloam, 2002).

"SPANK THE DOG!"

by Douglas Weiss, PhD

EVERYONE KNOWS WHO a man's best friend is, right? His dog. Dogs are unquestionably great creatures, but unfortunately they do come with one incredible deficit. These benevolent creatures we love to love have accidents. Throughout history, I am sure that dog owners wrestled with what to do about this problem, and then *eureka*! On the day newspapers were invented, the answer became clear. You roll up the newspaper, and when Fuzzy has an accident, you spank the dog. It works!

Now let me take the paradigm of spank the dog, break it down, and apply it to getting a grip on out-of-control behavior in our lives. Nobody likes pain. We try to avoid pain at all costs.

That's why God has allowed many consequences for improper behavior to be painful. As a counselor looking for ways to help people break out of the control of addictive behaviors, I saw the value in this principle, but I doubted if people would take too kindly being swatted with a rolled-up newspaper when their out-of-control behavior got the best of them! So one day when I was in my office and a sincere man asked how he should get rid of lustful thoughts, a technique one of my professors taught me about something else popped into my mind. The man in my office was lusting after, or objectifying, women. He didn't want to do this, but he felt helpless against his behavior. When he asked me for help, I got up, went to the outer office, and came back with the secret weapon for lust: *a rubber band.*

You are probably thinking, "How does a rubber band become a secret weapon against lust?" Well, that's what my client thought as well. I instructed my client to place the rubber band on his wrist, and every time he lusted, he was to snap his wrist with the rubber band. He did what his therapist said. Within a few weeks he reported that his lustful thoughts were reduced significantly. Instead of his brain getting a rush for lusting, it was now getting pain. Even after just a few days, the brain began to want to avoid lusting. You might think this is off the wall, but it really works.

In case you're still not sure what I'm talking about, I'll explain it this way. Whatever is controlling your life can be defined by behaviors. Once you identify these behaviors and take steps for getting a grip on these behaviors, you can also assign a negative consequence to the out-of-control behaviors.

Douglas Weiss, *Get a Grip* (Lake Mary, FL: Siloam, 2006), 206–208.

HEALTHY RELATIONSHIPS

THE VALUE OF FRIENDS AND FAMILY

by David B. Biebel, DMin, and Harold Koenig, MD

TO BE IN a relationship with someone is one of the greatest gifts we are given in this world, and our relationships with other people are often key ingredients in our ability to live happier, healthier lives.

Good relationships are good for you—physically, psychologically, socially, and spiritually. "There's a good deal of research showing that people who have strong, enduring social support have better health outcomes," said Frank Baker, PhD, vice president for behavioral research at the national office of the American Cancer Society in Atlanta. "Friends and relatives are important because they help you deal with the adversities of life; you're likely to have better health and be happier."[1]

Emotional support from family and friends buffers stressful life events and reduces the risk of (and speeds recovery from) depression.[2] When you've had a bad day, it always helps to have a friend to call for a heart-to-heart talk or just to take you out to do something fun or silly. People with these kinds of strong relationships—including marriage, other family members, and friends—live longer.[3] In fact, they may even be more resistant to infection due to better immune system functioning.[4] Social support is also associated with less cigarette smoking, less alcohol abuse, a healthier diet, more exercise, and better sleep quality.[5]

Social support also helps people recover from illness. Research on people with cardiovascular diseases suggests that close relationships help protect heart attack survivors against future cardiovascular problems. British researcher Dr. Francis Creed and his colleagues focused on 583 men and women, all about age sixty, all hospitalized with heart attacks. Each patient was asked about emotional issues, including what social support they had. The patients also took tests to determine whether they were anxious or depressed. A year later, those who had a close personal confidant had 50 percent less risk of dying from heart disease than those without a close confidant. In describing his findings, Dr. Creed explained, "It's the degree of intimacy of close relationships—not the number of social contacts—that appears to protect heart health." A close confidant, he said, is "usually a spouse or partner, but not necessarily. It may be a very, very close friend or relative."[6]

Let's face it: you were created to be in relationship with other people, and the more you "connect" with others, the happier and healthier you will be.

David B. Biebel and Harold G. Koenig, *Simple Health* (Lake Mary, FL: Siloam, 2005), 99–101.

SOUL MATES—THE JOY OF EMOTIONAL INTIMACY

by Douglas Weiss, PhD

I LIKEN THE SOUL of a person to a sponge inside the body. This sponge needs regular watering (or praise) to stay soft and alive. If a spouse decides to withhold that praise, the sponge begins to dry out. Over the years, if the sponge is not nurtured, that person will become brittle inside. The sponge gets hard and seems to break easily. This will show up in sarcasm, anger, bitterness, rigidity, and a lesser ability to give love to the spouse who is withholding the nurturing.

What is nurturing? *Nurturing* is the skill or ability to put praise and affirmation into our spouse's heart. Many of us did not grow up with parents who modeled this ability toward each other. Some of us grew up with little or no praise at all from our parents. Many of us cannot recall one positive thing that our mother or father said to us. They may have lacked the skill or were simply negligent in this area of nurturing our souls.

Personally, I can't recall such positive modeling of adult nurturing in my own family, either. Nevertheless, my past has not and will not determine my present or my future.

I can and have learned a new set of skills. You too have learned skills throughout your own lifetime. No doubt you have received some level of education, and you have also chosen to do many things differently than your parents did. Learning to nurture others can be just one more thing that you can educate yourself about and create differently for yourself in Christ Jesus. Trust me, if I can learn how to nurture—and my educational experience did not teach me this—then anyone can.

HONORING EMOTIONS

To acquire the skills necessary for emotional intimacy we must learn to honor emotions. By doing this, you assert that they are a real, valuable, precious part of the person you love. These feelings are an essential part of your spouse's being.

As human beings we can think and behave differently than we feel, but we can't feel differently than we feel. If I feel tired, then I am tired. That is who I am at that microsecond of time. Now here is the tricky part. Feelings may be real and a real part of who I am, but they are not necessarily truth, and they change constantly.

Learning to honor your spouse's feelings places you in a precarious balance. When you hear your spouse's feelings, you must honor them immediately. They are precious offerings to you at the time of sharing. However, you must resist the temptation to change, alter, or rationalize away what he or she may be feeling at the moment. Our spouses will not feel any one particular feeling forever. Feelings change, and being honored and heard are very important.

Your spouse and his or her emotions are ever changing. Honoring your spouse's emotions without feeling the need to fix them or fix the situation will produce enormous positive fruit in your relationship. So make a decision to honor your spouse's emotions and cherish the person he or she is on the inside.

Douglas Weiss, *Intimacy* (Lake Mary, FL: Siloam, 2001), 17–28.

FIVE MYTHS ABOUT MARRIAGE

by Linda Mintle, PhD

Myth: I can change my spouse.

Do you think you can change your spouse? If you do, you are headed for trouble. You can't force another person to change. Change is up to the willingness of each person, and an unwilling heart is a root cause of divorce.

Truth: You can change only your part in the dance.

You can change something in your relationship by changing *your* response, *not* your partner's. Change your behavior, and the interaction can't stay the same. Become part of the correction, not someone who reinjures.

Myth: We are too different.

Since no two families are the same, no two people will get along perfectly. Coming to marriage from your unique family system insures you will have differences with your spouse. Unless you clone yourself, you will be in a relationship with someone who thinks, feels, and acts differently.

Truth: Incompatibility or differences do not kill a relationship. How you work out those differences is what counts.

To enjoy a healthy marriage you need a compatible style of dealing with differences. There are couples where both people are fighters or both people are avoiders, but they will likely stay married because they have compatible styles of dealing with their differences. Other couples are mixed up with one being a fighter and the other being an avoider. However, they must work to have compatible styles of dealing with conflict.

If you are an avoider, you may have to force yourself to bring up problems. If you are a fighter, you may have to calm down, take five, watch your mouth, and speak in a reasonable tone. The styles of handling conflict must work for both people.

Myth: I've lost that loving feeling, and it's gone, gone, gone!

When positive exchanges outweigh negative ones, relationships do well. Relationships, when placed under stress, can deteriorate because of failed expectations, lack of understanding, inappropriate blame, acting out, and other destructive emotions and behaviors. When a partner allows the above to translate into ongoing negative exchanges, the relationship is in trouble.

Truth: That loving feeling can be restored.

Focus on the positive aspects of your relationship. If you love to ride bikes, go ride them. If you give good back rubs, give them often. If you love to hear you are loved, say it. Keep the friendship part of your relationship strong. Spend time together, laugh, and create happy memories. Most importantly, pray together as a couple. The spiritual unity that comes from praying together is powerful. Spiritual unity brings intimacy.

Myth: A more traditional marriage will save us.

Gender is a hot button for most couples. Arguments can be traced to core assumptions each partner has about how men and women are supposed to relate. Should husbands help out in the kitchen? Should wives run family finances? When marital problems arise, the assumption is that the more traditional the family becomes, the stronger the marriage will be.

Truth: God's intention is gender equality.

Before industrial America, the home was a place of living and working together in which all family members shared responsibility. By being renewed through the power of Jesus Christ, both genders need to be liberated from culturally assigned gender boxes. Couples must clarify role expectations and not lord power over one another. Mutual respect and affirmation are needed.

Myth: There has been an affair. We need to divorce.

Infidelity is destructive and causes great damage to marriages. Some think that an affair demands divorce. After all, adultery is a biblical out. So why not take it? You've been wronged. Why stay with someone who betrays you? You deserve better. You're entitled to a divorce.

Truth: Affairs are serious and damaging, but they are not beyond repair and reconciliation.

An affair needn't be a death sentence, and divorce is not always inevitable in the face of an affair. Divorce is never commanded or even encouraged in the Bible. But forgiveness and reconciliation are. Because you experience forgiveness from a loving heavenly Father, you can forgive your spouse, but more is needed. Beyond forgiveness is reconciliation. Both parties must be willing to talk about the affair and want reconciliation.

Linda Mintle, *I Married You, Not Your Family* (Lake Mary, FL: Charisma House, 2008).

IT'S A PACKAGE DEAL

by Linda Mintle, PhD

CONSIDER THIS LOVELY thought—there are at least six people in your marital bed! Now don't go checking for bodies. They aren't there physically. (If they are, we *really* need to talk.) Two families are emotionally present—you and your parents, and your spouse and his/her parents. And if your spouse has siblings, the bed is even more crowded—there is an entire family system joining you in marriage.

You probably didn't pay that much attention to your spouse's family when you married. If you did, no doubt it was only for a second. If you were like me, you didn't concern yourself at all with how the extended family behaved. After all, you were enamored with your new love. You only had to put up with the larger group on special occasions.

It takes great skill to be your own unique person while still remaining attached to the larger extended family. The better you are able to separate emotionally and still keep your family connection, the better marital partner you will make. It is necessary to develop a strong sense of self. Otherwise you'll expect your partner to complete the missing parts.

But some people confuse independence with emotional cut-off. People who cut off have little involvement with their original families. They usually do their own thing and don't turn to family members for support. Cut-off is an extreme reaction to the problem of balancing the emotional and intellectual self.

The other extreme is being raised in a family in which you never develop a sense of self because everyone has the same "groupthink." The family message is that you aren't supposed to have independent thoughts. Loyalty to the family is demanded. Excessive closeness is the glue that sticks everyone together.

How do you balance togetherness and separateness? Start by deciding where you fall on a continuum from cut-off to sticky.

If you find yourself cut off from your family, force yourself to be more involved. Learn to resolve conflicts. Share activities and interests. Turn to your family for support and problem solving. If you are cut off from your family because of abuse, don't accept the abusive behavior. You may be able to make a new appropriate connection.

If you are too connected with your extended family, find your voice. Do things apart from them, and set boundaries. Don't look to them for approval. Think, and don't let your emotions overpower you.

Remember that you have the power to make changes in your life. You are not a victim of your family, but recognize their powerful influence on you.

Linda Mintle, *I Married You, Not Your Family* (Charisma House: Lake Mary, FL, 2008), 45–65.

DATING YOUR SPOUSE

by Douglas Weiss, PhD

DATING IS IMPORTANT, and without it you will be forfeiting much of the potential that your marriage holds. So let's define what a date is and what it is not.

Dating is simply planning to spend anywhere from three to five hours together—just you and your spouse. Occasionally you may select to do something with another couple, but let that comprise no more than 25 percent of the time. A date is to be a fun time with your spouse, and it is best to have some agreed-up boundaries for dating.

1. No problem discussions

The first boundary for making dating successful is this: you must not discuss problems and personal issues that you are having with your spouse or children. In other words, never let this become a "gripe at your spouse" time about what he or she did or didn't do or how he or she is not meeting your needs. Remember, dating is supposed to be fun, and listening to your spouse whine and complain about you is not fun. You can discuss these issues during the other six and a half days of the week. But you must protect your date time from personal problems.

2. No money discussions

The second boundary for dating: you may not discuss money.

This boundary is particularly hard for the self-employed, especially if a couple works together for the company. Try to avoid talking about "the business" or financial issues related to the house or office. You have sixteen hours a day for six days a week to discuss these very important business issues. Don't do it at the time of the week that you get to celebrate your partner.

3. No errands

The third boundary for a couple developing a successful dating ritual is this: do not use this time to run errands. Dating is not a time to trap your spouse in a car and go to Target, Home Depot, the cleaners, or the bank. Running errands is not dating.

4. Limit shopping

The fourth boundary, and the last, involves shopping during dating. Ladies, most men don't like shopping, and not too many women want to spend a romantic evening in the power tool aisle at Home Depot. Shopping falls under the category of errands. Now, some couples may decide to use a date night to do some Christmas shopping, but I really caution couples against shopping dates in general.

I strongly encourage dating your husband or wife as much as possible. Personally, I could easily excuse myself from dating because of being busy with a practice, writing books and articles, speaking at conferences, and other routine media activities. But for me, the choice of dating is like the choice of tithing. Once you have decided to do it, the "how to do it" will always follow.

Douglas Weiss, *Intimacy* (Lake Mary, FL: Siloam, 2001), 182–186.

RECONNECTING EMOTIONALLY

by Douglas Weiss, PhD

CONNECTING IS FUNDAMENTAL to having and maintaining emotional intimacy. Many of us grew up unskilled emotionally. As a teenager in my home, I can remember that we seemed to express only three emotions. The first emotion we communicated was anger. The second emotion we were allowed to display was "really angry." This was when doors were slammed or something was thrown. The last permitted emotion was what I call "other." *Other* means, "Leave me alone!" "I'm going for a walk, a drive, or a drink." This emotion found some other way to avoid or not process what we felt.

I grew up truly emotionally illiterate. I felt as if I had all these feelings locked up inside of me, but I only had these three exit doors: door number 1—anger; door number 2—really angry; and door number 3—other. I went all the way through Bible college and partially through seminary before I really understood that I didn't have a clue as to what I was feeling inside.

I admit that at times I thought it rather odd that I was in this great counseling program but still wasn't being taught how to know and express my own feelings. Many of us have grown up without the ability or skill to identify our feelings.

It is critical that you understand how to express your feelings. Your feelings are like a large engine-powered ocean liner. This engine provides the ship's energy. It pushes it in whatever direction the rudder directs. The rudder is our rational mind. Our emotions have great energy and pressure our minds. If not properly understood, emotions can drive us in such a way that they cause us to crash and be destroyed.

Men in particular have more difficulty just sharing feelings instead of trying to solve problems. But as you grow in the skill of sharing, hearing, and honoring the feelings of your spouse, the quality of emotional intimacy soars. When I feel safe and honored as I share my feelings, I am more likely to keep sharing them with others as well.

When you decide to honor your spouse emotionally on a regular basis, you will begin to see your spouse as the best person on earth to be with. I know that I can share any feelings with Lisa and still feel accepted by her. When she honors my emotions, it makes me feel special, important, and loved by my wife.

Your spouse and his or her emotions are ever changing. Honoring your spouse's emotions without feeling the need to fix them or fix the situation will produce enormous positive fruit in your relationship.

Douglas Weiss, *Intimacy* (Lake Mary, FL: Siloam, 2001), 22–23, 28.

THE THREE DAILIES

by Douglas Weiss, PhD

PRAYER

Prayer is an absolute necessity in your marriage. I am constantly amazed when couples tell me that the last time they really prayed together, not including praying over food or a good-night prayer with children, was years ago. Sometimes they say, "We both pray, just not together."

That's fine, but prayer as a couple is not optional: "Unless the LORD builds the house, its builders labor in vain" (Ps. 127:1, NIV). The Lord must be part of building your house. Prayer is an active way to include the Lord as part of the building plan of your marriage.

Prayer is one of the priorities that must be set in place by a couple desiring more intimacy. Remember, intimacy is three-dimensional, involving spirit, soul, and body. As we grow together spiritually, our intimacy in the other two areas will grow as well.

FEELINGS

Emotional intimacy is the second important aspect couples need to develop and maintain throughout their relationship. Early in their dating relationship and in their marriage, they readily share with one another their feelings about life situations, people, God, and their dreams. Often they can't remember exactly what happened to their feelings later on, but those of many couples appear to go into hiding. Life gets more complicated, and their conversations get more managerial. Discussions become limited to "Who does this?" "How will that get done?" or "That needs to get paid."

Emotions are an important part of who both of you are. They encompass your spouse's personality and influence the way in which he or she processes life events. Many couples don't see each other for eight to ten hours a day.

As you sow emotional intimacy into your marriage, in time you will reap emotional intimacy.

PRAISE AND NUTURING

This is the last of the three daily exercises you must practice with your husband or wife. This exercise addresses the God-given need for nuturing and praise that each one of us has.

Praising and nuturing one another are essential ingredients for a vibrant, ongoing intimate relationship. As you practice praising and nurturing, you will become increasingly skilled and comfortable with giving and receiving it. It will be more difficult for some husbands and wives to give praise than others. For others, receiving or acknowledging the praise that is given will be hard. Still others will struggle with both aspects of giving and receiving praise.

As you practice praise, the oil of intimacy will drip into your soul and heal areas of dryness that you didn't even know existed.

Douglas Weiss, *Intimacy* (Lake Mary, FL: Siloam, 2001), 154, 156–159, 168–169.

FORGIVENESS

by Don Colbert, MD

O NE OF THE secret causes of stress plaguing millions of people is unforgiveness. People rehash the wrong that was done to them, or that they misperceive was done to them, and their body immediately has a stress response. Your brain actually does not distinguish between short-term and long-term memories when it produces a biochemical stress response. It thinks the offense, which may have occurred decades ago, is happening right now.

Years ago I had a very well-known actor come to my office to be seen as a patient. Although he was not scheduled for a visit, I worked him into the schedule as a courtesy. On this particular day, however, I had seen some very sick patients who required hospitalization, which took more of my time than normal. By the time I saw this man, I was a couple of hours late. A few weeks later I learned through a friend of his that he was highly offended and thought that I had deliberately caused him to wait, which was not the case at all. However, he perceived this offense to be real even though he had no way of knowing that I was treating such gravely ill patients.

When you feel you have been wronged or that life has not been fair to you, resist the urge to allow this to turn into an offense. Be determined not to allow one or more negative events to define who you are. Instead choose to forgive and "let it go."

The apostle Paul wrote, "Make allowance for each other's faults, and forgive anyone who offends you. Remember, the Lord forgave you, so you must forgive others" (Col. 3:13, NLT).

To forgive does not mean that you didn't get hurt. Rather, it's choosing not to live in the feeling of unforgiveness. You can trust God to deal with the offense and the offender. Forgiving in its simplest form is letting go of old hurts and releasing people and situations into God's hands.

If you continue to hold on to unforgiveness toward someone else, you do not hurt that other person; rather, you damage your own health. Therefore, you should release your anger and bitterness for the sake of self-preservation. When you forgive, you release your right to judgment, punishment, and revenge related to the person who angered you.

Don Colbert, *The Seven Pillars of Health* (Lake Mary, FL: Siloam, 2007), 248–250.

THE FORGIVENESS EXERCISE

By Douglas Weiss, PhD

THIS EXERCISE GUIDES you through the process so that you can forgive and have a place in time to mark when your offense was released from your soul. First, you need to make a list of those individuals who have offended you. Then, walk through this exercise with all those on your offender list. It might include your dad and mom, your spouse, and any others who have hurt you.

This exercise has three steps to it. So select one offender, and go through this exercise while you are home alone. You will need two kitchen chairs.

1. Assume the role of the offender.

Place the two chairs facing each other. Pick a chair and sit facing the other chair. We'll call the chair in which you are sitting "chair A."

While you are sitting in chair A, role-play your offender. You are now this person. As you role-play this individual, have him or her apologize and ask for forgiveness for all that they have done to you. They are hypothetically confessing to you in the other chair (chair B). If I were doing this exercise about my dad, I would sit in chair A as I role-played my dad. I would verbally own my sin, apologize, and ask for forgiveness for the things I did and didn't do to Doug in chair B.

As I role-play my dad, I might say, "Doug, I need you to forgive me of…" Now since I am playing my dad, I can say what he needs to say to me in order to own and apologize for his sin against my life.

2. Role-play your response as the one offended.

Now I have played my dad as he asked forgiveness for several offenses against Doug, who was symbolically sitting in chair B. Yet as the one offended, I heard my dad own his sin and ask forgiveness. Now I can start step two.

I begin by physically moving to sit in chair B, now role-playing myself.

After hearing my dad ask for forgiveness, I now decide how I will respond. Above all, be honest. If you are not ready to forgive your offender, tell him or her.

You could say, "I'm just not ready to do this yet, but I will try again in a few weeks."

Whatever you do when you play yourself, don't be a phony or do what you think you *should* do. Do what is real.

If you are able to forgive your offender, then tell him or her. In our example, Doug is now talking to Dad in the opposite chair.

I could say, "Dad, I forgive you."

I could really release him from his abuse and neglect of my soul and the impact his actions had on my life.

If you forgave your offender, move to step three. If at this time you are not able to forgive your offender, get out your calendar and set up a date in about three to four weeks when you will try this exercise again. Do this every month to measure your progress until you are able to forgive.

3. Role-play the offender's response to forgiveness.

In our example, Doug has forgiven Dad. Now I physically get up and sit down in chair A again and play the role of my dad. Now it is Dad's turn to respond to Doug's forgiveness.

Dad (role-played by Doug) might say, "Thanks, Doug." When Dad is done talking to Doug, the exercise is over.

Let's review:

1. Start in chair A as the offender asking for forgiveness.
2. Now sit in chair B as yourself and honestly respond to your offender's request for forgiveness.
3. If you have forgiven him or her, go back to chair A and play the offender responding to the forgiveness.

In all these exercises, each offender gets his or her time in the chair with you. You must role-play each one and receive an individual apology from each. Don't role-play more than one offender in a day.

As you do these exercises and move through forgiveness, especially toward your spouse, you can once again feel free to give, trust, and build. That's what it is about—removing all the roadblocks to intimacy. As you do this, the door will swing open to an entirely new and refreshing way of life.

Let's pray together:

> *Lord, help me to process my woundedness and to apply these exercises to my life. Comfort me, Lord, and lead me to still waters where I can drink of the intimacy that You have for me. In Jesus's name, amen.*

Douglas Weiss, *Intimacy* (Lake Mary, FL: Siloam, 2001), 63–66.

HEALING THE ROOTS OF ANGER

by Douglas Weiss, PhD

SMALL INFRACTIONS CAUSED by a couple's sins and unresolved conflicts during the course of a marriage create roadblocks to intimacy. The onslaught of trauma experienced by other couples causes deep, destructive rifts.

Neglect and abuse, which accompany addictions to alcohol, drugs, sex, food, and work, can seriously damage the spouse married to an addict. Lies, empty promises, and the roller-coaster rides that typify these addictive marriages create truly indescribable pain.

The scarring of physical and mental abuse causes more than just a buildup of painful events—it often causes legitimate rage. The effects of sexual infidelity, rape, and child abuse will most certainly traumatize any marriage, even those appearing to be very religious. Although such things "should" not happen in Christian marriages, I know they do.

On the other side of abuse is neglect. Neglect is more common in Christian marriages seeking help. Prayerlessness in a Christian couple's relationship is definitely a form of neglect. I cannot tell you how many women have come to my office over the years complaining about the lack of connection with their spouse.

Refusing to share your heart, coupled with an absence of prayer and praise over the decades, will create a silent anger, an internal rage within your spouse. This serious roadblock stunts the growth of trust and intimacy and can create real problems down the road for the couple who remains together.

Adulterous situations throw a spouse into a traumatic situation that he or she must then attempt to handle. To expect the spouse in an adulterous situation to simply move on and put the matter behind him or her minimizes the trauma. Adultery affects the spirit, soul, and body, creating deep wounds in one or both spouses.

In many relationships, trust has been broken, decency has been violated, and healing must take place in the soul of the wounded spouse. This individual is thrust into a paradoxical situation. Unfortunately, the person whom he or she loves the most may also be the one with whom he or she is most angry, and for good reason. This is an internal controversy that says "I love you" and "I'd like to pound you!" all at the same time.

Anger is a familiar problem in many marriages, and it must be taken seriously as you strive to be intimate with your spouse. Only when wounds inside a relationship are identified and addressed biblically can healing begin to take place. Silent anger about your wounds can block intimacy, even when you long for it in your marriage.

If you are a wounded spouse, the perpetrator is responsible for your feelings. Yet the responsibility to heal is yours. If I happened to walk outside and a sniper randomly shot me, I would be responsible to heal and repair from the damage of this event. I'm the one who would have to do what the doctor or physical therapist advised if I wanted to be restored.

Regardless of the past, healing can take place. It requires work and patience, but the results are nothing short of marvelous. As a Christian counselor I have witnessed the healing of deep wounds and broken marriages. I have watched as couples reclaimed intimacy and once again became vibrant and sexually passionate. We serve a great God, and as a colaborer with Him, all things are possible.

Douglas Weiss, *Intimacy* (Lake Mary, FL: Siloam, 2001), 47–51.

HEALTHY KIDS

THINGS THAT CREATE A PATTERN OF WORRY IN CHILDREN

by Gregory L. Jantz, PhD, with Ann McMurray

A CHILD WITH A sense of security looks out across the gulf to adulthood and sees a broadly supported expanse with plenty of room to move and solid railings. There's no need to focus on the abyss below because there is no fear of falling. Instead, the child has a wide-open view of the wonders that await. A child with a sense of insecurity looks out across the gulf to adulthood and sees a gap-filled, narrow track hemmed in on all sides by frayed, untrustworthy ropes. Forget looking up and out; there's an absolute need to focus on the abyss below because each fearful step forward contains the potential for falling. What starts out in childhood translates into adulthood. There are a variety of situations and conditions that can lead to this kind of insecurity growing up.

- *Abandonment by a parent.* When a parent basically discards a child through abandonment, damage occurs. In a death, a child learns all is not right with the world. In abandonment, a child assumes all is not right with him or her. *A child learns how much one person can hurt another.*
- *Rejection by a parent.* This is different from abandonment and is when a parent intentionally chooses to reject a child, whether or not there is a physical leaving. *A child learns that no matter what, they just aren't good enough.*
- *Frequent moves.* Often parents view a move as a positive change, due to a new house or new job. Children, however, have different priorities, and the one thing they cherish, such as a friend, a teacher, a school, an activity, or even a pet, can be sacrificed in the decision to relocate. *A child learns favorite things can be taken away by those who love them.*
- *Difficulties in school.* Children often worry about their work in school, but they also worry about other issues, such as social interactions. A child who is unpopular, bullied, unsuccessful, or simply unnoticed learns to distrust what could happen tomorrow. *A child learns what it feels like on the outside.*
- *Excessive criticism or negativity by a parent or significant adult.* Adults are supposed to be a child's biggest teacher and cheerleader. Sadly, too often what they teach isn't very cheery. The child then lives with a critical, negative adult who specializes in blame. This pattern is then internalized by the child and often emulated. *A child learns they are the problem.*
- *Family alcoholism or drug abuse.* When alcohol or drug abuse is present in the home, it becomes a home of calm and crisis. There are lulls between violent storms, whose appearance is not so much a matter of *if* but *when*. A child learns to survive within the chaos of crisis and to never take anything for granted. A calm sky only means a storm is coming. *A child learns up is down and down is up.*
- *A fearful or insecure parent or significant adult.* Some parents communicate hostility and negativity that damage the self-esteem of their children. Other parents or adults can be more passively damaging through a pattern of constant doubt, fear, worry, and anxiety. *A child learns the world is a scary place not to be trusted.*
- *Chronic medical conditions.* Imagine the concern of a child who never knows if a parent is going to have some sort of medical issue, from diabetic shock to an epileptic episode. Children, of course, can be instructed on how to cope with these health challenges in

a loved one and even in themselves, but the potential exists for the child to develop an excessive concern about an event reoccurring. *A child learns how quickly things can change.*

- *Perfectionism in the family.* This is one of the most pervasive ways a child is taught to worry. No one can be perfect all the time, so every task, every expectation has a built-in guarantee of failure. Even if the child believes something is right, it's not his or her opinion that counts. *A child learns it's never good enough.*

- *Overinvolved parenting.* When a child is smothered by a parent, he or she is not allowed to experience the world outside of the parental cocoon. Negative consequences are immediately treated as crises and whisked away by the parent. Instead of being strengthened by learning to deal with natural consequences and adversity, a coddled child is weakened and unprepared for the realities of a life detached from the parent. *A child learns the thoughts of others are more important than their own.*

Gregory L. Jantz with Ann McMurray, *Happy for the Rest of Your Life* (Lake Mary, FL: Siloam, 2009), 74–79.

LEAVING A HEALTHY INHERITANCE FOR THE NEXT GENERATION

by Kara Davis, MD

T HE LAW OF MOSES included specific instructions regarding inheritance. Along with material possessions, the father was to pass down an inheritance of virtue, teaching his children the laws of God and modeling for them, through the example of his own life, the importance of obedience. The notion of receiving an inheritance was so ingrained in the *natural* that the concept was used by David to describe his *spiritual* rewards: "The boundary lines have fallen for me in pleasant places; surely I have a delightful inheritance" (Ps. 16:6, NIV).

Most adults have an innate desire to pass on a blessing to future generations. People don't usually say, "I want my children to experience greater adversity than I did." Instead, we work hard and plan well, hoping our efforts will mean our children will be spared some of our own life's struggles.

But let's consider what we are passing on to future generations in regard to their health, a "commodity" that would be considered by many to be more precious than land or money. If we had an inheritance report card, then our grade would be an F. Some experts predict this generation will be the first in U.S. history to have a shorter life expectancy than their parents. In terms of health, we are failing our posterity.

Certainly many things are contributing to this crisis, but I'd like to focus on just three: television viewing, eating at home, and soft drink consumption. Let the facts speak for themselves.

Television viewing

- In preschool children, the risk of obesity increases by 6 percent for every hour of television watched per day.[1]
- Children aged two through eleven see on average twenty-three food advertisements per day, the vast majority for sugary cereal, fast food, candy, and snacks.[2]

Eating at home

- The more days per week children eat dinner at home, the more likely they are to have healthy eating habits.[3]
- Children who frequently eat meals with their families tend to do better in school.[4]

Soft drink consumption

- Soft drinks are now the leading source of added sugar in the American teenager's diet.[5]
- Approximately 60 percent of middle and high schools sell soft drinks in vending machines.[6]

The Book of Psalms tells us the value of children: "Sons are a heritage from the LORD, children a reward from him. Like arrows in the hands of a warrior are sons born in one's youth. Blessed is the man whose quiver is full of them. They will not be put to shame when they contend with their enemies in the gate" (Ps. 127:3–5, NIV). Our children are valuable in the sight of God. We have a responsibility to leave them an inheritance of good health.

Kara Davis, *Spiritual Secrets to Weight Loss* (Lake Mary, FL: Siloam, 2002, 2008), 134–137.

OBESE CHILDREN

by Scott Hannen, DC

A N ENTIRE GENERATION is being impacted by the carboholic culture we have created: Obesity in children has tripled in the past twenty years. A staggering 50 percent of adolescents in some minority populations are overweight. There is an epidemic of type 2 (formerly "adult-onset") diabetes in children, and heart attacks may become a disease of young adults.[1]

Why is the health of our children deteriorating on such a scale? In 1995 the American Academy of Pediatrics stated that advertising to young children is inherently deceptive and exploitative. Yet each year the food industry spends an estimated $10 billion to influence the eating behavior of children. The average child sees ten thousand food advertisements per year, 95 percent of them for fast food, soft drinks, candy, and sugared cereals—all high-profit and nutrition-poor products.[2]

I can't help wondering how the media would respond if obesity were any other illness that was impacting the health of an entire generation so drastically. I think it would be posted on the front page of every newspaper and given headlines in every news broadcast across the country. Is it possible that advertising promoting obesity with junk food pays the bills of the media, which is more important than our national health concerns? Or do we just think that the new body size is OK? People seem to be happy and adjusted to their larger size, and some show no concern for the health risk those extra pounds present.

For many of our children, the average breakfast consists of a toaster pastry and a glass of milk. You may think that sounds pretty harmless. However, the sugar content in those pastries sends the child into hyper drive like a rocket into orbit ("rocket fuel"). Milk allergies and sensitivities are highly prevalent in children, which many parents never figure out.

I watched a video presentation in graduate school of a kindergarten child who was sitting in class drawing a picture of a house. He was very docile and well behaved. The teacher gave him a glass of milk to drink, and fifteen minutes later he went crazy. It was like watching a Jekyll and Hyde movie. The child started scratching his crayons across the paper violently. His entire demeanor changed as he became highly irritated and hyperactive, all because he drank a glass of milk, "Hyde potion."

We then send these children to school full of "rocket fuel" and "Hyde potion" and then forbid the teacher to teach them Bible principles such as the Ten Commandments or the Golden Rule. Neither children nor teachers are allowed to pray. Teachers cannot use any kind of corporal discipline (spanking) to correct a child's misbehavior, yet doctors can put them on potentially harmful drugs to control them, and that seems to be OK. There is something badly wrong here that seems unreasonable to me. Does it to you?

Unfortunately, we have become a society at risk, forfeiting our long-term health for carboholic diets that are promoted by billions of dollars of media advertising.

Scott Hannen, *Healing by Design* (Lake Mary, FL: Siloam, 2003, 2007), 41–43.

TIPS FOR GETTING KIDS TO EAT HEALTHILY

by Don Colbert, MD

ALL PARENTS AND grandparents know what a challenge it can be to get kids to enjoy healthy foods at times. But in light of the epidemic of childhood obesity we're facing, teaching kids to eat living foods is one of the most important things parents can do.

GET THEM INVOLVED

One of the easiest ways to get your kids to try new foods is to get them involved in selecting the foods at the grocery store and preparing the foods at mealtime. Let your child be in charge of picking out one new fruit or vegetable a week. Teach them to read food labels, and make a game out of finding the healthiest bread, pasta, or cereal product. At home, make kids part of meal preparations by having them, wash fruits and vegetables being prepared, tear up lettuce for salads, snap green beans, shuck corn on the cob, mash potatoes with an old-fashioned potato masher, or break off broccoli and cauliflower florets.

GET "FRESH"!

If cooked veggies have been turning your kids off, don't fall into the trap of slathering them with butter or cheese to make them more palatable. Try serving them raw or steamed, such as carrots, snap peas, broccoli, and cauliflower. It's surprising how many people discover they love the fresh version of the same vegetables they thought they hated.

MAKE IT FUN

A quick trip down the cereal aisle at your local grocery store will tell you that children are drawn in by colorful packaging. Use this to your advantage! Purchase some fun storage containers and store fruits, vegetables, whole-grain cereals, and snack bars in these containers. Put them on a special shelf, and have him pull out his "special snack" container and help himself.

AVOID MEALTIME BATTLES

If mealtime is a stressful battleground at your house, don't use this time to start adding healthy foods to your child's diet. Try working them in as snacks throughout the day. Associate eating these foods with things she enjoys doing, and she's much more likely to accept them.

MOVE IT!

Healthy eating is not enough; it must be accompanied by an active lifestyle. If your child spends inordinate amounts of time on the couch or playing video or computer games, don't just tell him to go ride his bike—do it with him! Here are some other activities kids and parents can do together:

- Walk the family pet.
- Take a picnic lunch to the park.
- Play catch with a softball or baseball.
- Play some backyard volleyball, kickball, or badminton.
- Join a local YMCA or health club with family-style fitness programs.

Don Colbert, *Eat This and Live!* (Lake Mary, FL: Siloam, 2009), 170–171.

ADD AND HYPERACTIVITY

by Don Colbert, MD

I F YOUR CHILD has attention deficit disorder (ADD) and ADHD, you do not have to resort to heavy drug treatments that affect the unique, God-given personality of your precious child. Through practical natural methods, faith, prayer, and God's Word, your ADD or ADHD child can live a perfectly normal life free from the harmful effects of long-term drug treatments.

To overcome ADD, it's important to first gain wisdom about it. The Scriptures say, "Wisdom is a tree of life to those who embrace her; happy are those who hold her tightly" (Prov. 3:18, NLT).

ADD can occur with or without hyperactivity. ADD with hyperactivity is also called ADHD, or attention deficit hyperactivity disorder.

DOES YOUR CHILD HAVE ADD?

Fill out this ADD/ADHD quiz to find out if your child or loved one may have ADD or ADHD. (The symptoms must have started before age seven and must have been evident for six months.) Check the appropriate boxes.

Inattention

- ❑ Often fails to give close attention to details or makes careless mistakes in schoolwork, work, or other activities
- ❑ Often has difficulty sustaining attention in tasks or play activities
- ❑ Often does not seem to listen when spoken to directly
- ❑ Often does not follow through on instructions and fails to finish schoolwork, chores, or duties in the workplace
- ❑ Often has difficulty organizing tasks and activities

Hyperactivity

- ❑ Often fidgets with hands or feet or squirms in seat
- ❑ Often leaves seat in classroom or in other situations in which remaining seated is expected
- ❑ Often runs about or climbs excessively in situations in which it is inappropriate (in adolescents or adults, may be limited to subjective feelings of restlessness)
- ❑ Often has difficulty playing or engaging in leisure activities quietly
- ❑ Is often on the go or acts as if driven by a motor

If you have checked more than half of the boxes in either category, your child or loved one may be experiencing ADD or ADHD and should be evaluated by a professional.

Parents of children with ADD and ADHD need to understand their child's learning style. Here are a few suggestions for helping to create a better classroom environment for your child:

- Visit your child's classroom during class to observe your child.
- Moving your child closer to the teacher and away from distractions can help him focus.
- What kind of temperament does his teacher have? Is she rigid, irritable? Does she seem to take her frustrations out on the children?

- Schedule regular periodic meetings with the teacher to discuss your child's special learning needs.
- Many schools permit parents to eat lunch with their children. Join your child regularly for lunch.

God's rich love for your child includes blessing your youngster's life with natural, truly wholesome and nourishing foods. God says, "But I would feed you with the finest wheat. I would satisfy you with wild honey from the rock" (Ps. 81:16, NLT). Healthy, nutritious food is a major component to your natural solution to ADD and ADHD.

BRAIN FOOD

Several key neurotransmitters are critically important for focusing, learning, and memory. These most important neurotransmitters include acetylcholine, norepinephrine, serotonin, and dopamine. What your child eats every day forms these essential brain chemicals. Make sure you include these foods in your child's diet: organic eggs, almonds, almond butter, whole-grain products, seafood, poultry, sunflower seeds, veggies, fruit, and good fats such as fish oil, flaxseed oil, and extra-virgin olive oil.

Many children with ADD and ADHD have multiple food sensitivities. These kids' behavior can dramatically improve when certain foods are identified and eliminated from their diets. Many children have adverse reactions to sugars, corn syrup, junk food, food dyes, preservatives, additives, and artificial colors and sweeteners

As you learn and develop new habits, ask God to help you. Never forget how much He loves your child and how much He loves you too! He will give you the patience, discipline, and wisdom you need. All you need to do is ask.

Don Colbert, *The Bible Cure for ADD and Hyperactivity* (Lake Mary, FL: Siloam, 2001).

VACCINATIONS

by Leslie Ann Dauphin, PhD

O NE WAY TO prevent the spread of infectious diseases is through vaccines. Vaccines are administered orally, by injection, and, more recently, by inhalation. They are strongly recommended and should be administered according to the prescribed schedules to prevent unnecessary infections.

The media have done an effective job of scaring most parents about the dangers of childhood vaccinations, but I am going to debunk some of those myths. Here are three of the common misconceptions about vaccines.

1. Vaccines can cause severe side effects, disease, and can even lead to death.
2. Most people who get diseases have already been vaccinated.
3. The incidence of disease has decreased due to improvements in sanitation, not vaccines.

But the truth of the matter is vaccines are actually quite safe, and the side effects are usually very mild. Some examples are a low-grade fever or sniffles for a day or two, which are, of course, preferable to the actual disease symptoms. Vaccines that are given to children routinely have been shown to be effective in 85 to 95 percent of the children who receive them.[1]

Although the number of cases is considerably low, there have been some reports of serious illness and even death associated with vaccine use. For this reason the Vaccine Injury Compensation Act was passed in 1986. It awards cash benefits to families that have children who have suffered from severe injury such as brain damage or death due to vaccination.

A recent area of concern of vaccines has been a potential link to autism. The Department of Education reports that from school years 1991–1992 to 2001–2002 the number of children in the United States diagnosed with autism increased from 5,415 to 118,602.[2] The increase for cases of autism was greater than that for all other disabilities in general. Some groups have suggested that the MMR (mumps, measles, and rubella) vaccine and thimerosal, a mercury-based preservative, are linked to autism. These claims have not been supported by definitive experimental data. Also, there have been no harmful effects reported for thimerosal used at the doses recommended for vaccines.

Since 1999, the number of thimerosal-based vaccines has been decreased. To date there is no clear explanation for the increase in cases of autism, nor is there a clear understanding as to what causes the condition.

There should be some comfort in knowing that it is not easy to get a vaccine approved for widespread use. The FDA requires that vaccines be tested extensively to ensure safety before licensure for general use. It may take from ten to fifty years from the time a vaccine is discovered until the time it is approved. If approved for licensure and placed on the market, the FDA continues to monitor its safety. As the number of vaccinated people increases, research studies are conducted involving larger numbers to measure its efficacy and safety. Finally, the Vaccine Adverse Events Reporting System (VAERS) is used by the FDA and CDC to gather information about licensed vaccines. This system is designed so that doctors, patients, and others may report any unusual reactions, symptoms, or complications associated with a vaccine. The FDA views weekly VAERS reports for unusual reports about vaccines that are currently in use.

Leslie Ann Dauphin, PhD, *The Germ Handbook* (Lake Mary, FL: Siloam, 2005), 77–83.

VITAMIN and HERBAL SUPPLEMENTS

HOW TO CHOOSE

by Don Colbert, MD

I N A PERFECT world, the human body would indeed get all the nutrients it needs from food. The vitamins and minerals our bodies need to thrive should come through the foods we eat. However, processed foods have been stripped of much of their nutrient content. Cooking and storage are also reasons why our food loses more nutrients. Our toxic environment and toxins in our food, water, and air, as well as our overstressed lifestyles, have increased our nutrient requirements. Even if we were to eat adequate fruits and vegetables, the nutrient content in them has decreased due to our depleted soils.

What constitutes a good multivitamin? The answer is the same things that make living food healthy. Nature never produces nutrients in isolation. Oranges, for example, contain much more than vitamin C. Carrots contain much more than beta-carotene. When you eat them, you get a myriad of vitamins, phytonutrients, flavonoids, and more that interact in ways that are not fully understood but that we recognize to be healthy.

The healthiest supplements combine enzymes, coenzymes, trace elements, antioxidants, activators, phytonutrients, vitamins and minerals, and many other elements, which all work together synergistically. These supplements are called whole-food supplements and are generally what I recommend.

Nutritionist Paavo Airola, MD, PhD, in his book *How to Get Well*, stated, "When you take natural vitamins, as for instance in the form of rose hips, brewer's yeast, or vegetable oil, you get all the vitamins and vitamin-like factors that naturally occur in these foods. That is, all those that are already discovered as well as those that are not discovered yet."[1]

Whole-food supplements combine portions of the plants we know are healthy and those portions we have not yet discovered to be healthy. I believe it's wise to do this because medical knowledge is expanding so quickly that it gets outdated practically every few years. A nutrient we hadn't heard of a year ago can suddenly be discovered to protect against certain kinds of cancer or disease.

You need a comprehensive multivitamin, made from living ingredients and combined with living nutrition. I usually recommend supplementation with both pancreatic enzymes and/or HCL, especially for patients over fifty years of age. I prefer that nutritional supplements be in vegetable capsules, be excipient (filler) free, and nonirradiated.

Don Colbert, *The Seven Pillars of Health* (Lake Mary, FL: Siloam, 2007), 181, 222–223.

BASICS FOR ADULTS

by Don Colbert, MD

MY GOAL IS to simplify your life, not complicate it. When choosing a supplement, you should look for a multivitamin that contains all thirteen vitamins and seventeen to twenty-two minerals with 100 percent of daily values. Also, you need omega-3 fats and a phytonutrient powder. *That's it!*

When choosing a supplement, here is what I recommend for everyone, regardless of age:

1. Choose a comprehensive multivitamin that has at least 100 percent of the daily value (DV) or reference daily intake (RDI).

COMPONENTS OF A COMPREHENSIVE MULTIVITAMIN
Vitamins: A, B$_1$ (thiamine), B$_2$ (riboflavin), B$_3$ (niacin), B$_5$ (pantothenic acid), B$_6$ (pyridoxine), B$_{12}$, biotin, folic acid, C, D, E, K
Minerals: boron, calcium, chromium, cobalt, copper, iodine, iron, magnesium, manganese, molybdenum, phosphorus, potassium, selenium, silicon, sodium, sulfur, vanadium, zinc

Start slowly because they may upset your stomach. Start with half the recommended amount and space them out during the day after meals. You may increase the amount as tolerated, but do not take over 100 percent of the daily value.

2. Choose a high-quality omega-3 fat to take daily. Start slowly with one a day and increase as tolerated.

3. Choose a phytonutrient powder. This powder should contain a combination of colorful organic fruits and vegetables such as red, yellow, green, orange, and purple. Start slowly with just a teaspoon a day, and increase the amount as tolerated. Living foods may cause gas and bloating as your body adjusts to them.

High-quality fish oils, or omega-3 fats, are vitally important for good health. Realize that many deadly degenerative diseases are inflammatory, such as cancer, heart disease, Alzheimer's disease, arthritis, autoimmune disease, and so on. Fish oil is able to decrease inflammation significantly. I believe omega-3 fats are special fats the body needs as much as it needs vitamins. Much of the research on these powerful fats was done in the 1980s after realizing the Inuit Indians, who are Eskimos, rarely developed heart attacks or rheumatoid arthritis, yet their diet contained an enormous amount of fat from fish, seals, and whales, which are all high in omega-3 fats.

Phytonutrients are biologically active substances that give fruits and vegetables their color, flavor, smell, and natural disease resistance. They can have major health benefits for your body. There are so many different phytonutrients that it can be quite confusing! That's why I like to simply group them by color. Our goal should be to include as many colors as possible in our daily diet. Think of phytonutrients as a "rainbow of health," God's promise to you to keep you healthy.

Don Colbert, *The Seven Pillars of Health* (Lake Mary, FL: Siloam, 2007), 205–206, 223–224.

FOR THOSE OVER FIFTY

by Don Colbert, MD

I F YOU ARE over fifty years of age, you will probably need extra antioxidants, extra calcium and vitamin D, sublingual B_{12}, and maybe digestive enzymes. If you already have a disease or simply want more protection, start taking extra antioxidants after the age of forty.

1. Vitamin E (mixed tocopherols and tocotrienols), 200 to 400 IU a day (may be present in a multivitamin). Be careful not to take over 400 IU of vitamin E a day.
2. Vitamin C, 250 mg twice a day (may be present in a multivitamin)
3. Coenzyme Q_{10}, 100 mg a day
4. R-form alpha-lipoic acid or R-DHLA, 100 mg a day
5. N-acetyl-cysteine (NAC), 250 to 500 mg a day, or Recancostat (glutathione), one capsule once or twice a day
6. Turmeric and synergistic herbs (such as Protandim), one a day
7. Calcium and vitamin D: calcium, 400 mg three times a day, and vitamin D, 1,000–2,000 IU a day. Men generally only need 400 mg of calcium twice a day.
8. Digestive enzymes and/or HCL, one after each meal
9. Sublingual B_{12}, 1,000 mcg a day

I recommend a sublingual B_{12} supplement for patients over fifty years of age. After age fifty, many Americans do not produce adequate amounts of hydrochloric acid, which is required for binding B_{12} to a substance called intrinsic factor for absorption in the ileum, which is the last part of the small intestines.[1]

Opinions will always differ on what vitamins and minerals to take and on the amounts necessary. Before making any dramatic changes in the amount of vitamins or minerals you add to your daily diet, always consult your personal physician. There are other nutritional supplements that are important, including carnosine, glucosamine sulfate, vitamin K_2, and supplements for prostate health. Also, natural, bioidentical hormone replacement therapy is extremely important for women and men, especially over the age of fifty.

As more research is done on nutritional supplements, we will find that some supplements may be healthier than we thought, and others may be less healthy. It is impossible to banish all confusion regarding supplements, so we must do the best we can with the information we are given for the moment.

Don Colbert, *The Seven Pillars of Health* (Lake Mary, FL: Siloam, 2007), 224–227.

WARNINGS
by Don Colbert, MD

I F YOU HAVE ever walked into a health food store, you probably felt the same way many people do: overwhelmed by shelf after shelf crammed with thousands of multivitamins and minerals and individual supplements, each claiming to be the key to your health. Nutritional supplements have become big business, and confusion reigns for the poor consumer.

Now that nutritional supplements have become big business, many pharmaceutical companies have jumped on the bandwagon and are manufacturing multivitamins, omega-3 fats (fish oil pills), and many others that are sold in huge quantities at discount stores and supermarkets.

Most mass-produced nutritional supplements contain poor-quality synthetic nutrients, which are not nearly as healthy for you as are natural nutrients and may, in fact, be harmful.[1] These man-made multivitamin and mineral supplements are usually made from mineral salts, which are poorly absorbed by your body and therefore vastly less effective but very inexpensive. The manufacturers seem to believe that they can standardize, process, and manufacture vitamins in the same way they manufacture prescription drugs, which, by the way, is not a natural process. Some big pharmaceutical companies even use ingredients such as toxic partially hydrogenated soybean oil as fillers for their soft gels, which may have been extracted from coal tar, and put them in their tablets and capsules. A friend of mine calls these "toxic tagalongs."

One of the worst offenders is in fish oil supplements. Fish oils and omega-3 supplements can be good for you, but much of the fish oils in supplement form are rancid. Taste it and see for yourself. The fats oxidize quickly and become toxic, causing even more free-radical damage to your body. Some fish oils will not even have a rancid odor and taste, yet still contain high amounts of lipid peroxides.[2]

This may shock you, but the unhealthiest people I see are the ones who are mega-dosing on supplements. They are using supplements the way doctors use some drugs—to treat symptoms but not the cause. Sometimes these patients don't want to make other lifestyle and dietary changes, so they rely on pills from the health food store.

Like anything else in life, too much of a good thing may eventually harm your body. Mega-dosing on one type of vitamin or mineral is no different. For example, megadoses of vitamin B_6 can lead to neuropathy or damage to nerves in your arms and legs.[3]

When it comes to supplements, more is not necessarily better. You must remember that supplements are just that—to supplement a healthy diet. They are not the diet itself. As long as you eat a healthy diet, you don't have to meet all your nutritional needs with supplements.

Don Colbert, *The Seven Pillars of Health* (Lake Mary, FL: Siloam, 2007), 215–217, 219–221.

TOP FIVE LIFE-ENHANCING SUPPLEMENTS

by Janet Maccaro, PhD, CNC

A SET OF TOOLS you will find very effective in building your healthy body includes the following five life-enhancing supplements. Consider the brief description of their function, and learn to use them as needed to strengthen your personal health.

5-hydroxytryptophan (5-HTP) is an intermediate in the natural synthesis of the essential amino acid tryptophan to serotonin. 5-HTP is derived from the *Griffonia Simplicifolia* plant and is an important neurotransmitter involved in the regulation of brain activity responsible for emotion, appetite, and wake/sleep/wake cycles. By feeding your brain 5-HTP, your serotonin level rises, which in turn causes emotional well-being, appetite control, and better sleep quality. Suggested dose: 50-mg capsule once a day before a meal. *Do not use if you are pregnant or lactating.*[1]

Resveratrol promotes cardiovascular health by its antioxidant action and its ability to modulate platelet aggregation and arachidonic acid metabolism. Resveratrol is a compound that is often associated with the health benefits of red wine because of its powerful antioxidant and cardioprotective properties. It is derived from *Polygonum cuspidatum*, an herb that has been used for centuries for its nutritional benefits. Suggested dose: 200-mg capsule daily.[2]

Coenzyme Q$_{10}$ is a necessary component of cellular energy production and respiration. It enhances energy levels in every cell of the body, providing increased energy and exercise tolerance and optimal nutritional support of the cardiovascular system. It is especially supportive of tissues that require a lot of energy, such as periodontal tissue, the heart muscle, and the cells of the body's defense system. Suggested dose: two to four capsules per day in divided doses with meals. Take with vitamin E for enhanced benefit.[3]

Melatonin is a hormone that regulates the body's wake/sleep/wake cycle. The hormone is secreted in a circadian rhythm by enzymes, which are activated by darkness and depressed by light. Nightly melatonin supplementation can boost the performance of immune systems that are compromised by age, drugs, or stress during sleep. Suggested dose: one 3-mg capsule one-half to one hour before bedtime. *Do not take if you are pregnant or lactating.*[4]

Phosphatidylserine is found in all cells, but it is most heavily concentrated in brain cells. This brain nutrient improves cognitive function, emotional well-being, and behavioral performance by restoring cell membrane composition. Mental acuity is positively affected by supplementation with phosphatidylserine. Suggested dose: three 100-mg capsules daily in divided doses with meals.[5]

Janet Maccaro, *Natural Health Remedies* (Lake Mary, FL: Siloam, 2003, 2006), 38–41.

HERBAL REMEDIES FOR COMMON MALADIES

by Janet Maccaro, PhD, CNC

Heart disease
- Cayenne
- Garlic
- Hawthorn berry

High blood pressure
- Feverfew
- Garlic
- Valerian

Impotence
- Gingko biloba

Insomnia
- Astragalus
- Gotu kola
- Valerian

Liver problems
- Ginseng
- Milk thistle
- Turmeric

Memory
- Gingko biloba
- Gotu kola

Migraines
- Feverfew

Motion sickness
- Ginger

Nausea
- Ginger

Nervousness
- Chamomile
- Kava kava
- Passionflower
- Valerian

Pain
- Cayenne
- Peppermint
- White willow bark

Prostate problems
- Echinacea
- Goldenseal
- Saw palmetto

Sore throat
- Ginger
- Goldenseal
- Licorice

Sunburn
- Aloe

Upset stomach
- Chamomile
- Peppermint

Vein problems
- Chamomile
- Gotu kola

Viral disease
- Astragalus
- Garlic

Janet Maccaro, *90-Day Immune System Makeover* (Lake Mary, FL: Siloam, 2000, 2006), 194.

ABOUT THE AUTHORS

Lisa Bevere is the best-selling author of *Fight Like a Girl, Out of Control and Loving It! Kissed the Girls and Made Them Cry, Be Angry but Don't Blow It!* and *You Are Not What You Weigh*. In addition to speaking at national and international conferences, she is a frequent guest on Christian television and radio shows. Lisa is also the cohost of the weekly television program *The Messenger*, which broadcasts to 214 nations. She and her husband, John Bevere, also a best-selling author, make their home in Colorado with their four sons.

David B. Biebel, DMin, has been the editor of *Today's Christian Doctor*, a publication of the Christian Medical & Dental Associations, since 1992. He has authored, coauthored, and produced more than a dozen books, including the best seller *If God Is So Good, Why Do I Hurt So Bad?* and *New Light on Depression*, a Gold Medallion–winner that Biebel coauthored with Dr. Harold Koenig.

Lorriane Bossé-Smith is the author of seven books (*I Want My Life Back, Leveraging Your Communication Style, Leveraging Your Leadership Style, Fit Over 50, Finally FIT!* and *A Healthier, Happier You*). Lorraine has written for several magazines as well as newspapers and currently writes on assignment for *American Fitness*. She has shared her heart with radio listeners across the country and has been on live television shows. Lorraine is a certified human behavior consultant, speaker, life coach, and personal trainer and is listed in the 2000 Who's Who of Entrepreneurs and the 2005 Who's Who Among Female Executives. She holds a BS in business administration with minors in marketing and communication. Her mission: to improve the quality of YOUR life!

Reginald Cherry, MD, has practiced diagnostic and preventative medicine/alternative medicine in his clinic for over thirty years. Frustrated with the limited number of people he could help, he was led to expand his outreach through ministry with weekly television, a monthly newsletter, books, and other materials. The television program, *The Doctor and the Word*, now reaches millions of homes each week, and the medical newsletter, "Pathway to Healing," goes to thousands of partners. Dr. Cherry is the author of *The Bible Cure, Bible Health Secrets,* and *The Doctor and the Word*.

Joseph Christiano, ND, CNC, a naturopathic doctor and certified nutritional counselor, has spent forty years developing individualized diet and exercise programs for Hollywood celebrities, major media personalities, and swimsuit winners in the Miss America, Miss USA, and Mrs. America pageants. The former Mr. Florida and Mr. USA runner-up has been featured in national publications, including *Iron Man, Woman's World,* and *Women's Health and Fitness,* and has authored several books, including *My Body, God's Temple* and the best seller *Bloodtypes, Bodytypes, and You*. As founder of Dump the Junk America, Dr. Joe has developed a nationwide campaign for helping kids with obesity and related illnesses and poor academics.

Don Colbert, MD, is board certified in family practice and anti-aging medicine. He is the medical director of the Divine Health Wellness Center in Orlando, Florida, where he has treated over forty thousand patients. Dr. Colbert is an internationally known expert and prolific speaker on integrative medicine (a combination of traditional and alternative medicine). Dr. Colbert has also become affectionately known as "The doctor to God's generals." Dr. Colbert has been featured on *FOX News, NBC Nightly News,* and BBC, and in publications such as *The Atlanta Journal Constitution, Readers Digest, Newsweek, Prevention,* and many others. He is the best-selling author of over forty books, including the Bible Cure series, *What Would Jesus Eat?* as well as *The Seven Pillars of Health* (a *New York Times* best seller), that together have sold more than four million copies. Dr. Colbert's books are required reading at many medical schools around the world. Dr. Colbert is also the president of Divine Health Inc., which distributes and sells nutritional supplements and vitamins at www.drcolbert.com.

Francisco Contreras, MD, oversees the Oasis of Hope Hospital, a cancer-care facility in Mexico widely known for integrative treatment methods. Dr. Contreras is a lecturer and author of *Fighting Cancer 20 Different Ways*, *The Hope of Living Cancer Free*, and *Health in the 21st Century*.

Leslie Ann Dauphin holds a PhD in microbiology from North Carolina State University. Currently she is a microbiologist at the Centers for Disease Control and Prevention in Atlanta, Georgia. She has taught biological sciences for over ten years and speaks annually at national scientific conferences.

Kara Davis, MD, is a board-certified physician of internal medicine who practices in the Chicago suburbs. She previously served as an assistant professor of clinical medicine at the University of Illinois at Chicago, and she maintains an appointment at that institution. Dr. Davis regularly sees patients with diseases influenced by lifestyle and who suffer the many related consequences. Her interactions and observations with these patients planted the seed for her book, *Spiritual Secrets to Weight Loss*, and for national workshops and seminars that she now leads. In addition to her medical career, she is a pastor's wife and the mother of four wonderful children.

Hans Diehl, DrHSc, MPH, FACN, holds a doctorate in health science with an emphasis on lifestyle medicine and nutrition. He is the founder of the renowned Coronary Health Imporvement Project (CHIP) and founder and director of the Lifestyle Medicine Institute in Loma Linda, CA. He is much in demand as a world-class speaker, educator, motivator, and coauthor of *Dynamic Health: A Simple Plan to Take Charge of Your Life*.

Terry Dorian, PhD, wife, mother, author of the book *Total Health and Restoration*, radio/television personality, and popular conference speaker is considered one of the most discerning health researchers on the scene today. An expert on the role of organic whole foods in the prevention and cure of degenerative diseases, she counsels medical doctors and health practioners across the country. Terry Dorian received her PhD from Louisianna State University, her MA from West Virginia University, and her BA from Stephens College. Dr. Dorian has been a health researcher for more than twenty years.

Scott Farhart, MD, is an obstetrician/gynecologist with more than twenty years of experience treating women and advising them to make healthy choices from a Christian perspective. He is the author of *Intimate and Unashamed: What Every Man and Woman Need to Know* and *The Christian Woman's Complete Guide to Health*, which he coauthored with Dr. Elizabeth King. He appears regularly on the TBN program *Doctor to Doctor* and is a regular contributor to *JHMagazine*, the bimonthly magazine of John Hagee Ministries. He and his wife, Sandy, have been married since 1983 and have two children.

James P. Gills, MD, is the founder and director of St. Luke's Cataract and Laser Institute in Tarpon Springs, Florida. In addition to earning a reputation as the most experienced cataract surgeon in the world, he has dedicated his life to restoring more than physcical vision. Dr. Gills has been an active author about spiritual topics for many years. His books include *God's Prescription for Healing*, *A Biblical Economics Manifesto*, *Darwinism Under the Microscope*, *Come Unto Me*, *Rx For Worry*, and *Love: Fulfilling the Ultimate Quest*.

Scott K. Hannen, DC, is a licensed chiropractic physician and ordained minister who has clinically attended patients for more than fifteen years. He is a graduate of Life University, where he earned his doctorate in chiropractic medicine. His postgraduate studies include completing more than three hundred hours in the field of clinical neurology at the Carrick Institute for Graduate Studies. He also attended Capitol University of Integrative Medicine. Dr. Hannen is the author of *Healing* *by Design* and a frequent guest on Christian television networks, including *Doctor to Doctor*, and he has hosted TBN's worldwide *Praise the Lord: Doctor's Night*. Originally from Orlando, Florida, he currently lives in Ozark, Alabama, where he serves as the senior pastor of Glory to Him Family Church.

Gregory L. Jantz, PhD, is the founder of The Center for Counseling and Health Resources, Inc., and is known internationally for whole-person care. He is the author of twenty books, including *Happy for the Rest of Your Life* and *The Body God Designed*. Dr. Jantz brings his whole-person vision of hope to audiences around the country through speaking, seminars, conferences, radio, and television.

Ron Kardashian, NSCA-CPT, is a fitness expert with a private practice in Los Gatos and San Francisco, California, that serves corporations, churches, and clients nationwide. One of the nation's up-and-coming spiritual leaders, Kardashian is author of the book *Getting in Shape God's Way* and is also a licensed minister, educator, conference speaker, author, life coach, and host of the international television broadcast *Getting in Shape God's Way*. He lives in California with his beautiful wife, Tia, and their little girl. For information visit www.ronkardashian.tv.

Daniel E. Kennedy is the chief executive officer of the Oasis of Hope Hospital and has couseled cancer patients since 1993, emphasizing the emotional, psychological, and spiritual strategies for fighting cancer. He holds degrees in counseling, ministry, economics, and business. He and his uncle Dr. Francisco Contreras coauthored the book *Fighting Cancer 20 Different Ways*.

Elizabeth King, MD, graduated from Texas A & M College of Medicine and has been practicing medicine since July 2005. A popular obstetrician/gynecologist in San Antonio, she is the coauthor of *The Christian Woman's Complete Guide to Health* and has been featured in several local health-related television interviews. She resides in the San Antonio area with her husband, Aaron, a physician specializing in diabetes, and their son, Daniel.

Harold G. Koenig, MD, MHSC, founder and codirector of the Center for Spirituality, Theology and Health at Duke University Medical Center, is the nation's foremost authority on the healing power of faith. He is the author of twenty-nine books for Christian and mainstream publishers.

Aileen Ludington, MD, a board-certified physician, is an internationally known health educator and author with twenty-five years of experience and research in lifestyle changes with patients suffering from circulatory and degenerative diseases. She serves as the medical director of the Lifestyle Medicine Institute and is the coauthor of *Dynamic Health: A Simple Plan to Take Charge of Your Life*.

Janet Maccaro, PhD, CNC, is a respected lecturer, author, and radio/television personality. She has doctorates in nutrition and natural healing and is also a leading expert in natural progesterone supplementation. Internationally recognized for her knowledge in women's health, Janet Maccaro has written books that include *Fabulous at 50, A Woman's Body Balanced by Nature, The 90-Day Immune System Makeover, Breaking the Grip of Dangerous Emotions, Midlife Meltdown*, and *Natural Health Remedies*.

Ed McClure is an award-winning restauranteur, having created, opened, and managed gourmet restaurants and hotels for thirty-two years. After tipping the scales at over 460 pounds, he discovered weight-loss principles that allowed him not only to drop 198 pounds but also to keep the weight off. He and his wife, Elisa, are the coauthors of *Eat Your Way to a Healthy Life*. Ed continues to reach out to others to inspire, motivate, and share his knowledge and experience in battling obesity.

Elisa McClure, ND, CNC, CNHP, is extensively trained in a variety of modalities in the fields of naturopathy, nutrition, homeopathy, aromatherapy, culinary arts, and, in particular, weight loss. Elisa is also a dynamic teacher and avid researcher who delights in sharing her knowledge of nutrition through instructional cooking videos with those seeking a healthier lifestyle. She is the director of ZOE 8's innovative food ideas and has created hundreds of recipes for the ZOE 8 Total Health Program and the McClures' restaurant. Elisa and Ed have coauthored the book *Eat Your Way to a Healthy Life* and have opened Health Journey Wellness Center on the grounds of their inn in Boerne, Texas.

Linda S. Mintle, PhD, is a nationally recognized writer, speaker, licensed clinical social worker, and licensed marriage and family therapist who specializes in eating disorders. An assistant professor of clinical pediatrics in the Department of Pediatrics, Easten Virginia Medical School, Dr. Mintle also serves as a national news contributor for CBN News. She is the author of sixteen books, including *I Married You, Not Your Family; Breaking Free From Compulsive Overeating; Lose It for Life; Raising Healthy Kids;* and *Press Pause Before You Eat.* While Dr. Mintle's book *I Married You, Not Your Family* carries the Charisma House logo, it was originally written for and published by Siloam. The timely and critical information it provides add a wholeness to truly living a healthy life—mind, body, and spirit.

Dino Nowak is a physical fitness expert who has trained and consulted high-profile artists in the entertainment industry in both mainstream and Christian markets. He writes and produces a weekly radio program and is a frequent contributor to several fitness magazines. Nowak is certified through the American College of Sports Medicine, the American Council on Exercise, and the Cooper Institute.

Pamela M. Smith, RD, is a nationally known nutritionist, energy coach, culinary consultant, and best-selling author. She provides wellness coaching to professional, corporate, and life athletes—from the NBA's Shaquille O'Neal, Orlando Magic, and LA Clippers, and the PGA's Larry Nelson and Brad Faxon to the executives and culinary development teams at Darden Restaurants, Walt Disney World, Hyatt Hotels and Resorts, and many more. Pam creates menus and recipes for some of America's best restaurants, including the hot new restaurant Seasons 52—all with a focus on great food that is great for you. Smith has inspired hundreds of thousands through her books, private practice, Web site, seminars, workshops, and radio. She is the author of twelve books and many articles and columns for magazines, newspapers, and Web sites.

Douglas Weiss, PhD, is a licensed psychologist and the executive director of Heart to Heart Counseling Center in Colorado Springs. The author of numerous books, including *Sex, Men and God; Intimacy; The Seven Love Agreements;* and *Get a Grip,* he is a regular guest on national television (both secular and Christian) as well as radio.

NOTES

SECRET #3: FAITH AND DIVINE HEALING

1.   F. F. Bosworth, *Christ the Healer* (Grand Rapids, MI: Fleming H. Revell, 2001).

SECRET #11: AVOIDING GERMS

1.   Centers for Disease Control and Prevention, "An Ounce of Prevention Keeps the Germs Away," http://www.cdc.gov/ounceofprevention/docs/oop_brochure_eng.pdf (accessed August 4, 2009).

SECRET #13: MANAGING A GOOD NIGHT'S SLEEP

1.   M. Billiard and A. Bentley, "Is Insomnia Best Categorized as a Symptom or a Disease?" *Sleep Medicine* 5, suppl. 1 (2004): S35–40; A. D. Krystal, "Depression and Insomnia in Women," *Clinical Cornerstone* 6, suppl. 1B (2004): S19–28; M. Novak et al., "Increased Utilization of Health Services by Insomniacs—an Epidemiological Perspective," *Journal of Psychosomatic Research* 56, no. 5 (2004): 527–536; D. Foley et al., "Sleep Disturbances and Chronic Disease in Older Adults: Results of the 2003 National Sleep Foundation Sleep in America Survey," *Journal of Psychosomatic Research* 56, no. 5 (2004): 497–502; C. L. Drake et al., "Insomnia Causes, Consequences, and Therapeutics: An Overview," *Depression and Anxiety* 18, no. 4 (2003): 163–176; C. H. Schenck et al., "Assessment and Management of Insomnia," *Journal of the American Medical Association* 289, no. 19 (2003): 2475–2479.

SECRET #16: WHY WHOLE GRAINS ARE BETTER THAN PROCESSED FOODS

1.   Whole Grain Council, "Easy Ways to Enjoy Whole Grains," http://www.wholegrainscouncil.org/whole-grains-101/easy-ways-to-enjoy-whole-grains (accessed September 8, 2008).

2.   Steve Koenning and Gary Payne, "Mycotoxins in Corn," *Plant Pathology Extension*, North Carolina State University, September 1999, http://www.ces.ncsu.edu/depts/pp/notes/Corn/corn001.htm (accessed August 6, 2009).

SECRET #17: THE TEN COMMANDMENTS OF HEALTHY EATING AND DRINKING

1.   Office of the Surgeon General, "U.S. Surgeon General Releases Advisory on Alcohol Use in Pregnancy," press release, February 21, 2005, http://surgeongeneral.gov/pressreleases/sg02222005.html (accessed August 5, 2009).

2.   M. B. Engler et al., "Flavonoid-Rich Dark Chocolate Improves Endothelial Function and Increases Plasma Epicatechin Concentrations in Healthy Adults," *Journal of the American College of Nutrition* 23 (June 2004): 197–204.

SECRET #20: WATER—HOW MUCH?

1.   Ion Health, "How Much Water Should You Drink," http://www.ionhealth.ca/id70.html (accessed September 9, 2008). Also, Health4youonline.com, "Dehydration—the Benefits of Drinking Water," http://www.health4youonline.com/article_dehydration.htm (accessed September 9, 2008).

SECRET #21: IS BOTTLED WATER SAFE?

1.   Beverage Marketing Corporation, "Bottled Water Continues As Number 2 in 2004," International Bottled Water Association, http://www.bottledwater.org/public/Stats_2004.doc (accessed September 9, 2008).

2.   Ibid.

3.   NSF International, "Bottled Water Fact Kit: Five Facts to Know About Bottled Water," http://www.nsf.org/consumer/newsroom/pdf/fact_water_five.pdf (accessed September 9, 2008).

4.   Natural Resources Defense Council, "Bottled Water: Pure Drink or Pure Hype?" http://www.nrdc.org/water/drinking/bw/exesum.asp (accessed September 9, 2008).

5.   Ibid.

6.   John Stossel, "Is Bottled Water Better Than Tap?" ABC News, May 6, 2005, accessed via http://abcnews.go.com/2020/Health/story?id=728070&page=1 (accessed September 9, 2008).

7.   Natural Resources Defense Council, "Bottled Water: Pure Drink or Pure Hype?"

Secret #24: The Top Ten Heart-Healthy Foods

1.   G. E. Fraser et al., "A Possible Protective Effect of Nut Consumption on Risk of Coronary Heart Disease," *Archives of Internal Medicine* 152 (1992): 1416–1424; L. Brown, "Nut Consumption and Risk of Recurrent Coronary Heart Disease" (abstract), *FASEB Journal* 13, no. 4–5 (1999): A538.

2.   D. Steinberg and A. Lewis, "Oxidative Modification of LDL and Atherogenesis," *Circulation* 95 (1997): 1062–1071.

3.   S. V. Nigdikar et al., "Consumption of Red Wine Polyphenols Reduces the Susceptibility of Low-density Lipoproteins to Oxidation in Vivo," *American Journal of Clinical Nutrition* 68 (1998): 258–265.

4.   J. M. Geleijnse et al., "Tea Flavonoids May Protect Against Atherosclerosis: The Rotterdam Study," *Archives of Internal Medicine* 159 (1999): 2170–2174.

5.   M. Woodward and H. Tunstall-Pedoe, "Coffee and Tea Consumption in the Scottish Heart Study Follow-up: Conflicting Relations With Coronary Risk Factors, Coronary Disease, and All Cause Mortality," *Journal of Epidemiology Community Health* 53 (1999): 481–487.

6.   A. L. Waterhouse, J. R. Shirley, and J. L. Donovan, "Antioxidants in Chocolate," *The Lancet* 348 (1996): 384.

7.   J. X. Kang and A. Leaf, "Prevention of Fatal Arrhythmias by Polyunsaturated Fatty Acids," *American Journal of Clinical Nutrition* 71, Supplement (2000): 202S–207S.

Secret #27: High-Fructose Corn Syrup

1.   United States Department of Agriculture Economic Research Service, http://www.ers.usda.gov/data/foodconsumption/foodavailqueriable.aspx (accessed May 1, 2008).

2.   S. J. Nielsen and B. M. Popkin, "Changes in Beverage Intake Between 1977 and 2001," *American Journal of Preventive Medicine* 27, no. 3 (2004): 205–210.

3.   Emma Hitt, "Fructose but Not Glucose Consumption Linked to Atherogenic Lipid Profile," Medscape Medical News, http://www.medscape.com/viewarticle/559344 (accessed May 1, 2008).

Secret #28: Cautions About Dairy

1.   Educate-Yourself.org, "Dairy Products," Nutrition, the Key to Energy, http://www.educate-yourself.org/nutrition/#dairyproducts (accessed September 9, 2008).

2.   George Mateljan Foundation, "Pasteurization," http://www.whfoods.com/genpage.php?tname=george&dbid=149#answer (accessed September 9, 2008).

3.   U.S. Department of Agriculture, "The Dangers of Raw Milk," *FoodFacts*, October 2006; Cornell University, "Why Pasteurize? The Dangers of Consuming Raw Milk," *Dairy Science Facts*, 1998.

Secret #29: Cautions About Meat

1.   C. A. Daley et al., "A Literature Review of the Value-Added Nutrients Found in Grass-fed Beef Products," California State University–Chico, draft manuscript, June 2005, http://www.csuchico.edu/agr/grassfedbeef/health-benefits/index.html (accessed September 9, 2008).

2.   Associated Press, "Red Meat Raises Breast Cancer Risk," MSNBC.com, February 7, 2007, http://www.msnbc.com/id/15702642/print/1/displaymode/1098/ (accessed October 17, 2008).

3.   James Buchanan Brady Urological Institute, "Racemase: A New Marker for Cancer and More," *Prostate Cancer Update*, Winter 2003, http://urology.jhu.edu/newsletter/prostate_caner67.php (accessed October 17, 2008).

Secret #31: Tips for Healthy Shopping

1.   Additives that always contain MSG: hydrolyzed protein, hydrolyzed plant protein, hydrolyzed vegetable protein, hydrolyzed oat flour, plant protein extract, sodium caseinate, calcium caseinate, textured protein, yeast extract, autolyzed yeast. Additives that frequently contain MSG: malt extract, malt stock, various flavorings, spices, various seasonings, bouillon, broths, "natural flavoring."

Secret #33: When Organic Produce Is Not Available

1.   ConsumerReports.org, "When Buying Organic Pays (and Doesn't)," June 2, 2008, http://blogs.consumerreports.org/baby/2008/06/organic-food.html?resultPageIndex=1&resultIndex=1&searchTerm=buying%20organic (accessed September 8, 2008).

Secret #38: Eat for Your Blood Type

1.   Steven M. Weissberg and Joseph Christiano, *The Answer is in Your Bloodtype* (Lake Mary, FL: Personal Nutrition USA, 1999), 154.

2.   Ann Louise Gittleman with James Templeton and Candace Versace, *Your Body Knows Best* (New York: Pocket Books, a div. of Simon and Schuster, Inc., 1996), 126–127.

3.   Weissberg and Christiano, *The Answer is in Your Bloodtype*, 155.

4.   Gittleman, *Your Body Knows Best*, 127.

5.   Weissberg and Christiano, *The Answer is in Your Bloodtype*, 127.

6.   Ibid., 124.

7.   Ibid.

8.   Ibid., 155.

Secret #49: Bariatric Surgery

1.   This article first appeared in the July/August 2008 issue of *Today's Christian Woman* magazine.

2.   C. L. Ogden et al., "Prevalence of Overweight and Obesity in the United States, 1999–2004," *Journal of the American Medical Association* 295 (2006): 1549–1555.

Secret #50: Weight-Loss Medications

1.   U.S. Food and Drug Administration Center for Drug Evaluation and Research, "Questions and Answers About Withdrawal of Fenfluramine (Pondimin) and Dexfenfluramine (Redux)," http://www.fda.gov/cder/news/phen/fenphenqa2.htm (accessed April 28, 2008).

2.   CenterWatch, "Drugs Approved by the FDA: Drug Name: Redux (Dexfenfluramine Hydrochloride)," http://www.centerwatch.com/patient/drugs/dru129.html (accessed April 28, 2008).

3.   U.S. Food and Drug Administration, "FDA Announces Withdrawal of Fenfluramine and Dexfenfluramine," http://www.fda.gov/cder/news/phen/fenphenpr81597.htm (accessed April 28, 2008).

4.   U.S. Food and Drug Administration, "FDA Approves Orlistat for Over-the Counter Use," February 7, 2007, http://www.fda.gov/NewsEvents/Newsroom/PressAnnouncements/2007/ucm108839.htm (accessed August 6, 2009).

5.   Y. Waknine, "International Approvals: Accomplia and Abraxane," Medscape Medical News, http://www.medscape.com/viewarticle/537382 (accessed April 28, 2008).

6.   S. Wood, "Unanimous 'No' to Rimonabant: Safety Not Demonstrated, FDA Advisory Panel Says," Medscape Medical News, http://www.medscape.com/viewarticle/558224 (accessed April 28, 2008).

7.   M. E. J. Lean et al., "Sibutramine: A Review of Clinical Efficacy," *International Journal of Obesity* 21, no. 1 (1997): S30–S36.

8.   L. Sjöström et al., "Randomised Placebo-Controlled Trial of Orlistat for Weight Loss and Prevention of Weight Regain in Obese Patients," *The Lancet* 352, no. 9123 (1998): 167–172.

Secret #51: Stress Can Make You Fat

1.   R. Pasquali et al., "Hypthalamic-Pituitary-Adrenal Axis Activity and Its Relationship to the Autonomic Nervous System in Women with Visceral and Subcutaneous Obesity: Effects of the Corticotrophin-Releasing Factors-Arginine-Vasopressin Test and of Stress," *Metabolism* 45 (1996): 351–356.

Secret #52: Drinking on the Pounds

1.   Megan Patrick, "Starbucks Tries Pouring Out the Calories and Fat," *Seattle Post*, June 30, 2004.

2.   Center for Science in Public Interest, "Highlights From Liquid Candy: How Soft Drinks Are Harming Americans' Health," http://www.cspinet.org/sodapop/highlights.htm (accessed November 24, 2004).

3.   M. Gibney et al., "Consumption of Sugars," *American Journal of Clinical Nutrition* 62 (1995): 178S–195S.

Secret #53: Body Fat Distribution

1.   J. A. Simpson et al., "A Comparison of Adiposity Measures as Predictors of All-cause Mortality: The Melbourne Collaborative Study," *Obesity* 15 (2007): 994–1003.

2.   P. L. Lutsey et al., "Dietary Intake and the Development of the Metabolic Syndrome," *Circulation* 117 (January 22, 2008): 754–761.

Secret #55: Basic Nutrition and Exercise Guidelines

1.   Lutsey et al., "Dietary Intake and the Development of the Metabolic Syndrome."

Secret #62: The Glycemic Index

1.   BestDietTips.com, "Glycemic Index List of Foods," http://www.bestdiettips.com/html/glycemic_index.php (accessed September 8, 2008).

Secret #66: The Power of Positive Words

1.   Adapted and expanded from Don Colbert, *Stress Less* (Lake Mary, FL: Siloam, 2005).

Secret #69: Toxic Onslaught

1.   Dr. Paul Yanick, *Quantum Repatterning Technique—II* (n.p.: Quantafoods, LLC, 2006).

2.   Lynn Goldman, "A Special Report on Toxic Chemicals and Children's Health in North America," Commission for Environmental Cooperation of North America, March 2004.

3.   Duff Conacher and Associates, *Troubled Waters on Tap: Organic Chemicals in Public Drinking Water Systems and the Failure of Regulation* (Washington DC: Center for Study of Responsive Law, 1988).

4.   WebMD, "Liver Failure," Digestive Disorders Health Center, http://www.webmd.com/digestive-disorders/digestive-diseases-liver-failure (accessed August 6, 2009); Lauran Neergaard, "Accidental Acetaminopen Poisonings Rise," *USA Today*, December 26, 2005, http://www.usatoday.com/news/health/2005-12-26-tylenol_x.htm (accessed August 6, 2009).

Secret #75: Go Ahead—Sweat It!

1.   Department of Health and Human Services, Substance Abuse and Mental Health Services Administration Drug Testing Advisory Board, scientific meeting notes for "Drug Testing of Alternative Specimens and Technologies," http://www.health.org/workplace/dtabday2.aspx (accessed February 21, 2006).

2.   JigsawHealth.com, "Sweat," http://www.jigsawhealth.com/sweat.aspx (accessed February 21, 2006).

Secret #82: Know Your Heart Rate Training Zone

1.   "Essentials of Strength Training and Conditioning," *Essentials of Personal Training Symposium, Section V: Aerobic Exercise Prescription* (NSCA Certification Commission, 1997), 6–7.

2.   Ibid.

Secret #88: The Battle Between Your Ears

1.   *Webster's New Collegiate Dictionary*, 9th ed., s.v. "equanimity."

Secret #89: What Is Heart Disease?

1.   *World Book Encyclopedia*, software version 1.0, 1998, s.v. "heart."

2.   The Franklin Institute, "Arterial Disease," http://www.fi.edu/learn/heart/healthy/art-dis.html (accessed August 17, 2009).

3.   Ibid.

4.   Charles A. Andersen, "Understanding Your Atherosclerosis and Living With It," *Iowa Health Book: Internal Medicine*, www.vh.org/patients/ihb/intmed/cardio/athero/atherosclerosis.html.

Secret #90: Symptoms of Blocked Arteries

1.   Barry L. Zaret, Marvin Moser, Lawrence S. Cohen, eds., *Yale University School of Medicine Heart Book* (New York: William Morrow and Company, Inc., n.d.), 136.

2.   Ibid.

Secret #92: High Cholesterol

1.   Karen Cicero, "Heart-Smart Snacks," *Prevention*, as viewed at Yahoo! Health, http://health.yahoo.com/other-other/heart-smart-snacks/prevention--17580.html (accessed August 19, 2009).

Secret #93: Lower Blood Pressure

1.   L. A. Ferrara et al., "Olive Oil and Reduced Need for Antihypertensive Medications," *Archives of Internal Medicine* 160, no. 6 (May 27, 2000): 837–842.

2.   J. C. Witterman et al., "A Prospective Study of Nutritional Factors and Hypertension Among U.S. Women," *Circulation* 80, no. 5 (November 1989): 1320–1327; A. Ascherio et al., "A Prospective Study of Nutritional Factors and Hypertension Among U.S. Men," *Circulation* 86, no. 5 (November 1992): 1475–1484.

Secret #94: Prevent Hardening of the Arteries

1.   American Heart Association, *Heart Disease and Stroke Statistics—2003 Update* (Dallas, TX: American Heart Association, 2002).

Secret #96: Twenty Ways to Fight Cancer

1.   For information on the Hallelujah Diet, visit the Hallelujah Diet Web site, http://www.hacres.com/diet/diet.asp.

Secret #97: Diabetes

1.   Centers for Disease Control and Preventions "National Diabetes Fact Sheet: General Information and National Estimates on Diabetes in the United States, 2000" (Atlanta, GA: U.S. Department of Health and Human Services, Centers for Disease Control and Prevention, 2002).

Secret #99: Crohn's Disease

1.   Linda Page, *Healthy Healing*, 11th ed. (n.p.: Traditional Wisdom, Inc., 2000), C360.

Secret #102: Irritable Bowel Syndrome

1.   M. H. Pittler and E. Ernst, "Peppermint Oil for Irritable Bowel Syndrome: A Critical Review and Metaanalysis," *American Journal of Gastroenterology* 93, no. 7 (1998): 1131–1135; J. H. Liu et al., "Enteric-Coated Peppermint Oil Capsules in the Treatment of Irritable Bowel Syndrome: A Prospective, Randomized Trial," *Journal of Gastroenterology* 32 (1997): 765–768; M. J. Dew, B. K. Evans, and J. Rhodes, "Peppermint Oil for the Irritable Bowel Syndrome: A Multicenter Trial," *British Journal of Clinical Practice* 38 (1984): 394–398.

2.   Dew, Evans, and Rhodes, "Peppermint Oil for the Irritable Bowel Syndrome: A Multicenter Trial."

3.   M. Camilleri, "Therapeutic Approach to the Patient With Irritable Bowel Syndrome," *American Journal of Medicine* 5A (1999); R. B. Lynn, "Current Concepts: Irritable Bowel Syndrome," *New England Journal of Medicine* 329 (1993); *Mayo Clinic Family Health Book* (n.p.: William Morrow & Co., 1996); *Applied Therapeutics: The Clinical Use of Drugs* (n.p.: Applied Therapeutics, 1995); *Micromedex Healthcare Series* (n.p.: Micromedix, Inc., 2001); *Washington Manual of Medical Therapeutics* (n.p.: Lippincott-Raven Publishers, 1998); *Griffith's 5-Minute Clinical Consult* (n.p.: Lippincott, Williams & Wilkins, Inc., 1999); *Sleisenger & Fordtran's Gastrointestinal and Liver Disease* (n.p.: W. B. Saunders Company, 1998).

Secret #104: Autoimmune Diseases

1.   Medline Plus, "Autoimmune Diseases," http://www.nlm.nih.gov/medlineplus/autoimmunediseases.html (accessed August 20, 2009).

2.   Carol and Richard Eustice, "Living Well With Autoimmune Disease," Arthritis.About.com, http://arthritis.about.com/cs/betterliving/fr/maryshomon.htm (accessed August 20, 2009).

Secret #106: Skin Disorders

1.   Acne Information Package, National Institute of Arthritis and Musculoskeletal and Skin Diseases, DHEW Publication N. (HRA) 76-1639.

2.   Joseph Pizzorno and Michael Murray, *Textbook of Natural Medicine*, vol. 2 (New York: Churchill Livingstone, 1999).

Secret #110: Sleep Disorders

1.   *Good Night America: Deep Sleep Reference Guide*, "Personalized Sleep Plan Checklist" (n.p.: Good Night America LLC, 1998).

Secret #112: Andropause (Male Menopause)

1.   Linda Page, *Healthy Healing*, 11th ed. (n.p.: Traditional Wisdom, Inc., 2000), H422.

Secret #113: Prostate Disease

1.   J. D. McConnell, "Epidemiology, Etiology, Pathophysiology, and Diagnosis of Benign Prostatic Hyperplasia," in P. C. Walsh et al., eds. *Campbell's Urology*, vol 2, 7th ed. (Philadelphia, PA: W. B. Saunders Company, 1998), 1429–1452.

Secret #119: Dental Problems

1.   Author interview with Michael T. Maccaro, DMD, in 2002.

2.   Ibid.

SECRET #128: HEALTHY BONES

1.   J. Y. Reginster et al., "Long-Term Effects of Glucosamine Sulfate on Osteoarthritis Progression: A Randomized, Placebo-Controlled Trial," *Lancet* 357 (2001): 251–256.

SECRET #130: Q&A ON AGING

1.   Robert M. Giller and Kathy Matthews, *Medical Makeover* (New York: William Morrow and Company, 1989), 236–252.

SECRET #131: ALZHEIMER'S—THE LONG GOOD-BYE

1.   James F. Balch and Phyllis Bach, *Prescription for Nutritional Healing* (Garden City, NY: Avery Publishing Group, 1997), 123.

SECRET #132: ZAPPING THE BIG EIGHT AGE-MAKERS—PART 1

1.   *Life Extension*, "Delaying the Onset of Degenerative Diseases," supplemental edition, December 2003, 34–36.

2.   Federico Parodi et al., "Oral Administration of Diferuloylmethane (Curcumin) Suppresses Proinflammatory Cytokines and Destructive Connective Tissue Remodeling in Experimental Abdominal Aortic Aneurysms," *Annals of Vascular Surgery* 20, no. 3 (May 2006): 360–368.

3.   F. Suarez et al., "Pancreatic Supplements Reduce Symptomatic Response of Healthy Subjects to a High Fat Meal," *Digestive Disease Sciences* 44, no. 7 (July 1999): 1317–1321; Brad Rachman, "Unique Features and Application of Non-Animal Derived Enzymes," *Clinical Nutrition Insights* 5, no. 10 (1997): 1–4; K. Odea, "Factors Influencing Carbohydrate Digestion: Acute and Long-Term Consequences," *Diabetes, Nutrition and Metabolism* 3 (1990): 251–258; J. Schick et al., "Two Distinct Adaptive Responses in the Synthesis of Exocrine Pancreatic Enzymes to Inverse Changes in Protein and Carbohydrate in the Diet," *American Journal of Physiology: Gastrointestinal and Liver Physiology* 24, no. 6 (December 1984): G611–G616.

4.   V. E. Kagan et al., "Dihydrolipoic Acid—a Universal Antioxidant Both in the Membrane and in the Aqueous Phase, Reduction of Peroxyl, Ascorbyl and Chromanoxyl Radicals," *Biochemical Pharmacology* 44, no. 8 (October 1992): 1637–1649.

SECRET #133: ZAPPING THE BIG EIGHT AGE-MAKERS—PART 2

1.   G. Tate et al., "Suppression of Acute and Chronic Inflammation by Dietary Gamma-Linolenic Acid," *Journal of Rheumatology* 16, no. 6 (June 1989): 729–734; T. H. Lee et al., "Effects of Dietary Fish Oil Lipids on Allergic and Inflammatory Diseases," *Allergy Proceedings* 12, no. 5 (September–October 1991): 299–303.

2.   S. Lee-Huang et al., "Anti-HIV Activity of Olive Leaf Extract (OLE) and Modulation of Host Cell Gene Expression by HIV-1 Infection and OLE Treatment," *Biochemical and Biophysical Research Communications* 307, no. 4 (August 2003): 1029–1037; T. H. Abdullah et al., "Enhancement of Natural Killer Cell Activity in AIDS With Garlic," *Dtsch Zsohr Onkol* 21 (1989): 52–53.

3.   L. A. Braam et al., "Vitamin K_1 Supplementation Retards Bone Loss in Postmenopausal Women Between 50 and 60 Years of Age," *Calcified Tissue International* 73, no. 1 (July 2003): 21–26; K. G. Jie et al., "Vitamin K Status and Bone Mass in Women With and Without Aortic Atherosclerosis: A Population-Based Study," *Calcified Tissue International* 59, no. 5 (November 1996): 352–356.

4.   E. P. Quinlivan et al., "Importance of Both Folic Acid and Vitamin B_{12} in Reduction of Risk of Vascular Disease," *Lancet* 359 (January 2002): 227–228.

SECRET #135: DIETARY KEYS TO LONGER LIFE

1.   Michael F. Roizen, MD, *Real Age Makeover* (New York: Harper Collins, 2005), 60–63.

SECRET #137: WAYS TO EXTEND YOUR DAYS—PART 1

1.   N. T. Telang et al., "Inhibition of Proliferation and Modulation of Estradiol Metabolism: Novel Mechanisms for Breast Cancer Prevention by the Phytochemical Indole-3-Carbinol," *Proceedings of the Society for Experimental Biology and Medicine* 216 (November 1997): 246–252.

2.   K. Zmilacher, R. Bettegay, and M. Gastpar, "L-5-Hydroxytryptophan Alone and in Combination With a Peripheral Decarboxylase Inhibitor in the Treatment of Depression," *Neuropsychobiology* 20, no. 1 (1988): 28–35.

3.   A. Kobayashi et al., "Effects of L-Theanine on the Release of A-Brain Waves in Human Volunteers," *Nippon Noegikagaku Kaishi* 72 (1998): 153–157.

4.   E. M. Duker et al., "Effects of Extracts From Cimicifuga Racemosa on Donadotropin Release in Menopausal Women and Ovariectomized Rats," *Planta Medica* 57, no. 5 (October 1991): 420–424.

5.   T. E. McAlindon, M. P. LaValley, and D. T. Felson, "Efficacy of Glucosamine and Chondroitin for Treatment of Osteoarthritis," *Journal of the American Medical Association* 284, no. 10 (September 2000): 1241; see also V. R. Pipitone, "Chondroprotection with Chondroitin Sulfate," *Drugs Under Experimental and Clinical Research* 17, no. 1 (1990): 3–7.

6.   O. Kucuk et al., "Lycopene Supplementation in Men With Prostate Cancer (PCa) Reduces Grade and Volume of Preneoplacia (PIN) and Tumor, Decreases Serum PSA and Modulates Biomarkers of Growth and Differentiation," Karmanos Cancer Institute, Wayne State University, Detroit, Michigan, 1999.

7.   B. Andallu and B. Radhika, "Hypoglycemic, Diuretic and Hypocholesterolemic Effect of Winter Cherry (Withania Somnifera, Dunal) Root," *Indian Journal of Experimental Biology* 38, no. 6 (June 2000): 607–609.

8.   E. Haak et al., "Effects of Alpha-Lipoic Acid on Microcirculation in Patients With Peripheral Diabetic Neuropathy," *Experimental and Clinical Endocrinology and Diabetes* 108, no. 3 (2000): 168–174.

9.   N. Crespo et al., "Comparative Study of the Efficacy and Tolerability of Policosanol and Lovastatin in Patients With Hypercholesterolemia and Noninsulin Dependent Diabetes Mellitus," *International Journal of Clinical Pharmacology Research* 19, no. 4 (1999): 117–127.

Secret #143: Your Annual Exam

1.   ClevelandClinic.org, "Thyroid Disease," http://www.clevelandclinic.org/health/health-info/docs/2000/2011.asp?index=8541 (accessed April 3, 2008).

Secret #145: Pregnancy: The First Trimester

1.   American College of Obstetricians and Gynecologists, *Your Pregnancy and Birth* (Washington DC: American College of Obstetricians and Gynecologists, 2005), 84–85.

Secret #146: Abnormalities During Pregnancy

1.   A. J. Wilcox et al., "Incidence of Early Loss of Pregnancy," *New England Journal of Medicine* 319 (1988): 189–194.

2.   Centers for Disease Control and Prevention, "Current Trends Ectopic Pregnancy—United States, 1990–1992," *Morbidity and Mortality Weekly Report* 44, no. 3 (January 27, 1995): 46–48, http://www.cdc.gov/mmwr/preview/mmwrhtml/00035709.htm (accessed April 18, 2008).

3.   J. C. Smulian et al., "Birth Defects Surveillance," *New Jersey Medicine* 99, no. 12 (2002): 25–31.

Secret #147: Pregnancy: The Second Trimester

1.   American College of Obstetricians and Gynecologists, *Your Pregnancy and Birth* (Washington DC: American College of Obstetricians and Gynecologists, 2005), 84–85.

Secret #149: Childbirth

1.   American College of Obstetricians and Gynecologists, "Episiotomy," *Obstetrics and Gynecology* 107 (2006): 957–962.

Secret #150: Infertility: Causes and Treatments

1.   National Institute of Child Health and Human Development, "Understanding Klinefelter Syndrome," http://www.nichd.nih.gov/publications/pubs/klinefelter.cfm (accessed April 18, 2008).

2.   Maria G. Essig, MS, ELS, "Semen Analysis: Test Overview," February 20, 2007, http://health.yahoo.com/reproductive-diagnosis/semen-analysis/healthwise--hw5612.html (accessed April 18, 2008).

Secret #151: Birth Control

1.   Robert Hatcher et al., *Contraceptive Technology*, 17th ed. (New York: Ardent Media, 1998), 215–218.
2.   Ibid., 516.

Secret #152: STDs

1.   National Institute of Allergy and Infectious Diseases, "Pelvic Inflammatory Disease," Fact Sheet, July 1998.

2.   National Institute of Allergy and Infectious Diseases, "Workshop Summary: Scientific Evidence on Condom Effectiveness for Sexually Transmitted Disease (STD) Prevention," July 20, 2001, http://www3.niaid .nih.gov/research/topics/STI/pdf/condomreport.pdf (accessed April 4, 2008).

SECRET #153: HPV—HUMAN PAPILLOMAVIRUS

1.   Centers for Disease Control and Prevention, "Genital HPV Infection—CDC Fact Sheet," March 2008, http://www.cdc.gov/std/HPV/STDFact-HPV.htm (accessed April 4, 2008).

2.   Association of Professors of Gynecology and Obstetrics, "Sexually Transmitted Infections: The Ob-Gyn's Role," three-part teaching module in the APGO Educational Series on Women's Health Issues, 2003.

3.   Centers for Disease Control and Prevention, "Genital HPV Infection—CDC Fact Sheet."

SECRET #154: HIV AND AIDS

1.   Centers for Disease Control and Prevention, "Trends in HIV/AIDS Diagnoses—33 States, 2001–2004," *Morbidity and Mortality Weekly Reports* 54, no. 45 (November 18, 2005): 1149–1153, http://www.cdc .gov/mmwr/preview/mmwrhtml/mm5445a1.htm (accessed April 7, 2008).

2.   American College of Obstetricians and Gynecologists (ACOG), "Human Immunodeficiency Virus Infections in Pregnancy," *ACOG Educational Bulletin* 232 (1997).

3.   Centers for Disease Control and Prevention, "Mother-to-Child (Perinatal) HIV Transmission and Prevention," October 2007, http://www.cdc.gov/hiv/topics/perinatal/resources/factsheets/perinatal.htm (accessed April 7, 2008).

SECRET #157: A WOMAN'S GASTROINTESTINAL SYSTEM

1.   DicQie Fuller, *The Healing Power of Enzymes* (New York: Forbes, Inc., 1998), 118.

2.   *Stop Improper Digestion, Renew Life*; 2076 Sunnydale Blvd., Clearwater, FL 33765.

SECRET #159: A WOMAN'S CARDIOVASCULAR SYSTEM

1.   National Heart, Lung, and Blood Institute, "What Are High Blood Pressure and Prehypertension?" http://www.nhlbi.nih.gov/hbp/hbp/whathbp.htm (accessed March 27, 2006).

SECRET #167: VARICOSE VEINS

1.   T. E. Bienlanski and Z. H. Piotrowski, "Horse Chestnut Seed Extract for Chronic Venous Insufficiency," *Journal of Family Practice* 48, no. 3 (March 1999): 171–172; H. Bisler et al., "[Effects of Horse Chestnut Seed Extract on Transcapillary Filtration in Chronic Venous Insufficiency]," *Deutsche Medizinische Wochenschrift* (Stuttgart) 111, no. 35 (August 29, 1986): 1321–1329.

2.   U. Siebert et al., "Efficacy, Routine Effectiveness, and Safety of Horse Chestnut Seed Extract in the Treatment of Chronic Venous Insufficiency. A Meta-Analysis of Randomized Controlled Trials and Large Observational Studies," *International Angiology* (Torino) 21, no. 4 (December 2002): 305–315; M. H. Pittler and E. Ernst, "Horse Chestnut Seed Extract for Chronic Venous Insufficiency. A Criteria-Based Systematic Review," *Archives of Dermatology* 134, no. 11 (November 1998): 1356–1360; C. Diehm et al., "Comparison of Leg Compression Stocking and Oral Horse Chestnut Seed Extract Therapy in Patients With Chronic Venous Insufficiency," *Lancet* 347, no. 8997 (February 3, 1996): 292–294.

SECRET #170: THE HEALING POWER OF OPTIMISM

1.   Michael D. Lemonick, "The Biology of Joy," *TIME*, January 17, 2005.

SECRET #177: DEPRESSION

1.   Diagnostic criteria from the *Diagnostic and Statistic Manual of Mental Disorders*, fourth edition (Washington DC: American Psychiatric Press, 1994).

SECRET #180: THE VALUE OF FRIENDS AND FAMILY

1.   Elaine Zablocki, "Love's Not Only Good for the Soul," WebMD Health News, February 14, 2001, http://www.webmd.com/sex-relationships/news/20010214/loves-not-only-good-for-soul (accessed August 25, 2009).

2.   S. Cohen and T. A. Willis, "Stress, Social Support, and the Buffering Hypothesis," *Psychological Bulletin* 98 (1985): 310–357; L. K. George, "Social Factors and the Onset and Outcome of Depression," in K. W. Schaie et al., eds., *Aging, Health Behaviors, and Health Outcomes* (Hillsdale, NJ: Lawrence Erlbaum Associates, 1992), 137–159; L. K. George et al., "Social Support and the Outcome of Major Depression," *British Journal of Psychiatry* 154 (1989): 478–485.

3.   L. F. Berkman and S. L. Syme, "Social Networks, Holds Resistance, and Mortality," *American Journal of Epidemiology* 109 (1979): 186–204; T. M. Vogt et al., "Social Networks as Predictors of Ischemic Heart Disease, Cancer, Stroke, and Hypertension," *Journal of Clinical Epidemiology* 45 (1992): 659–666; J. S. House et al., "Social Relationships and Health," *Science* 241 (1988): 540–545.

4.   J. K. Kiecolt-Glaser et al., "Stressful Personal Relationships: Immune and Into Credit Function," in R. Glaser and J. Kiecolt-Glaser, *Handbook of Human Stress and Immunity* (San Diego, CA: Academic Press, 1994), 321–329; S. Cohen et al., "Social Ties and Susceptibility to the Common Cold," *Journal of the American Medical Association* 277 (1997): 1940–1944.

5.   L. F. Berkman and L. Breslow, *Health and Ways of Living: The Alameda County Study* (New York: Oxford University Press, 1994).

6.   C. Dickens, *Heart* 90 (April 2004): 518–522, as referenced in Jeanie Lerche Davis, "Close Relationship Helps Heart," WebMD Health News, April 14, 2004, http://www.webmd.com/heart-disease/news/20040414/close-relationship-helps-heart (accessed August 25, 2009).

SECRET #191: LEAVING A HEALTHY INHERITANCE FOR THE NEXT GENERATION

1.   B. A. Dennison, T. A. Erb, and P. L. Jenkins, "Television Viewing and Television in Bedroom Associated With Overweight Risk Among Low-Income Preschool Children," *Pediatrics* 109 (2002): 1028–1035.

2.   L. M. Powell et al., "Exposure to Food Advertising on Television Among US Children," *Archives of Pediatric and Adolescent Medicine* 161, no. 16 (2007): 553–560.

3.   M. W. Gillman et al., "Family Dinner and Diet Quality Among Older Children and Adolescents," *Archives of Pediatric and Adolescent Medicine* 9 (2000): 235–240.

4.   M. E. Eisenberg et al., "Correlations Between Family Meals and Psychosocial Well-Being Among Adolescents," *Archives of Pediatric and Adolescent Medicine* 158 (2004): 792–796.

5.   G. Block, "Foods Contributing to Energy Intake in the US," *Journal of Food Composition and Analysis* 17 (2004): 439–447.

6.   M. Nestle, "Soft Drink 'Pouring Rights': Marketing Empty Calories to Children," *Public Health Reports* 115, no. 4 (July/August 2000): 308–319.

SECRET #192: OBESE CHILDREN

1.   Kelly D. Brownell and David S. Ludwig, "Fighting Obesity and the Food Lobby," *Washington Post*, June 9, 2002, B7.

2.   Ibid.

SECRET #195: VACCINATIONS

1.   U.S. Food and Drug Administration, "Vaccine Safety Questions and Answers," http://www.fda.gov/BiologicsBloodVaccines/SafetyAvailability/VaccineSafety/ucm133806.htm (accessed August 26, 2009).

2.   F. Edward Yazbak, MD, "Autism in the United States: A Perspective," United States Department of Education, http://www.jpands.org/vol8no4/yazbak.pdf (accessed November 18, 2004).

SECRET #196: HOW TO CHOOSE

1.   Paavo Airola, MD, PhD, *How to Get Well* (Scottsdale, AZ: Health Plus Publishers, 1974), in Jane Sheppard, "The Baffling World of Nutritional Supplements," Healthy Child Online, http://www.healthychild.com/supplements-for-children/the-baffling-world-of-nutritional-supplements/ (accessed August 26, 2009).

SECRET #198: FOR THOSE OVER FIFTY

1.   MayoClinic.com, "Vitamin B12," http://www.mayoclinic.com/print/vitamin-B12/Ns_patient-vitaminb12/METHOD=print (accessed February 8, 2006).

SECRET #199: WARNINGS

1.   Dr. Ben Kim, "Synthetic vs. Natural Vitamins," Life Essentials Health Clinic, http://chetday.com/naturalvitamin.thm (accessed February 23, 2006).

2.   Dominique Patton, "Oxidised Fish Oils on Market May Harm Consumer, Warns Researcher," NutraIngredients.com/Europe, October 20, 2005, http://www.nutringredients.comnews/ng.asp?id=63341-fish-oil-antioxidant (accessed February 23, 2006).

3.   A. Ohnishi, H. Ishibashi, K. Ohtani, K. Matsunaga, and T. Yamamoto, "[Peripheral Sensory Neuropathy Produced by a Megadose of Vitamin B6,]" [article in Japanese] *J Uoeh* 7, no. 2 (June 1, 1985): 201–205.

SECRET #200: TOP FIVE LIFE-ENHANCING SUPPLEMENTS

1.   K. Zimlacher et al., "L-5-Hydroxytrptophan Alone and in Combination With a Peripheral Decarboxylase Inhibitor in the Treatment of Depression," *Neuropsychobiology* 20 (1988): 25–35.

2.   C. R. Pace-Asciak et al., "The Red Wine Phenolics Transresveratrol and Quercertin Block Human Platelet Aggregation and Eicosanoid Synthesis: Implications for Protection Against Coronary Heart Disease," *Clinica Chimica ACTA* (Amsterdam) 235 (March 31, 1995): 207–219.

3.   H. Langsjoen et al., "Usefulness of Coenzyme Q_{10} in Clinical Cardiology: A Long-Term Study," *Molecular Aspects of Medine* 15 Suppl (1994): S165–S175.

4.   M. E. Attenburrow et al., "Low Dose Melatonin Improves Sleep in Middle-aged Subjects," *Psychopharmacology* 126 (July 1996): 179–181.

5.   Cenacchi et al., "Cognitive Decline in the Elderly: A Double-Blind, Placebo-Controlled Multi-Center Study on Efficacy of Phosphatidylserine Administration," *Aging* (Milano) 5 (April 1993): 123–133.

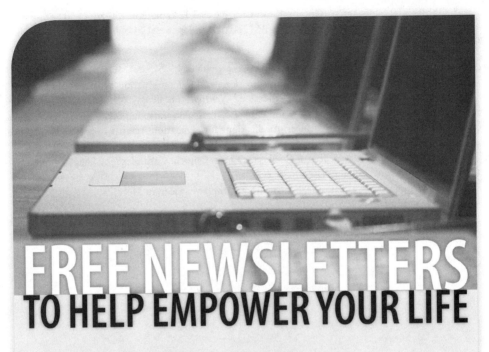

FREE NEWSLETTERS
TO HELP EMPOWER YOUR LIFE

Why subscribe today?

☐ **DELIVERED DIRECTLY TO YOU.** All you have to do is open your inbox and read.

☐ **EXCLUSIVE CONTENT.** We cover the news overlooked by the mainstream press.

☐ **STAY CURRENT.** Find the latest court rulings, revivals, and cultural trends.

☐ **UPDATE OTHERS.** Easy to forward to friends and family with the click of your mouse.

CHOOSE THE E-NEWSLETTER THAT INTERESTS YOU MOST:

- Christian news
- Daily devotionals
- Spiritual empowerment
- And much, much more

SIGN UP AT: **http://freenewsletters.charismamag.com**

8178